ABC of
Prehospital Emergency Medicine

ABC series

An outstanding collection of resources for healthcare professionals

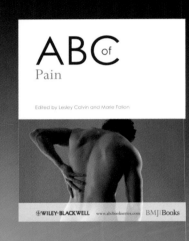

ABC of Pain

Edited by Lesley Colvin and Marie Fallon

WILEY-BLACKWELL www.abcbookseries.com BMJ|Books

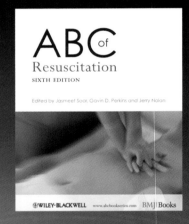

ABC of Resuscitation

SIXTH EDITION

Edited by Jasmeet Soar, Gavin D. Perkins and Jerry Nolan

WILEY-BLACKWELL www.abcbookseries.com BMJ|Books

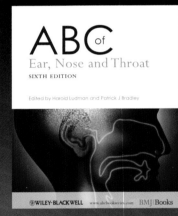

ABC of Ear, Nose and Throat

SIXTH EDITION

Edited by Harold Ludman and Patrick J Bradley

WILEY-BLACKWELL www.abcbookseries.com BMJ|Books

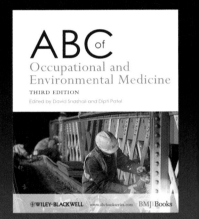

ABC of Occupational and Environmental Medicine

THIRD EDITION

Edited by David Snashall and Dipti Patel

WILEY-BLACKWELL www.abcbookseries.com BMJ|Books

The *ABC* series contains a wealth of indispensable resources for GPs, GP registrars, junior doctors, doctors in training and specialised healthcare professionals

▶ **Highly illustrated, informative and a practical source of knowledge**

▶ **An easy-to-use resource, covering the symptoms, investigations, treatment and management of conditions presenting in day-to-day practice and patient support**

▶ **Full colour photographs and illustrations aid diagnosis and patient understanding of a condition**

For more information on all books in the *ABC* series, including links to further information, references and links to the latest official guidelines, please visit:

www.abcbookseries.com

BMJ|Books

WILEY Blackwell

ABC of

Prehospital Emergency Medicine

EDITED BY

Tim Nutbeam

Consultant in Emergency Medicine
Derriford Hospital
Plymouth Hospitals NHS Trust
Plymouth;
Midlands Air Ambulance
Cosford;
West Midlands Ambulance Service Medical Emergency Response Incident Team (MERIT), UK

Matthew Boylan

Consultant in Military Emergency Medicine and Prehospital Care
Royal Centre for Defence Medicine
University Hospitals Birmingham
Birmingham;
Midlands Air Ambulance
Cosford;
West Midlands Ambulance Service Medical Emergency Response Incident Team (MERIT);
Mercia Accident Rescue Service (MARS) BASICS, UK

WILEY Blackwell

BMJ Books

Library of Congress Cataloging-in-Publication Data
ABC of prehospital emergency medicine / edited by Tim Nutbeam, Matthew Boylan.
       p. ; cm. – (ABC series ; 258)
   Includes bibliographical references and index.
   ISBN 978-0-470-65488-0 (pbk. : alk. paper) – ISBN 978-1-118-59228-1 (ePdf) – ISBN 978-1-118-59229-8 (eMobi) –
ISBN 978-1-118-59230-4 (ePub)
   I. Nutbeam, Tim., editor of compilation. II. Boylan, Matthew, editor of compilation. III. Series: ABC series (Malden, Mass.)
   [DNLM: 1. Emergency Medicine – methods. 2. Emergency Medical Services – methods. WB 105]
   RC86.7
   616.02′5 – dc23
                                                                                          2013017945

A catalogue record for this book is available from the British Library.

Wiley also publishes its books in a variety of electronic formats. Some content that appears in print may not be available in electronic books.

Cover image: Courtesy of Shropshire Fire & Rescue Service
Cover design by Meaden Creative

Set in 9.25/12 Minion by Laserwords Private Limited, Chennai, India
Printed in Singapore by Ho Printing Singapore Pte Ltd

1   2013

Contents

v

Contributor list

Peter Aitken

Associate Professor, Anton Breinl Centre for Public Health and Tropical Medicine, James Cook University;

Senior Staff Specialist, Emergency Department, The Townsville Hospital, Townsville, QLD;

Acting Clinical Director Counter Disaster, Retrieval Services Queensland, QLD, Australia

Keith Allison

Consultant Plastic Surgeon, The James Cook University Hospital, Middlesbrough, UK

Peter Anthony Berlac

Medical Director of Prehospital Emergency Medicine, University of Copenhagen, Copenhagen, Denmark

Tracy-Louise Appleyard

Consultant in Obstetrics and Gynaecology, Southmead Hospital, Bristol, UK

Neil Ballard

Senior Staff Specialist, Aeromedical and Retrieval Services, Ambulance Service of New South Wales;

Senior Staff Specialist, Emergency Medicine, Prince of Wales Hospital, Randwick, NSW;

Medical Coordinator, Careflight Queensland, Robina, QLD;

Senior Lecturer, School of Public Health, James Cook University, Townsville, QLD, Australia

Jennifer Bard

Professor of Law and Director, Health Law Program and J.D./M.D. Dual Degree Program, Texas Tech University School of Law;

Professor (Adjunct), Department of Psychiatry, Texas Tech University School of Medicine, Lubbock, TX, USA

Anna Barnard

Plastic Surgery Specialist Trainee, The James Cook University Hospital, Middlesbrough, UK

Clare Bosanko

Specialty Doctor Emergency Medicine, University Hospital of North Staffordshire, Stoke-On-Trent;

Midlands Air Ambulance, Cosford;

West Midlands Ambulance Service Medical Emergency Response Incident Team (MERIT), UK

Martin Botha

Chairman, Resuscitation Council of Southern Africa, Regional Training Manager and part-time Lecturer, International SOS and University of the Witwatersrand, Johannesburg, South Africa

Matthew Boylan

Consultant in Military Emergency Medicine and Prehospital Care,

Royal Centre for Defence Medicine, University Hospitals Birmingham, Birmingham;

Midlands Air Ambulance, Cosford;

West Midlands Ambulance Service Medical Emergency Response Incident Team (MERIT), UK

Mercia Accident Rescue Service (MARS) BASICS, UK.

Adam Bystrzycki

Emergency Physician, Alfred Hospital;

Senior Lecturer, Monash University, Melbourne, VIC, Australia

Vic Calland

Independent General and Prehospital Practitioner;

Honorary Secretary, British Association for Immediate Care (BASICS), UK

Tudor A. Codreanu

Senior Medical Practitioner, Critical Care Directorate, Emergency Department, Bunbury and Busselton Hospitals, South West Health Campus, Bunbury, WA, Australia;

Professor of Disaster Medicine, Vrije Universiteit Brussels, Belgium

MAJOR R. J. Dawes

Specialist Registrar in Anaesthetics and Intensive Care, Defence Medical Services, UK

Tim Draycott

Consultant Obstetrician and Gynaecologist, Research into Safety & Quality Group, Southmead Hospital, Bristol, UK

Mark Elcock

State Medical Director, Retrieval Services, Queensland, Brisbane, QLD;

Associate Professor, Anton Breinl Centre for Public Health and Tropical Medicine, James Cook University, Townsville, QLD, Australia

Anna Fergusson

Specialist Trainee in Anaesthetics, Birmingham School of Anaesthesia, Birmingham, UK

Lynn Gerber Smith

Clinical Nurse, Trauma Resusciatation Unit, R Adams Cowley Shock Trauma Center, University of Maryland Medical Center, Baltimore, MD, USA

Clare Hammell

Consultant Anaesthetist, Leighton Hospital, Crewe, UK

Tim Harris

Consultant in Emergency Medicine and Prehospital Care, Royal London Hospital;

Consultant in Intensive Care Medicine, Newham University Hospital, London, UK

LT COL Jeremy Henning

Consultant in Anaesthesia & ICU, The James Cook University Hospital, Middlesbrough;

Defence Lecturer in Critical Care, Royal Centre for Defence Medicine, University Hospitals Birmingham, Birmingham, UK

Per Kristian Hyldmo

Consultant in Anesthesiology, Air Ambulance Department, Sorlandet Hospital, Kristiansand, Norway

Matt Hooper

Executive Director, MedSTAR Emergency Medical Retrieval Service;

Associate Professor, Anton Breinl Centre for Public Health and Tropical Medicine, James Cook University, Townsville, QLD, Australia

Tim Hooper

Specialist Registrar, London HEMS & Defence Medical Services, London, UK

Jonathan Hulme

Consultant in Anaesthesia & Intensive Care Medicine, Sandwell & West Birmingham Hospitals NHS Trust, City Hospital, Birmingham;

Medical Director, West Midlands Central Accident Resuscitation & Emergency (CARE) Team, Birmingham;

West Midlands Ambulance Service Medical Emergency Response Incident Team (MERIT);

Midlands Air Ambulance, Cosford, UK

Fiona Jewkes

Clinical Author, NHS Pathways Connecting for Health, Leeds, UK

Alex Jones

Plastic Surgery Specialist Trainee, The James Cook University Hospital, Middlesbrough, UK

Dennis Jones

Critical Care Flight Nurse, The Johns Hopkins Hospital, Baltimore, MD, USA

Christopher A. Kahn

Assistant Professor of Clinical Emergency Medicine,

Director, Emergency Medical Services and Disaster Medicine Fellowship

Base Hospital Medical Director

Emergency Preparedness and Response Medical Co-Director

Department of Emergency Medicine

University of California, San Diego, CA, USA

Damian Keene

Specialist Trainee, Department of Anaesthetics, Royal Centre For Defence Medicine, University Hospitals Birmingham, Birmingham, UK;

West Midlands Ambulance Service Medical Emergency Response Incident Team (MERIT);

Midlands Air Ambulance, Cosford, UK

David Kloeck

Paediatric Intensive Care Fellow, Paediatric Intensive Care, Chris Hani Baragwanath Academic Hospital, Soweto;

University of the Witwatersrand, Johannesburg, South Africa

Walter Kloeck

President Emeritus, College of Emergency Medicine of South Africa, Rondebosch, South Africa

Craig M. Klugman

Professor and Chair, Department of Health Sciences, DePaul University, Chicago, IL, USA

Kristi L. Koenig

Professor of Emergency Medicine, Director, Centre for Disaster Medicine, Director of Public Health Preparedness, Director, International Disaster Medical Sciences Fellowship, University of California at Irvine, Orange, CA, USA

Efraim Kramer

Adjunct Professor and Head, Division of Emergency Medicine, University of the Witwatersrand, Johannesburg, South Africa

Mark Little

Emergency Physician and Clinical Toxicologist, Cairns Base Hospital, Cairns, QLD;

Associate Professor, Anton Breinl Centre for Public Health and Tropical Medicine, James Cook University, Townsville, QLD, Australia

David Lockey

Consultant, North Bristol NHS Trust and London's Air Ambulance, Hon Professor, University of Bristol, Bristol, UK

Adam Low

Specialist Registrar in Anaesthetics, West Midlands Deanery, Birmingham;

West Midlands Ambulance Service Medical Emergency Response Incident Team (MERIT), UK

Rod Mackenzie

Consultant in Emergency Medicine and Prehospital Emergency Medicine, Clinical Director, Major Trauma Service, Cambridge University Hospitals NHS Foundation Trust, Cambridge, UK

Assiah Mahmood

Clinical Governance Manager, Magpas Helimedix, St. Ives, UK

Kristyn Manley

Registrar Obstetrics and Gynaecology, Southmead Hospital, Bristol, UK

Suzanne Mason

Professor of Emergency Medicine, Health Services Research, School of Health and Related Research (ScHARR), University of Sheffield, Sheffield, UK

Stefan Mazur

Prehospital and Retrieval Physician and Operations Lead Consultant, MedSTAR, South Australian Emergency Medical Retrieval Service;

Emergency Physician, Royal Adelaide Hospital, Adelaide, QLD;

Associate Professor, School of Public Health and Tropical Medicine, James Cook University, Townsville, QLD, Australia

Lucas A. Myers

Assistant Professor of Emergency Medicine, Mayo Clinic Medical Transport, Mayo Clinic, Rochester, MN, USA

Ian Norton

Director, Disaster Preparedness and Response, National Critical Care and Trauma Response Centre (NCCTRC), Royal Darwin Hospital;

Emergency Physician, Emergency Department, Royal Darwin Hospital, Darwin, NT, Australia

Tim Nutbeam

Consultant in Emergency Medicine, Derriford Hospital, Plymouth Hospitals NHS Trust, Plymouth;

Midlands Air Ambulance, Cosford;

West Midlands Ambulance Service Medical Emergency Response Incident Team (MERIT), UK

Matt O'Meara

Registrar in Critical Care, Queens Medical Centre, Nottingham;

Honorary Lecturer, Academic Department of Traumatology, University of Birmingham, Birmingham, UK

Andrew Pearce

Clinical Director Training and Standards South Australian Statewide Retrieval Service, Royal Adelaide Hospital, Adelaide, SA, Australia

Keith Porter

Professor of Clinical Traumatology, University of Birmingham, Birmingham, UK

Harvey Pynn

Military Consultant in Emergency Medicine, Bristol Royal Infirmary;

Honorary Consultant in Prehospital Emergency Care, Great Western Air Ambulance;

Senior Medical Instructor, Wilderness Medical Training, Kendal, UK

Keith Roberts

Specialist Registrar, Hepatobiliary Surgery, University Hospitals Birmingham, Birmingham, UK

Anders Rostrup Nakstad

Consultant in Anaesthesiology, Air Ambulance Department, Oslo University Hospital, Oslo, Norway

Christopher S. Russi

Assistant Professor of Emergency Medicine, Mayo Clinic Medical Transport, Mayo Clinic, Rochester, MN, USA

Malcolm Q. Russell

Medical Director, Kent Surrey & Sussex Air Ambulance Trust;

Emeritus Helicopter Physician, London's Air Ambulance;

Mercia Accident Rescue Service (MARS);

West Midlands Ambulance Service NHS Trust;

United Kingdom International Search and Rescue (UK ISAR)

Mårten Sandberg

Professor in Prehospital and Emergency Medicine, University of Oslo, Oslo, Norway

Claire Scanlon

Specialist Trainee, Anaesthetics, City Hospital Birmingham, Birmingham, UK

Suzanne Sherwood

Clinical Nurse, R Adams Cowley Shock Trauma Center, University of Maryland Medical Center, Baltimore, MD, USA

Peter Shirley

Consultant, Intensive Care and Anaesthesia, Royal London Hospital, London, UK

A. Niroshan Siriwardena

Professor of Primary and Prehospital Health Care, University of Lincoln, Lincoln, UK

Julian Sandell

Consultant in Paediatric Emergency Medicine, Poole Hospital NHS Foundation Trust, Poole, UK

Wayne Smith

Head Disaster Medicine – Provincial Government Western Cape;

Senior Honorary Lecturer, Division of Emergency Medicine, University of Cape Town, Cape Town, South Africa

Andrew Thurgood

Consultant Nurse & Immediate Care Practitioner, Mercia Accident Rescue Service (MARS), UK

Jason van der Velde

Prehospital Physician, MEDICO Cork Research Fellow, Cork University Hospital, Cork, Ireland

Lee Wallis

Professor and Head, Division of Emergency Medicine, University of Cape Town, Cape Town, South Africa

Pete Williams

Consultant in Emergency & Paediatric Emergency Medicine, Dr Gray's Hospital, Elgin, UK

Foreword

Until recently, training in advanced prehospital care relied on seeking out experts and hassling them for snippets of wisdom, and applying for a post on one of the few existing helicopter emergency medical services. No single written resource was available for study, and the preparation for the Diploma in Immediate Medical Care required assimilation of several disparate texts.

Recent years have seen the modernization and some standardization of practice, an explosion of services able to provide prehospital critical care, and the hard won recognition of the subspecialty of Prehospital Emergency Medicine (PHEM), with dedicated training schemes for PHEM practitioners. The need is greater than ever to collate an overview of recommended practice into a single publication.

This book covers a comprehensive spectrum of prehospital topics written by the 'hard-hitters' in the field: specialists at the forefront of civilian and military practice. It will guide PHEM trainees, help in postgraduate immediate care exam preparation, and assist any prehospital provider wanting an update in the current state of the art.

This is the book I wanted as a trainee but never had. I am thrilled at its publication, and am heartened that I now have the pleasure of recommending it to my own trainees.

Dr Cliff Reid
Senior Staff Specialist and Director of Training
Greater Sydney Area Helicopter Emergency Medical Service
Ambulance Service New South Wales;
Clinical Associate Professor in Emergency Medicine
University of Sydney
Sydney, NSW, Australia

Preface

The *ABC of Prehospital Emergency Medicine* began life in 2009 as a collaborative project in response to joint frustrations over the lack of a concise, single resource capable of delivering the essential knowledge and key practical techniques required for effective Prehospital Emergency Medicine (PHEM) practice.

We began the project with two clear aims:

- to present accessible, cutting edge, expert opinion on core PHEM topics
- to provide the reader with the practical knowledge and resources to put this knowledge into clinical practice.

Throughout our own training and ongoing practice in PHEM we have been inspired and informed by a number of experienced prehospital practitioners both in the UK and abroad. We are grateful that many of these individuals have agreed to share their knowledge and experience more widely by contributing to this text. Our expert authors represent the wide range of healthcare practitioners to which we hope this text is both accessible and useful.

Over the last 4 years the project has been forced to evolve and grow in response to exciting developments in clinical care and prehospital governance. The most welcome of these has been the formal recognition of PHEM as a subspecialty within the UK and the development of a comprehensive PHEM curriculum. It is our hope that this text will serve as a useful educational tool for PHEM trainees, as well as a useful revision aid for the seasoned prehospital practitioner.

We must thank the team at Wiley Blackwell, our supportive (and tolerant) families and our expert team of authors without all of whom this project would never have happened. Finally we would like to dedicate this text to the hundreds of prehospital practitioners who have dedicated many hundreds of thousands of hours of their own time to make the speciality what it is today.

Tim Nutbeam
Matthew Boylan

CHAPTER 1

Prehospital Emergency Medicine

Matthew Boylan[1] and Tim Nutbeam[2]

[1]Royal Centre for Defence Medicine, University Hospitals Birmingham, Birmingham, UK
[2]Derriford Hospital, Plymouth Hospitals NHS Trust, Plymouth, UK

Introduction

'Prehospital care' is the term given to the provision of medical care outside of the hospital or alternative fixed healthcare setting. In the developed world, the provision of prehospital care is usually the responsibility of a regional ambulance or emergency medical service (EMS). A number of agencies may operate in support of the ambulance service including private ambulance companies, rescue organizations (e.g. mountain rescue, air ambulance services), the voluntary aid societies (e.g. Red Cross) and immediate care practitioners (e.g. British Association of Immediate Medical Care, BASICS).

Prehospital emergency medicine

Prehospital emergency medicine (PHEM) is a field within prehospital Care (Figure 1.1). PHEM's evolution has been triggered by the demand to meet new challenges imposed by the regionalization of specialist medical and trauma services. Many of the critically injured or unwell patients that prove to benefit most from these new systems of care are paradoxically those less likely to tolerate extended transfer without advanced critical care support. As a result, there is a need to provide a body of prehospital practitioners capable of providing advanced clinical assessment and critical care intervention at the scene of an incident, together with safe critical care retrieval to an appropriate centre of care. In most continents the enhanced skill set required to provide this level of care falls outside that deliverable by the ambulance service or its supporting bodies, and therefore requires the deployment of specially trained physician-led teams.

The role of the PHEM practitioner or team is to augment the existing prehospital response, not replace it. Their function is to provide an additional level of support for those patients with higher acuity illness and injury, both on scene and during transfer. In doing so they are also well placed to educate and enhance the skills of the prehospital providers they work alongside.

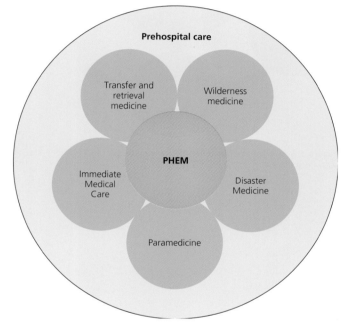

Figure 1.1 Prehospital emergency medicine.

Training in PHEM

An important move forward in the evolution of the field of PHEM in the UK has been its recognition as a new medical subspecialty led by the Intercollegiate Board for Training in prehospital Emergency Medicine (IBTPHEM). IBTPHEM has produced a curriculum that outlines the knowledge, technical skills and non-technical (behavioural) skills required to provide safe prehospital critical care and safe transfer. Links to the IBTPHEM and their curriculum can be found in the further reading section. The key themes of the curriculum are shown in Figure 1.2.

Similar prehospital training programmes exist across Europe (e.g. Germany) where they are firmly integrated into medical training and the emergency medical services (EMS). In Australasia, geography has been the driving force behind the development of retrieval medicine as a specialization. A number of retrieval services (e.g. Greater Sydney Area HEMS) have recognized the commonality between PHEM and retrieval medicine and have

ABC of Prehospital Emergency Medicine, First Edition.
Edited by Tim Nutbeam and Matthew Boylan.
© 2013 John Wiley & Sons, Ltd. Published 2013 by John Wiley & Sons, Ltd.

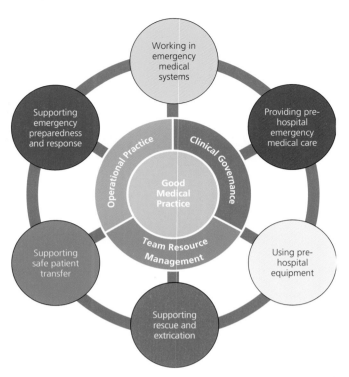

Figure 1.2 Prehospital emergency medicine curriculum themes (Courtesy of IBTPHEM).

moved towards delivering a combined model that provides both interfacility secondary transfer and primary prehospital retrieval. The experiences of many of these systems has helped mould the new PHEM subspecialty within the UK.

Summary

PHEM is a challenging and exciting development within the area of prehospital care. This book aims to provide some of the underpinning knowledge required for effective PHEM practice.

Further reading

IBTPHEM website: www.ibtphem.org.uk.

CHAPTER 2

Activation and Deployment

Andrew Thurgood[1] and Matthew Boylan[2]

[1]Mercia Accident Rescue Service (MARS), UK
[2]Royal Centre for Defence Medicine, University Hospitals Birmingham, Birmingham, UK

> **OVERVIEW**
>
> By the end of this chapter you should:
> - Understand how emergency calls are handled and prioritized
> - Understand the different types of dispatch
> - Understand the risks and benefits of deployment by road
> - Understand the risks and benefits of deployment by air.

Introduction

The first step in delivering high-quality prehospital care is the timely activation and deployment of prehospital resources. The initial aim is to get the right resource to the right patient in the right time frame. This process requires efficient call handling, robust call prioritization and intelligent tasking of resources. Prehospital practitioners may deploy to scene using a variety of different transport modalities. The choice of modality will be determined by the system in which they work and by the nature and location of the incident.

Activation of prehospital services

It is important for the prehospital practitioner to have an understanding of how emergency calls are processed and resources dispatched.

Call handling

In most developed countries there is a single emergency telephone number that members of the public may dial to contact the emergency services. The emergency number differs from country to country but is typically a three-digit number that can be easily remembered and dialled quickly, e.g. 911 in the USA, 999 in the UK and 000 in Australia. In the 1990s the European Union added 112 as the Global System for Mobile Communications (GSM)-approved common emergency telephone number.

Emergency calls from telephone and mobile phones pass to operators within designated Operator Assistance Centres (OACs)

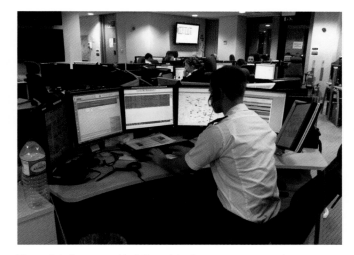

Figure 2.1 Computer-aided dispatch in the emergency control centre.

run by phone providers. Their function is to determine which emergency service is required and forward the caller details to the appropriate Police, Fire or Ambulance Emergency Control Centre (ECC). In the UK this information is passed electronically in the form of Caller Line Identification (CLI) via a system called Enhanced Information Service for Emergency Calls (EISEC). The data then appears automatically as an incident on the dispatchers computer-aided dispatch (CAD) screen in the ECC (Figure 2.1). While this automatic data transfer occurs, the caller is connected to a call taker at the ECC who will begin the process of call prioritization.

Call prioritization

There are a number of systems by which calls can be prioritized. The most common system used within the UK ambulance service is the Advanced Medical Priority Despatch System (AMPDS). Similar systems of Medical Priority Dispatch are in use within the USA and Australia. AMPDS uses a structured question–answer logic tree to allocate a dispatch priority: **Red – Category A** (immediately life threatening), **Amber - Category B** (urgent call), or **Green – Category C** (routine call). This mode of caller interrogation is known as systematized caller interrogation. AMPDS incorporates protocolized pre-arrival first aid instructions that are relayed by the call taker to the caller while they await the emergency response.

ABC of Prehospital Emergency Medicine, First Edition.
Edited by Tim Nutbeam and Matthew Boylan.
© 2013 John Wiley & Sons, Ltd. Published 2013 by John Wiley & Sons, Ltd.

In addition, each injury and injury mechanism is allocated a unique AMPDS code for audit purposes.

Although effective in prioritizing an ambulance service response, AMPDS has been shown to lack the sensitivity and specificity required to select calls that would benefit from enhanced prehospital emergency medicine (PHEM) intervention. In order to identify these cases, an additional tier of enhanced caller interrogation and dispatch criterion is required. For maximum efficiency this tier should be delivered by active PHEM practitioners (e.g. critical care paramedics or doctors) as they are in the best position to make accurate judgements about the likely need for advanced interventions. The use of non-clinical dispatchers in this role is associated with high rates of over-triage.

The model operated by London Helicopter Emergency Medical Service (HEMS) in the UK represents current best practice for enhanced call prioritization and dispatch. A dedicated HEMS dispatch desk within the Ambulance Control Centre is manned by an operational HEMS paramedic. They are responsible for scanning all the incoming cases and identifying those that would benefit from enhanced intervention. A set of evidence-based criteria known to be associated with severe injury are used to trigger the 'immediate dispatch' of the helicopter or car-based team (Box 2.1). Certain other cases undergo direct caller interrogation by the paramedic to assess whether enhanced intervention would be beneficial (Box 2.2). This is termed 'delayed dispatch'. The clinical knowledge and experience of the HEMS paramedic is critical in ensuring rapid and accurate identification and prioritization of these cases. The third form of dispatch is the crew request, which is treated as an immediate dispatch.

Box 2.1 **Immediate dispatch criteria (London HEMS)**

Fall from greater than 2 floors (>20 feet)
'One under' (fall or jumped in front of a train)
Ejected from vehicle
Death of a same vehicle occupant
Amputation above wrist or ankle
Trapped under vehicle (not motorcycle)
Request from any other emergency service.

Box 2.2 **Incident categories for interrogation (London HEMS)**

Shooting
Stabbing
Explosions
Road traffic collisions
Industrial accidents/incidents
Hanging
Drowning
Entrapments
Amputations
Burns/scalds
Building site accidents
Falls from height less than two floors
Impalement

Dispatch

While the call is being prioritized by the call taker, the dispatcher is responsible for allocating an appropriate resource(s) to the incident. Most modern CAD systems have an integral automatic vehicle location system (AVLS) which will automatically populate a list of the nearest available resources. The choice of resource will depend on the location, mechanism of injury, number of patients involved and the perceived severity of injury. Most ambulance services have now moved from VHF radio to digital data transmission (e.g. Airwave in the UK) as their primary mode of communication. Incident details are sent directly to vehicle-mounted data terminals with integrated satellite navigation systems that will automatically plot the route to the incident. Alternative modes of dispatch include activation via a base telephone landline, mobile phone or pager system. The activation and dispatch process is summarized in Figure 2.2.

Deployment of prehospital services

The ambulance service may deploy its resources to the scene of an incident in a number of different ways: foot, bicycle, motorbike, car, ambulance, helicopter or fixed wing aircraft. The decision to deploy a particular asset will be determined by the distance the asset is from the incident, the accessibility by road, known congestion and the required skill set of the responders. PHEM practitioners deployed to augment the ambulance service response will usually deploy by land vehicle or by helicopter.

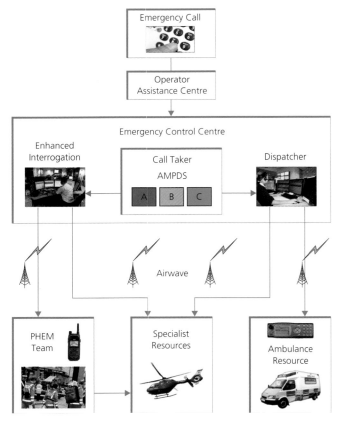

Figure 2.2 Overview of activation and dispatch process.

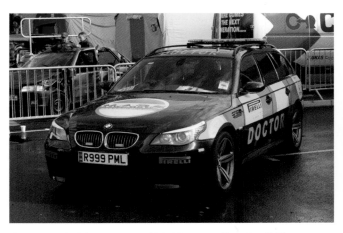

Figure 2.3 Physician response vehicle (Courtesy of Ivan Barefield).

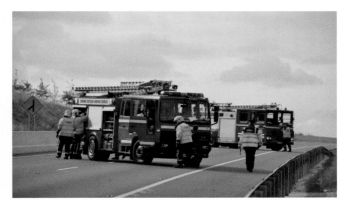

Figure 2.4 Fire tenders protecting the scene in the 'fend-off' position (Courtesy of Shane Casey).

Deployment by land vehicle

Many systems deploy their prehospital practitioners by rapid response vehicle (Figure 2.3). Land-based deployment is not restricted by weather or daylight hours in the same way that helicopter deployment is. They are ideal for operations in built-up urban areas as they are not limited by the need for an appropriate-sized landing site. Over short distances they also offer similar response times to helicopters because of the additional time taken by helicopters for take-off and landing.

Response vehicles must be roadworthy. A daily vehicle check is important and should include fuel and oil levels, water coolant, screen wash, electrics, lights and tyres (tread depth, inflation and damage). Medical equipment should be appropriately restrained and a lockable box available for CD storage. The vehicle should have visual and audible warning devices, as well as high-visibility markings. Drivers must be appropriately trained and insured for emergency response driving.

Activation may be via radio or mobile phone. If activation occurs while the vehicle is mobile, the driver should pull over at the next safe opportunity before further details of the incident are taken. Appropriate personal protective equipment should be donned at this point. Progression to scene should be made rapidly but safely with the full use of visible and audible warning devices. Parking at scene will usually be under the direction of the police. If the prehospital practitioner is first on scene at a road traffic accident, the fend-off position may be used to protect the incident scene (Figure 2.4). The vehicle should be positioned approximately 50 meters back from the incident and positioned to afford maximum use of rear visual devices and reflective high-visibility markings. The front wheels should be turned in a safe direction to reduce the risk of the vehicle being pushed into the incident if another vehicle collides with it. Keys should left in the ignition and the engine left running to prevent the battery draining flat. Once parked in a fend-off position, no one should return to the vehicle unless absolutely necessary.

Deployment by helicopter

In remote and rural areas, helicopters increase both the range and speed of PHEM team deployment and allow a single team

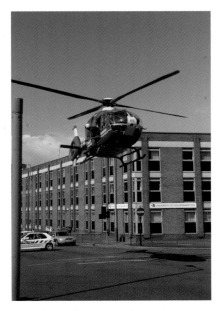

Figure 2.5 Urban HEMS (Midlands Air Ambulance).

to cover a large geographical area. Helicopters have also shown proven benefit in the urban setting where congestion may limit rapid deployment by road (Figure 2.5). Their use may be restricted by poor weather conditions, onset of darkness or the lack of an appropriate landing site.

Helicopter operations within Europe are regulated by the Joint Aviation Regulations Operations Specifications (JAR-OPS). Similar national regulations are in place in the USA and Australasia. JAR-OPS define a HEMS flight as a flight to facilitate emergency medical assistance, where immediate and rapid transportation is essential, by carrying either:

- medical personnel
- medical supplies (equipment, blood, organs, and drugs)
- ill or injured persons and other persons directly involved.

The HEMS designation is important as it carries with it alleviation from normal weather limits and exemption from certain Rules of

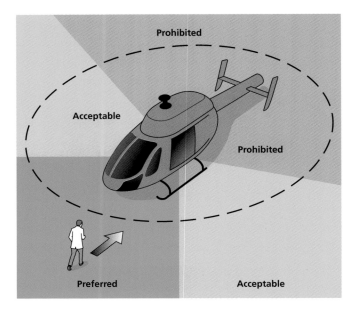

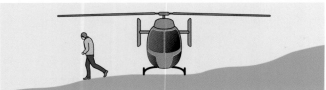

On sloping ground always approach or leave on the downslope side for maximum rotor clearance

Figure 2.6 Helicopter safety zones.

Air – in particular those relating to congested area overflight and landing. Medical personnel carried on HEMS flights fall into one of two categories:

1 **HEMS crew member** – an individual who has been specifically trained and assigned to the HEMS flight to provide medical assistance to the patient and assist the pilot during a mission with such roles as navigation or radio management.
2 **Medical passenger** – an individual who is carried during a HEMS flight whose primary roll is patient care. No specific training other than a pre-flight briefing is required, but they must be accompanied by a HEMS crew member.

Incidents that do not meet the JAR-OPS definition of HEMS are classified as air ambulance missions and cannot employ the same exemptions.

Deployment by helicopter provides a unique bird's-eye view of the incident scene on approach which may prove beneficial at large or major incidents. A landing site twice the diameter of the rotor blades is required and should be flat, free of debris and clear of any wires. Take-off and landing are the most hazardous periods of a HEMS flight therefore talking should be kept to a minimum during these phases unless a hazard is being noted. Once landing is complete, exit from the aircraft between the 2 and 10 o'clock position after gaining the pilots permission by a thumb up signal (Figure 2.6). This ensures avoidance of the aircrafts main hazard areas, i.e. engine exhausts and rotor blades. Care should be taken on sloping ground to avoid walking into the rotor disc by exiting downhill from the aircraft.

Tips from the field

- Use of PHEM practitioners for enhanced prioritization of emergency calls minimizes over-triage
- Always pull over safely before taking incident details or programming the sat-nav
- Always carry a set of maps as a back-up in case of sat-nav failure
- Take advantage of the bird's-eye view of the scene afforded by helicopter deployment – assess for hazards, mechanism and casualty locations.

Further reading

Brown JB, Forsythe RM, Stassen NA, Gestring ML. The National Trauma Triage Protocol: can this tool predict which patients with trauma will benefit from helicopter transport? *J Trauma* 2012;**73**:319–325.

Lin G, Becker A, Lynn M. Do pre-hospital trauma alert criteria predict the severity of injury and a need for an emergent surgical intervention? *Injury* 2012;**43**:1381–1385.

Ringburg AN, de Ronde G, Thomas SH, *et al.* Validity of helicopter emergency medical services dispatch criteria for traumatic injuries: a systematic review. *Prehosp Emerg Care* 2009;**13**:28–36.

Sherman G. *Report on Operating Models for NHS Ambulance Trust Control Rooms in England*, 2007. Manchester: Mason Communications Ltd.

CHAPTER 3

Personal Protective Equipment

Clare Bosanko[1] and Matthew Boylan[2]

[1]University Hospital of North Staffordshire, Stoke-On-Trent, UK
[2]Royal Centre for Defence Medicine, University Hospitals Birmingham, Birmingham, UK

OVERVIEW

By the end of the chapter you should be able to:

- Identify which items of personal protective equipment (PPE) should be part of the prehospital providers kit
- Describe what features (PPE) should have
- Describe what legislation and standards exist to define PPE.

Introduction

Is it safe to approach? First aid and basic life support training always starts with the premise that the rescuer should only approach a casualty if it is safe to do so. Healthcare providers working in the prehospital environment have an obligation to treat patients and if the risk cannot be completely removed it must be mitigated. Personal protective equipment (PPE) is the term used to describe those items worn or used to reduce risk where it cannot be entirely avoided. In recent years, healthcare-associated infections and chemical, biological, radiation and nuclear (CBRN) hazards have highlighted the importance of PPE for the safety of both the patient and the practitioner.

Legislation

Many countries have legislation defining the role of PPE in the workplace and the responsibilities of employers and employees. The primary need to control hazards and reduce risks to health and safety are highlighted in all these documents. Where changes to working practices alone are insufficient to protect employees from exposure to the hazard, PPE should be provided to lessen the risk.

In the UK, PPE provision is controlled by the Health and Safety Executive in the Personal Protective Equipment at Work Regulations, 1992. These define PPE as 'all equipment which is intended to be worn or held by a person at work and which protects him against one or more risks to his health or safety'. The regulations also govern assessment of suitability, maintenance, storage, instruction in and use of PPE. In the USA, the Occupational Health and Safety Administration publish similar guidelines (Table 3.1).

Table 3.1 International legislation pertaining to personal protective equipment provision

	Title of legislation	What it covers
UK	HSE: Personal Protective Equipment at Work Regulations 1992 Personal Protective Equipment Regulations 2002	Responsibilities for provision of PPE Quality assurance, CE marking
Europe	Council Directive 89/686/EEC	Quality assurance
USA	NFPA 1999: 2008	Quality assurance

EEC, European Economic Community; HSE, Health and Safety Executive; NFPA, National Fire Protection Agency.

PPE for prehospital providers is covered by the generic guidance for all industries but specific details regarding the requirements are not nationally or internationally defined. In the UK, responsibility is devolved to NHS trusts, and in the USA, Emergency Medical Services Authorities for each state produce guidance documents. The US Food and Drug Administration regulates the safety and efficacy of some forms of PPE, and the UK Health and Safety Executive provides quality assurance via the CE marking system (Table 3.2).

Table 3.2 International standards relating to items of personal protective equipment

	UK/Europe	USA
Gloves	BS EN 455–2: 2009	FDA
Work gloves		NFPA 1999
High-vis clothing	EN 471 89/686/EEC	ANSI/ISEA 107-2010
Footwear	EN 345	ANSI Z41-1999 OSHA
Hard hat	EN 397 EN 443	NFPA 1971: 2007 ANSI Z89.1: 2003 OSHA: 29 CFR 1910.135
Eye protection	BS EN 166: 2002	ANSI Z87.1
Respirator	EN 12941	NIOSH

ANSI, American National Standards Institute; BS, British Standard; CFR, Code of Federal Regulations; EN, European; FDA, Food and Drug Administration; ISEA, International Safety Equipment Organization; NFPA, National Fire Protection Agency; NIOSH, National Institute for Occupational Safety and Health; OSHA, Occupational Health and Safety Administration.

ABC of Prehospital Emergency Medicine, First Edition.
Edited by Tim Nutbeam and Matthew Boylan.
© 2013 John Wiley & Sons, Ltd. Published 2013 by John Wiley & Sons, Ltd.

The role of PPE

Prehospital providers work in an environment with risks from multiple sources; therefore, different items of personal protective equipment are required. Gloves, masks, eye protection, sleeve protectors and aprons guard against blood-borne pathogens and reduce transmission of infection to and from patients. In contrast helmets, boots and high-visibility clothing protect the wearer from injury, e.g. at the scene of a road traffic collision (RTC).

The PPE must be designed to allow the wearer to perform the risk-related activity without limitation, but with maximum protection. Clearly, for PPE to function properly the user must be trained in how to don, wear, remove and adjust their PPE, in addition to knowledge of its limitations, how it should be stored, cared for, maintained and disposed of.

There are also a number of specialist items of PPE, used by groups of providers with unique risks.

Essential personal protective equipment for prehospital practitioners

Helmet

Prehospital practitioners should wear head protection for all RTCs involving extrication, when working at height, during civil unrest, working on industrial sites and in any other designated 'hard hat' area. Increasingly, helmets are certified to fire fighting standards (e.g. EN443). They should have clear labelling of the wearer's job title and an integrated visor, the standard of which is separately regulated. Modern helmets are lightweight for comfort, with an adjustable headband and chin strap to ensure good fit (Figure 3.1).

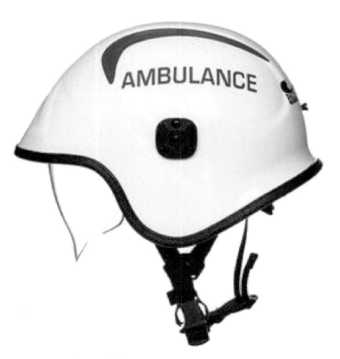

Figure 3.1 Pacific A7A helmet.

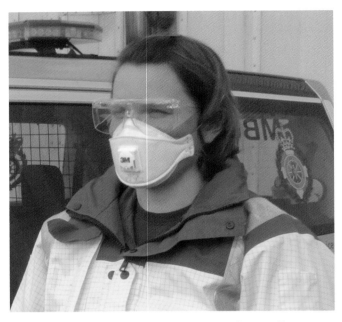

Figure 3.2 Eye protection and respiratory protection (FFP3 mask).

Eye protection

Eye protection should be worn when there is a risk of injury to the eye from debris, such as during cutting glass or metal at an RTC. Eye protection also protects against the risk of infection from splashes of body fluid or blood and respiratory secretions during airway management. Goggles, protective glasses (Figure 3.2), visors and full face splash guards are all available. Eyewear should include side protection and should fit over prescription glasses if necessary.

Ear protection

Hearing protection should be considered for noisy environments, e.g. helicopter emergency medical services (HEMS), motorsports, pop concerts, etc. Ear defenders provide the best attenuation of noise but are cumbersome and may not fit with the type of helmet worn. Ear plugs are a more practical alternative and can be easily stowed in a pocket of a jump suit when not in use.

Face masks

Masks provide respiratory protection against dust and fibres in the air and also prevent splashing of blood or body fluids onto the face. Specialist masks (e.g. the FFP3 mask) can be used to reduce transmission of airborne pathogens when caring for patients with known infectious diseases such as pandemic flu or TB (Figure 3.2). Masks are single patient use and should be replaced once moist or soiled. The manufacturer's instructions should be followed for maximum length of wear.

Clinical gloves

Clinical gloves are designed to protect the wearer from contaminants and reduce transmission of infection. They are manufactured from a range of materials including latex, nitrile and vinyl. Proteins in latex may cause allergy, particularly with repeated exposure among healthcare workers. As a result, nitrile and vinyl gloves, which are hypoallergenic, are becoming more common. Gloves should be worn if there is a risk of exposure to blood or body fluids, contact with mucous membranes or broken skin and when handling contaminated instruments. Nitrile gloves have the added benefit of some chemical resistance.

Hand washing should ideally be performed before and after the wearing of gloves. In the prehospital environment where this may not be possible, the use of detergent wipes and alcohol gel are acceptable alternatives.

Extrication gloves
Clinical gloves provide no protection against fragments of glass, jagged metal or hot surfaces. A set of heavy duty extrication gloves (Figure 3.3) should be worn in any situation where sharp or rough surfaces or a potentially high heat exposure is likely to be encountered, such as patient extrication.

High-visibility clothing
Prehospital providers working on or near a highway or in low-visibility settings should wear high-visibility clothing. EN 471 is the European standard, and Class 3 garments are required for any individual likely to be working on or near motorways or dual carriageways. These offer the highest level of visibility and must incorporate a minimum of $0.80\,\text{m}^2$ of fluorescent background material and $0.20\,\text{m}^2$ of retro-reflective materials. Whether on a jacket or a set of coveralls this usually takes the form of two 5-cm bands of reflective tape around the body, arms and braces over both shoulders (Figure 3.4). The most recent regulations from the USA also set minimum areas for reflective material in the shoulder area, or encircling the sleeves, consistent with the European standard.

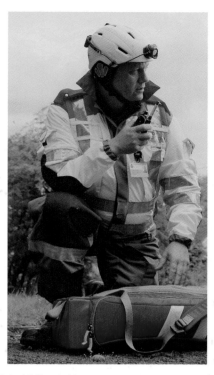

Figure 3.4 High-visibility clothing.

Boots
Footwear should be of the safety boot type. The European standard demands a toe cap able to withstand impact of up to 200 joules. The Occupational Health and Safety Administration and American National Standards Institute guidance recommends minimum height of 4 inches (10.2 cm), cut/puncture and abrasion resistance, and barrier protection with chemical resistance in addition to a safety toe.

Additional items
In addition to the items described above, each practitioner will identify equipment which he/she wishes to carry dependent on the requirements of his/her role. For example, a head torch, flood lights, vehicle hazard warning lights. Clearly the practitioner should ensure these items meet relevant safety regulations.

Specialist personal protective equipment

Helicopter Emergency Medical Services operations
Prehospital practitioners involved with HEMS operations require additional PPE as a result of their aviation role (Figure 3.5).

Flame-retardant flight suits made of Nomex or Kermel should be worn and are designed to protect against flash fire (4–5 seconds of flame). Most come with reflective strips, knee pads and a selection of pockets. The addition of full-length cotton undergarments will improve the flash fire protection rating of the suit significantly by preventing excessive heat soak to the underlying skin. Flight helmets have a role in both protection of the head and communication

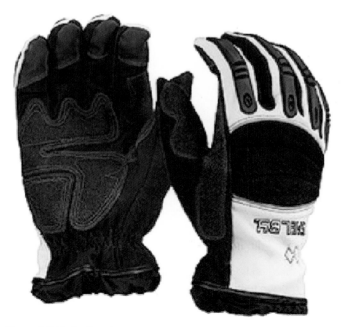

Figure 3.3 Extrication gloves.

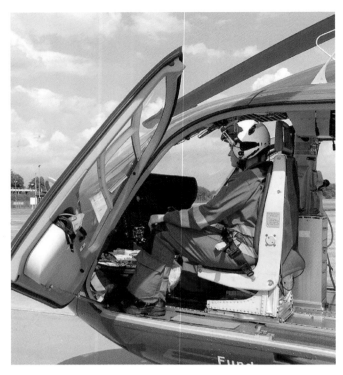

Figure 3.5 HEMS personal protective equipment.

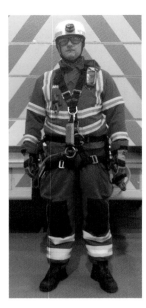

Figure 3.6 USAR personal protective equipment.

between crew members, and are deemed compulsory for HEMS work by the Civil Aviation Authority. The most common types in use are the 'Alpha Helmet' or 'Communica' style.

Urban search and rescue

Prehospital practitioners may be required to attend to patients in environments where there is a risk of a fall from height (e.g. scaffolding, cranes, pylons, hydraulic lifting platforms, etc.). It is essential that when working in such environments the practitioner is protected in the event of a fall by some form of fall arrest harness and helmet (Figure 3.6).

Tactical operations

Prehospital practitioners may be called to patients who have been shot or stabbed, or may be involved in providing medical support to police firearms teams. In both cases if the practitioner is deploying forward of a police rendezvous point then they should be wearing body armour and if necessary a Kevlar helmet (Figure 3.7). These items will protect against penetrating trauma from knives, handguns and fragmentation in the event of an explosion.

Water operations

When working on or around water there is a risk of falling or being knocked in. A personal flotation device (PFD) that triggers on contact with water should be worn by all prehospital personnel operating in this environment. Specialist medics trained in swift water rescue may attend with a greater level of PPE (Figure 3.8).

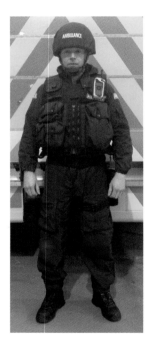

Figure 3.7 Tactical personal protective equipment.

CBRN/HAZMAT incidents

If a chemical, biological, radiological or nuclear (CBRN) incident or a release of hazardous materials (HAZMAT) is suspected the main priority for responding medical personnel is personal safety. Do not approach any further. Withdraw immediately (using personal issue escape hoods if necessary), contain where possible and report your suspicion immediately in order to obtain early expert help.

Personal issue escape hoods (Figure 3.9) are designed to allow the wearer to escape from an area of a suspected CBRN hazard and call for expert help. They provide temporary (approximately

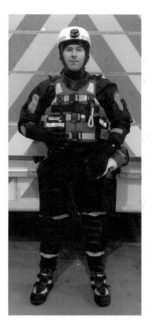

Figure 3.8 Swift water personal protective equipment.

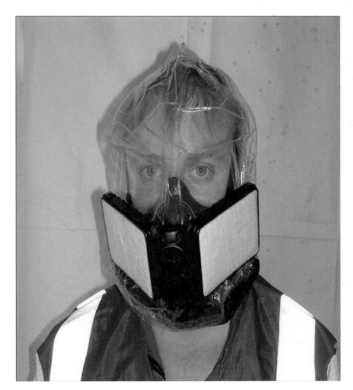

Figure 3.9 EH20 escape hood.

20 minutes) protection against airborne CBRN agents and facial liquid splashes. They are not effective in non-oxygen environments, e.g. smoke-filled room.

Personal issue electronic personal dosimeters (Figure 3.10) may help provide an early-warning signal to the wearer of dangerous

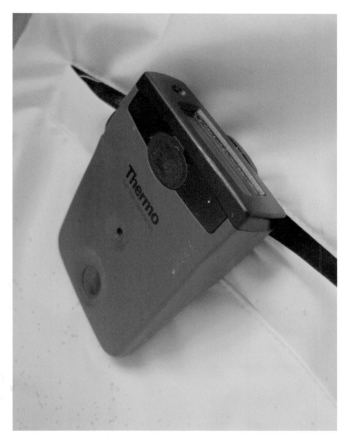

Figure 3.10 Electronic personal dosimeter.

levels of ionizing radiation in order that they may withdraw from the area and call for expert help. Their ability to record cumulative radiation exposure is useful in that they may facilitate the deployment of clinical personnel into the scene to treat casualties while at the same time monitoring their radiation exposure.

The UK Health Protection Agency provides a useful flowchart to help determine the level of PPE required for treatment of CBRN patients (Figure 3.11).

More detail on specialized chemical protection PPE can be found in Chapter 34.

Tips from the field

- PPE is there for your protection. Keep it in good working order and check it regularly for defects
- Be flexible and have different clothing options for different weather conditions. Performing CPR in the middle of summer wearing a thick high-visibility coat will rapidly lead to exhaustion of the rescuer. Most manufacturers will have lightweight versions which still meet the regulations
- Some items of PPE are used less frequently and therefore can become unfamiliar. Incorporate PPE into training and ensure regular revision of unfamiliar kit

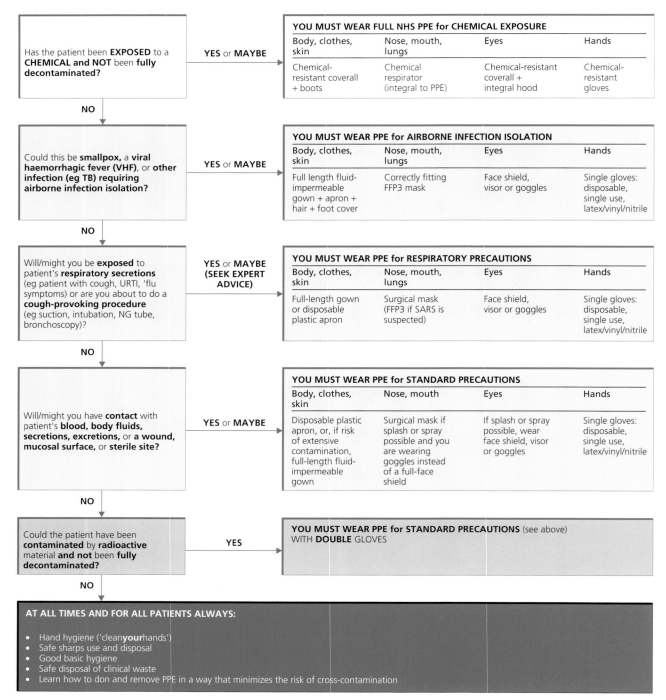

Figure 3.11 Health Protection Agency (UK) PPE Guide. (Source: http://www.hpa.org.uk/webc/HPAwebFile/HPAweb_C/1194947395416).

Further reading

Cox RD. Hazmat. eMedicine 2009. http://emedicine.medscape.com/article/764812-overview (accessed 25 February 2013). Accessed December 2010.

European PPE Guidelines. http://ec.europa.eu/enterprise/policies/european-standards/harmonised-standards/personal-protective-equipment/index_en.htm (accessed 25 February 2013).

HSE. A short guide to the Personal Protective Equipment at Work Regulations 1992. http://www.hse.gov.uk/pubns/indg174.pdf (accessed 25 February 2013).

Krzanicki DA, Porter KM. Personal protective equipment provision in prehospital care: a national survey. *EMJ* 2009; **26**: 892–895.

NFPA 1999. Standard on Protective Clothing for Emergency Medical Operations. http://www.nfpa.org.

NHS Healthcare Associated Infection and Cleanliness Division. Ambulance Guidelines. http://aace.org.uk/wp-content/uploads/2011/11/New-DH-Guidelines-Reducing-HCAIs.pdf (accessed 25 February 2013).

OSHA. PPE Information Booklet. http://www.osha.gov/Publications/osha3151.html (accessed 25 February 2013).

CHAPTER 4

Scene Safety and Assessment

Vic Calland[1] *and Pete Williams*[2]

[1]British Association for Immediate Care (BASICS), UK
[2]Dr Gray's Hospital, Elgin, UK

OVERVIEW

By the end of this chapter you should:

- Understand the immediate importance of personal and team safety at a scene
- Have a method of assessing a scene in an organized manner
- Understand the principles of 'reading' a scene.

Introduction

The safety of a scene is everyone's responsibility and begins long before the incident occurs. Not only is specific prehospital clinical training required, training in safety (and response driving if appropriate) within a properly governed system is essential (Box 4.1).

Box 4.1 **Training**

Clinical
Safety & environmental
Response driving
Governance

Although fire and rescue retain primacy regarding scene safety, it is up to all those present to ensure their own actions do not jeopardize the safety of the patient or other rescuers.

Arriving at the scene you need to have a strategy in your mind. One way is to use a mnemonic to take you through the key issues in a logical order (Box 4.2). These will now be considered in more detail.

Safety

Before entering the immediate vicinity of the scene rapidly but thoroughly assess for hazards and liaise with personnel already on scene. If the scene is not safe, you may need to stand off until fire

---

ABC of Prehospital Emergency Medicine, First Edition.
Edited by Tim Nutbeam and Matthew Boylan.
© 2013 John Wiley & Sons, Ltd. Published 2013 by John Wiley & Sons, Ltd.

Box 4.2 **Scene assessment**

S afety
C ommunicate
R ead the wreckage
E veryone accounted for?
A ssess the casualties
M ethod of extrication
E vacuation route
R ight facility

---

and rescue (or other service) can make the scene safe for you to approach. It is important to remember that the scene is a dynamic environment. What was once safe may become decidedly *unsafe* with the passage of time, the cutting of vehicles, the moving of structures or the leakage of fuel. Not only should you keep reassessing the casualty's condition, you should also reassess your environment for your own, your team's and your patient's safety (the 1–2–3 of safety).

Where is the danger?

Trauma is caused by the application of excessive energy to living tissue. Recognizing how energy interacted with your patient provides the basis of assessing the mechanism of injury, which in turn can help you predict the likely injuries sustained. Recognizing sources of unstable energy and taking action to limit their uncontrolled release is fundamental to scene safety. The most relevant types of energy are kinetic, potential, thermal, electrical and chemical (Table 4.1). Other significant hazards present on scene may include biological, radiological and nuclear sources.

Once the scene has been surveyed for potential hazards an assessment must be made regarding these. Some hazards, such as a long drop, cannot be removed but can however be mitigated by providing protection such as a barrier. It is important to realize that hazards will change during your time on scene. Stable wreckage, once cut, may become unstable, trivial spills may progress to produce fire, chemical or slip hazards, the weather may deteriorate and it is not uncommon for rescuers exercising in warm PPE not to notice their immobile shocked patient becoming progressively colder.

Table 4.1 Scene hazards

Scene	Kinetic	Potential	Thermal	Electrical	Chemical
Road or Motorsport	Other traffic	Undeployed airbags Seatbelt pretensioners Unstable vehicle	Exhaust systems Brakes Coolants	Battery Multi-fuel Roadside cables	Fuel Engine compartment leaks Cargo
Rail	Trains Points	Trip hazards	Brakes	High tension	Freight
Water	Moving water	Flood barrier giving way	Hypothermia	Disrupted cables	Pollution
Home	Pets Assailants	Trip hazards	Fire Kettles	Disrupted cables Faulty equipment	Kitchen Garage

Communicate

Control must be informed when you arrive on scene. The METHANE message format may be used to initiate an appropriate allocation of resources (Box 4.3).

Box 4.3 **METHANE message**

M y callsign
E xact location
T ype of incident
H azards
A ccess and egress
N umber of casualties
E mergency services required

Early communication with the other agencies on scene is vital, both to make them aware of your presence and to receive a briefing on their initial assessment, priorities and plan. Witnesses should also be spoken to in order to gain a better understanding of the events leading up to the injury or illness. Finally, good communication with the patient(s) is key to determining the location of injuries, appreciating changes to the level of consciousness and reducing fear, anxiety and pain.

Read the wreckage

Assessing the mechanism of injury can be likened to taking the history of a patient's presenting complaint. A thorough understanding of the mechanism allows the responder to predict what injuries a casualty has sustained and to question their clinical assessment when those predicted injuries have not been found.

Soon after an injury has occurred there may be little in the way of clinical signs to indicate a life-threatening problem. Pathology is in evolution and many of the classical signs seen in hospital emergency departments are yet to develop. Circulating catecholamines may complicate diagnosis further by masking pain and blood loss. Appreciating the mechanism will allow the responder to maintain a high index of suspicion in the face of an initial negative assessment. In most circumstances injuries sustained are highly predictable from the mechanism of injury by considering where the energy has gone.

The ability to predict pathology from the mechanism of injury is an important skill that must be developed in order to provide accurate medical guidance to the Fire Service during extrications.

Fire crews will not want to cause pain or exacerbate injury and so have traditionally been trained to remove the vehicle from around the casualty. This may result in avoidable delays, and with third-impact injuries any delay in getting to the operating theatre will adversely affect survival. Being able to advise the Fire Service appropriately needs understanding of good clinical skills, mechanisms of injury and extrication techniques.

Fall from height

Injury severity depends upon the height fallen and the compressibility of the surface onto which the person lands. Falls from greater than two storey (20 feet, 6 metres) onto non-compressible surfaces (e.g. concrete) will be associated with more severe injuries. Falling from height onto one's heels leads to a characteristic transmission of force through the body and predictable pattern of injury (Figure 4.1).

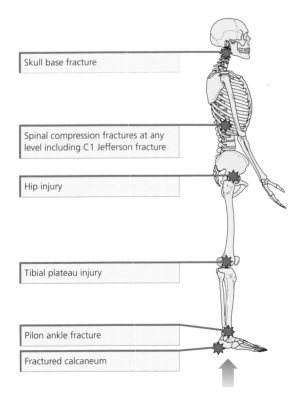

Skull base fracture

Spinal compression fractures at any level including C1 Jefferson fracture

Hip injury

Tibial plateau injury

Pilon ankle fracture

Fractured calcaneum

Figure 4.1 Fall from height.

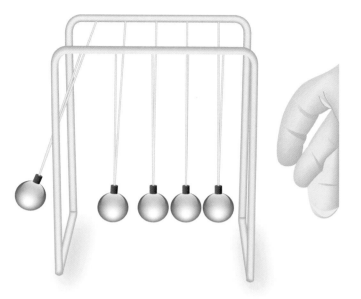

Figure 4.2 Newton's cradle.

Motor vehicle collisions

In any vehicle accident there are up to four impacts. The vehicle hits the object that stops it. The occupant hits the inside of the vehicle. The organs are then jerked to a halt, and then finally anything (or anyone) that is unrestrained within the vehicle can also hit them. Modern cars with crumple zones and restrain systems can mitigate the effects of most impacts up to about 40 mph. At greater speeds however the forces applied can cause fatal 'third-impact' injuries such as a ruptured liver or a torn aortic arch. It is important to remember the principle behind Newton's cradle (Figure 4.2).

It is the energy in one side that is transferred to the other. Thus if a lorry hits a car, the car receives the energy from the lorry and it is therefore obviously more seriously deformed. If however two cars of equal mass, both travelling at 50 mph collide head on, the effect will be the same as one car driving in to an immovable object at 50 mph, and not a 100-mph impact as might be imagined.

MVC frontal impact

Following a frontal impact unrestrained occupants will continue to move forward until they impact with the interior of the vehicle. These impact injuries and the resultant deceleration forces produce a predictable pattern of injury (Figure 4.3).

If the patient is wearing a seatbelt a different pattern of injury will be seen depending on the type of belt (three point or lap) and whether the shoulder strap was over the right shoulder or left. The line of injury will reflect the location and orientation of the belt straps worn. During extrication, seatbelts should be cut rather than unbuckled. This prevents re-use and also indicates permanently that it was fastened at the time of the accident. When cutting the belt, be aware that seat belt pretension systems that have fired during the impact may leave the casualty tightly secured by the belt. Appropriate support should be given to the casualty to prevent them slumping forward when this restraining force is released.

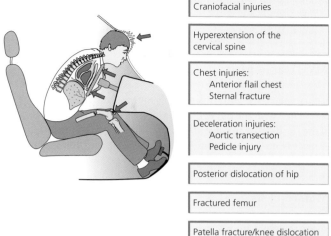

Figure 4.3 Frontal impact (unrestrained).

Craniofacial injuries

Hyperextension of the cervical spine

Chest injuries:
 Anterior flail chest
 Sternal fracture

Deceleration injuries:
 Aortic transection
 Pedicle injury

Posterior dislocation of hip

Fractured femur

Patella fracture/knee dislocation

Airbags will further modify the injury pattern. It is important to remember that the airbag is designed for the 'average' occupant and has drawbacks for both the very large and small.

MVC lateral impact

Motor vehicles are not well designed to tolerate lateral impacts, especially if the impacting force is concentrated over a small area of the vehicle such as with a lateral impact of car versus pole. The vehicle design is unable to dissipate the energy before the deforming force reaches the patient, and so significant passenger cell intrusion and associated injuries usually result. Naturally the side of the patient presented to the impacting force will sustain the greater degree of injury (Figure 4.4).

Right-sided impacts pose a threat to structures on the right of the body and vice versa. 44% of aortic injuries sustained in road accidents occur in side impacts. If the vehicle undergoes a rotational force the driver or the passenger may be turned out of the restraining diagonal strap of their seatbelt. If the occupant turns

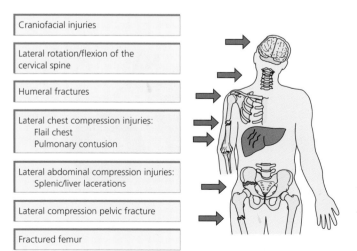

Craniofacial injuries

Lateral rotation/flexion of the cervical spine

Humeral fractures

Lateral chest compression injuries:
 Flail chest
 Pulmonary contusion

Lateral abdominal compression injuries:
 Splenic/liver lacerations

Lateral compression pelvic fracture

Fractured femur

Figure 4.4 Lateral impact.

to look at the oncoming impact they will substantially reduce the ability of the cervical spine to extend and therefore will be more prone to neck injury.

MVC rear impacts

Most healthcare professionals will have seen the classical whiplash injury associated with this type of impact. Low back injury is also associated with the impact. The injuries are likely to be more severe if the car they are in is fitted with a tow bar, because the force of the impact is not absorbed in the rear crumple zones but transmitted directly to the passenger shell.

Motorcyclists

Motorcyclists often also have three impacts. First they hit whatever stops their progress. They will tend to rise up off the bike and can sustain pelvic and femoral fractures as they hit the fuel tank and handlebars. They then progress rapidly to a second impact wherever they land, and their organs are forced to a halt a fraction of a second later.

Pedestrians

It is traditionally said that adult pedestrians turn away from an oncoming car whereas children turn towards it. This does not appear to be evidence based. However, Waddell's triad is a pattern of injury that does appear to be seen in pedestrian children who are struck by motor vehicles (Figure 4.5).

Everyone found?

Several times a year the emergency services attend accidents and leave without assessing all the casualties. It may be a child ejected from a vehicle, or someone who has staggered from the scene to collapse later. It can be the joy rider who flees to avoid arrest. You need to use multiple clues to determine how many people were involved.

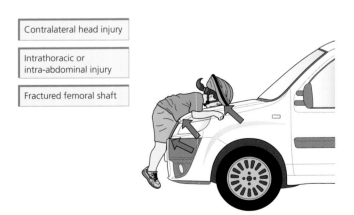

| Contralateral head injury |
| Intrathoracic or intra-abdominal injury |
| Fractured femoral shaft |

Figure 4.5 Waddell's triad.

Assessment of the patients

The number, location and acuity of all casualties should be assessed. Where more than one casualty is involved, triage should be performed to prioritize extrication, treatment and evacuation. A simple triage tool (e.g. triage sieve) may be used.

Clinical assessment of the individual patient must be made in the context of what the casualty was doing at the time of the injury and how soon the assessment was made. A jockey in a horse race may well be tachycardic and tachypnoeic from physical exertion. In this situation, trends in vital signs are of far greater significance than individual values. If a rider has a respiratory rate of 30/minute at first contact, dropping to 22 by 3 minutes after the incident and then increasing again to 26 by 5 minutes, these subtle changes can easily be missed. Careful monitoring of physiological trends is essential if these trends are to be detected.

Method of extrication

The Fire Service needs clinical support in determining the most appropriate method of extrication in relation to two key elements: time frame and route. This requires the prehospital provider to understand what can and what can't be achieved by the firefighters. If the patient is time critical, in order to achieve a rapid extrication, compromises may have to be made with regard to spinal immobilization, etc.

Evacuation

This merits some consideration. What is the most suitable way of getting the patient to hospital? Not all patients can travel by air ambulance, but it may be preferable to an ambulance ride down unmade farm tracks. Casualties have been evacuated from railways on board trains, from river banks in passing boats and even on quad bike.

Is the ambulance the correct side of the accident to go to the most appropriate hospital? Has the gate to the air ambulance landing point been unlocked? Consider the route before you take the patient along it.

Right hospital

It is not just about choosing between the cottage hospital or the trauma unit. Not only do you need to decide the most appropriate facility for the clinical care of your patient but you need to consider trying to keep families together (particularly if there are children), getting them closer to their home to make travelling easier for friends and relatives, and even if all other matters are equal, getting the crews back to their station more quickly. These are matters to discuss with the Ambulance Officer on scene. Make sure the crew knows where you want the patient to go, and make sure the police and relatives know where they went.

Tips from the field

- All incident scenes should be approached in a structured manner
- Liaise early with the Incident Safety Officer (usually Fire Service)
- Scene safety and an ability to 'read the wreckage' both require an understanding of the way energy is transferred
- The mechanism of injury may be the only clue to life threatening injury in the early stages following an accident
- Vehicle safety systems may produce their own hazards
- For anyone interested in active prehospital care work extensive exploration of this topic is essential.

Further reading

Calland V. *Safety at Scene: A Manual for Paramedics and Immediate Care Doctors*. St. Louis: Mosby, 2001

Watson L. *Mechanisms of Injury*. http://www.resqmed.com (accessed 25 February 2013).

CHAPTER 5

The Primary Survey

Tim Nutbeam[1] and Matthew Boylan[2]

[1] Derriford Hospital, Plymouth Hospitals NHS Trust, Plymouth, UK
[2] Royal Centre for Defence Medicine, University Hospitals Birmingham, Birmingham, UK

OVERVIEW

By the end of this chapter you will:

- Have an understanding of the role of the primary survey in patient assessment and management
- Understand that the primary survey may be customised to individual patient needs and practitioner skill set/experience.

Introduction

The primary survey is a systematic process by which life-threatening conditions are identified and immediate life-saving treatment is started.

Initially developed for the assessment of trauma patients, the principles of thorough protocol-led assessment, combined with immediate interventions can be equally applied to the medical patient.

Not every practitioner's 'primary survey' will be the same – there will be variations dependent upon:

- assessment tools availability and competency (e.g. the use of ultrasound)
- variations in interventions performed (e.g. many practitioners will not be in a position to perform RSI).
- practitioner experience.

The ABC system (or more recently the <C>ABC) system is the most commonly used in clinical practice (Table 5.1). It provides a stepwise and reproducible assessment tool which proceeds in a logical fashion, both in terms of clinical importance and anatomic region (Figure 5.1).

In reality it is unusual to perform these steps in isolation: a team approach allows for many of these steps to occur concurrently. Despite a team approach, a single clinician must take responsibility for the primary survey and ensure that all steps have been completed.

Table 5.1 CABC and ABC

<C>	Control of catastrophic haemorrhage
A	Airway (+ cervical spine control if indicated)
B	Breathing (+ oxygen if indicated)
C	Circulation with control of non-catastrophic external haemorrhage

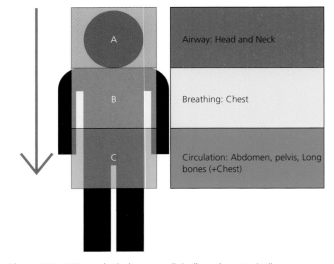

Figure 5.1 ABC as a logical process clinically and anatomically.

The primary survey is a not, as it names implies, a one-off process; it consists of multiple surveys. Triggers for repetition of the survey include:

- any acute change in clinical condition
- after intervention, e.g. performing RSI
- after patient movement, e.g. transfer to helicopter
- patient handover.

Other opportunities to repeat the primary survey will arise and should be taken, especially in the unstable patient.

In short the primary survey consists of:

<C>: Control of catastrophic external haemorrhage. This may involve the use of an assistant to control bleeding (elevation, pressure, indirect pressure, haemostatic) and the application of tourniquets.

ABC of Prehospital Emergency Medicine, First Edition.
Edited by Tim Nutbeam and Matthew Boylan.
© 2013 John Wiley & Sons, Ltd. Published 2013 by John Wiley & Sons, Ltd.

A: Airway assessment and intervention. This includes the identification and resolution (or at least temporisation) of the obstructed and obstructing airway. A neck assessment should also identify wounds and laryngeal injury as well as factors identifying a difficult (surgical) airway. Consideration should be given for C spine injury and immobilization device(s) applied as indicated.

B: Breathing assessment and intervention. Identify and treat life-threatening injuries (Table 5.2). Oxygen for hypoxaemia.

C: Circulation assessment and intervention. Intravenous (or intraosseous) access. Adjuncts including application of pelvic binder, reducing and splinting long bone fractures, stopping haemorrhage from wounds.

D: Assessment of disability. Intervention (e.g. airway management for low conscious level) if required. This is a good stage at which to establish an appropriate analgesic strategy.

E: Exposure: this includes assessment of temperature, and, if time and conditions allow, the secondary survey.

A modified primary survey for medical conditions can be found in Table 5.3.

The secondary survey is a thorough 'top to toe' assessment to identify any other injuries/stigmata which the primary survey may not have revealed. The prehospital environment may not always be where this should occur. Ongoing transfer arrangements, on scene time, scene conditions and patient instability will dictate the appropriateness of this.

Table 5.2 Life-threatening injuries requiring intervention in the primary survey

	Injury	Intervention
<C>	Catastrophic haemorrhage	Use of assistant/hameostatics/tourniquets
A	Actual or impending airway obstruction	Airway manoeuvres/adjuncts, suction, RSI, surgical airway
B	Tension pneumothorax	Decompression + thorocostomy
	Massive haemothorax	Thorocostomy (± drain)
	Open pneumothorax	Appropriate dressing (e.g. Ashermann chest seal)
	Flail chest	Awareness of need for IPPV
	Cardiac tamponade	Thoracotomy
C	Haemodynamic instability	Blood or blood products/tranexamic acid
	Pelvic fracture	Pelvic binder
	Long bone fracture	Reduction and splinting
D	Decreased GCS	Airway management/IPPV if indicated

Table 5.3 Life-threatening medical conditions requiring intervention in the primary survey

	Condition	Intervention
A	Actual or impending airway obstruction	Airway manoeuvres/adjuncts, suction, RSI, surgical airway. Adrenaline in presence of anaphylaxis
B	Tension pneumothorax	Decompression + thorocostomy
	Heart failure	GTN/CPAP if available
	Asthma/COAD	Nebulisers (salbutamol, ipatropium bromide, Mg^{2+}), titrate oxygen therapy
	Poor tidal Volumes	NIPPV, IPPV (RSI)
	Hypoxaemia	Titrate oxygen therapy
	Cardiac tamponade	Pericardocentesis (± thoracotomy)
C	Haemodynamic instability	Intravenous fluids, inotropes, vasopressors
	Cardiac arrest	Chest compressions
D	Low blood sugar	Sugar
	Decreased GCS	Airway management/IPPV if indicated
E	Sepsis	Antibiotics

Tips from the field

- Practice 'your' primary survey until it is automatic – you (and your patient) will rely on this at times of stress
- Work with your team; tasks can be delegated but one person must take responsibility for completion
- Repeat the primary survey whenever an opportunity arises – patient care is a dynamic process
- The first <C> is for Catastrophic haemorrhage – the remainder of the primary survey should not be delayed for slow bleeds/ooze/non-major wounds, etc.
- Get your hands on: assessment of 'breathing' through clothes is unreliable and potentially a fatal mistake.

Further reading

Committee on Trauma, American College of Surgeons. *ATLS: Advanced Trauma Life Support Program for Doctors*, 8th edn. Chicago: American College of Surgeons, 2008.
See individual Airway, Breathing, Circulation etc., chapters for further reading suggestions.

CHAPTER 6

Airway Assessment and Management

Mårten Sandberg[1,2], Anders Rostrup Nakstad[2], Peter Anthony Berlac[3], Per Kristian Hyldmo[4], and Matthew Boylan[5]

[1]University of Oslo, Oslo, Norway
[2]Oslo University Hospital, Oslo, Norway
[3]University of Copenhagen, Copenhagen, Denmark
[4]Sorlandet Hospital, Kristiansand, Norway
[5]Royal Centre for Defence Medicine, University Hospitals Birmingham, Birmingham, UK

OVERVIEW

By the end of this chapter you should know:

- The importance of a secure airway
- How to identify which patients need a secured airway
- How to predict a difficult airway
- The importance of simple measures in securing the airway
- The value of supraglottic airway devices
- The principles of basic and advanced airway techniques.

Introduction

Ensuring delivery of oxygenated blood to the brain and other vital organs is the primary objective in the initial treatment of the severely injured or ill patient: securing a patent and protected airway has priority over management of all other conditions (with the exception of catastrophic haemorrhage). Failure to identify the need for airway intervention may be just as disastrous as the inability of the prehospital care provider to perform the necessary interventions. Airway obstruction can occur at any level between the mouth and the carina (Box 6.1).

Box 6.1 **Causes of airway obstruction**

Pharynx
Maxillofacial trauma
Soft tissue swelling including the epiglottis
Liquid – secretions/blood/vomit
Tongue – swelling/unconsciousness

Larynx
Foreign body
Oedema (e.g. allergic reactions, inflammation, trauma, burns)
Laryngospasm
Laryngeal trauma

Subglottic
Foreign body
Swelling – bacterial tracheitis.

ABC of Prehospital Emergency Medicine, First Edition.
Edited by Tim Nutbeam and Matthew Boylan.
© 2013 John Wiley & Sons, Ltd. Published 2013 by John Wiley & Sons, Ltd.

Airway assessment

The awake, alert patient who is able to speak with a normal voice has no immediate threat to the airway. In contrast, the obtunded or unconscious patient requires rapid assessment and protection of the airway. An obstructed airway can be the cause or result of a decreased level of consciousness.

The following steps should be undertaken to assess the airway.

Look

Look at the face, neck, oral cavity and chest.
Assess for:

- obvious signs of maxillofacial or neck trauma
- foreign bodies, swelling, blood or gastric contents in the mouth
- paradoxical movement of the chest and abdomen – 'see-sawing'
- accessory muscle use (head bobbing in infants)
- suprasternal, intercostal or supraclavicular recession
- tracheal tug (downward movement of the trachea with inspiration)
- fogging of an oxygen mask with ventilation (rules out complete obstruction).

Listen

Listen for breath sounds.
Assess for:

- snoring sounds caused by partial occlusion of the pharynx by the tongue
- gurgling sounds indicative of fluid in the airway (e.g. secretions, blood, vomit)
- inspiratory stridor reflecting upper airway narrowing and obstruction
- absent breath sounds may indicate complete obstruction or respiratory arrest

Although listening for and interpreting breath sounds may be simple and potentially invaluable, ambient noise at an accident scene or in a moving ambulance can make this difficult and potentially inaccurate.

Feel

Feel for expired air against the back of your hand or on your cheek whilst listening for breath sounds and watching for chest movement.

Assess for:

- absent breathing may indicate complete obstruction or respiratory arrest.

Difficult airway assessment

The **HAVNOT** mnemonic may be useful in helping identify factors predictive of a difficult airway (Box 6.2). Features indicative of difficult airway rescue are equally important to recognize (Box 6.3). It is vital that these features are identified early in the assessment process as they may guide the level of intervention undertaken in the field and/or trigger early transfer to hospital for definitive airway management with advanced techniques (e.g. fibre optic intubation, gas induction, etc.).

Box 6.2 Predicting the difficult airway (HAVNOT)

H History of previous airway difficulties
A Anatomical abnormalities of the face, mouth and teeth (receding mandible, large tongue, buck teeth, high arched palate)
V Visual clues – obesity, facial hair, Age >55 years
N Neck immobility – short bull neck, MILS, arthritis
O Opening of the mouth <3 fingers
T Trauma – maxillofacial injury, burns and airway bleeding

Box 6.3 Predicting difficult airway rescue

Difficult mask ventilation (MOANS)
Mask Seal Difficulty – Beard/Facial trauma
Obesity/**O**bstetric/**O**bstructed (e.g. angioedema, abscesses)
Advanced Age (>55 years)
No teeth
Snorer/**S**tiff lungs e.g. severe asthma, pulmonary oedema

Difficult supraglottic airway (RODS)
Restricted mouth opening (less than 4–5 cm/3 fingers)
Obstruction at the larynx or below
Distorted airway – affects seal e.g. trauma/abscesses
Stiff lungs, e.g. severe asthma, pulmonary oedema
Stiff C spine, e.g. reduced movement, fixed flexion of neck

Difficult cricothyroidotomy (SHORT)
Surgery/**S**cars/**S**hort neck
Haematoma
Obesity
Radiotherapy
Trauma (laryngeal)/**T**umours

Airway management

Fortunately, most patients in the prehospital setting have a patent airway and may only require supplemental oxygen. In patients with a compromised or threatened airway, immediate action is needed. Prehospital care should start with simple, basic manoeuvres such as the chin lift or jaw thrust, proceeding to more complex measures if simple procedures prove insufficient. The level of intervention will be determined by the practitioner's skillset (Figure 6.1).

Caution is advised when manipulating the airway in patients with possible neck trauma because of the potential risk of spinal cord injury. Although airway management takes priority over spinal cord protection, measures can and should be taken to simultaneously immobilize and protect the neck using manual in-line stabilization (MILS) while securing the airway.

Patient positioning

Conscious patients will maintain themselves in the optimum position to maintain their airway and drain secretions/blood. This position should be maintained where possible and the patient should not be forced to lie supine. Obtunded or unconscious patients should be turned into the recovery position in order to prevent the tongue from falling back into the pharynx, obstructing the upper airway. This position also allows gastric contents and other fluids (blood, secretions) to flow freely out of the mouth, rather than into the lower airways. In unresponsive spontaneously breathing trauma patients, the *lateral trauma position* (Figure 6.2) should be used. A stiff neck collar is applied in the supine position and the patient log-rolled into the lateral position. The head and body are then supported in this position, e.g. with folded blankets.

Suction

Correct positioning with postural drainage is more important than suction in the presence of gross liquid contamination of the airway, e.g. torrential bleeding, active vomiting. When oral suction is required a wide-bore suction catheter (e.g. Yankauer) connected to a powered suction unit is preferable. Hand-held suction units should only be used as a back-up as they are less effective. Suction should be performed under direct vision and for no longer than 15 seconds in any patient. Flexible suction catheters may be inserted through oral or nasal airways to provide ongoing airway toilet. The appropriate size (French gauge) is numerically twice the internal diameter of the airway (mm).

Foreign body removal

Simply encouraging coughing in the alert patient will be enough to clear most foreign bodies from the upper airway. Should the patient collapse or become weak, back-slaps and abdominal thrusts should be attempted. In the event of a respiratory arrest CPR should be initiated and an attempt to remove the foreign body under direct vision using Magills forceps or a suction catheter should be tried. In extremis a surgical airway may be used to bypass the obstruction.

Facial fracture reduction

Bilateral mandibular fractures can result in an unstable anterior segment which can displace backwards obstructing the airway. Manually lift the displaced fragment forward to relieve the obstruction. Maxillary (Le Fort) fractures can result in a mobile mid-face segment which may displace backwards obstructing the airway. To reduce, the mobile segment should be grasped between the thumb and the index/middle finger (inserted into the patients mouth) and pulled forwards.

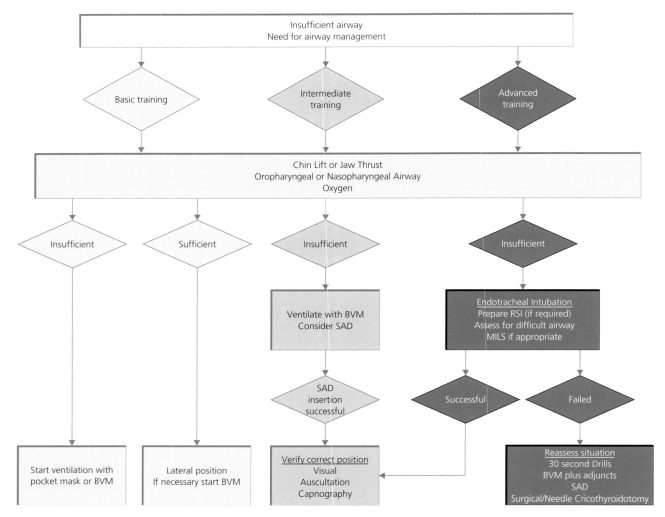

Figure 6.1 Airway management algorithm. (Source: Berlac P, Hyldmo PK, Kongstad P et al. Acta Anaesthesiol Scand. 2008 Aug;52(7):897–907).

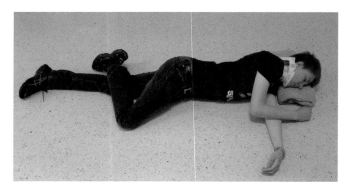

Figure 6.2 Lateral trauma position.

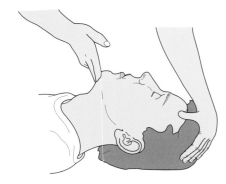

Figure 6.3 Chin lift.

Manual airway manoeuvres

The **chin lift** manoeuvre is performed by gripping the chin between the thumb and forefinger and lifting the mandible upwards (which in turn lifts the tongue off the posterior pharyngeal wall). In the non-trauma patient it may be combined with **head tilt** (Figure 6.3) to improve airway axis alignment (except in infants). Head tilt

should be avoided in trauma patients, since this manoeuvre may convert a cervical fracture without cord injury to one with cord injury.

The **jaw thrust** (Figure 6.4) manoeuvre is an alternative technique to chin lift and is preferred when spinal injury is suspected. The practitioner's fingers are placed under and behind the angle of the mandible and the jaw lifted forwards and upwards. Counter

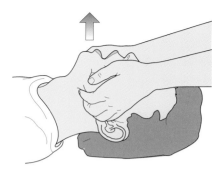

Figure 6.4 Jaw thrust.

pressure is applied over the maxilla using the thenar eminences (or thumbs) to prevent movement of the head. Simultaneous application of a face mask capable of delivering oxygen or ventilation is possible with this technique.

Basic airway adjuncts

The **oropharyngeal airway** (OPA) is designed to hold the tongue forward, preventing posterior displacement of the tongue and obstruction of the upper airway. The appropriate size is equivalent to the distance between the incisors to the angle of the jaw (Figure 6.5) or the corner of the mouth to the tragus. In adults and older children it should be inserted upside down into the mouth before being rotated 180 degrees when the soft palate is encountered. In children under 4 years the airway should be inserted without rotation after depressing the tongue with a tongue blade or laryngoscope. The OPA is not suitable for patients with an intact gag reflex, as it may provoke vomiting and laryngospasm. A patient who readily accepts an OPA will need endotracheal intubation either prehospitally if skills permit, or soon after arrival at the hospital.

The **nasopharyngeal airway** (NPA) serves the same purpose as the OPA, but is better tolerated in patients with intact airway reflexes. They are particularly useful in patients with limited mouth opening, e.g. trismus. The airway is made of soft malleable plastic to minimize risk of injury during insertion. After lubrication it should inserted through the nostril, along the floor of the nasal cavity and into the upper airway until stopped by the flange (Figure 6.6).

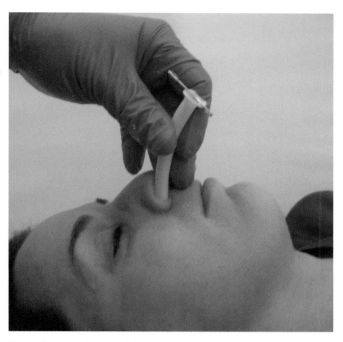

Figure 6.6 Nasopharyngeal airway insertion.

Slight rotation during insertion may be helpful. A size 6.0 airway should be used for adult females and a size 7.0 for adult males. Other sizes are available and the appropriate airway length is equal to the distance between the nostril and the angle of the jaw. The appropriate diameter should fit the nostril without causing sustained blanching. Profuse soft-tissue bleeding from the nasal cavity and nasopharynx can occur despite careful insertion. Caution must be employed in patients with head trauma, as a NPA could enter the cranial cavity through a skull base fracture if incorrectly inserted.

If there is difficulty in achieving a clear airway or where rescue ventilation is required as part of a failed airway drill, a combination of two NPAs and an OPA should be employed (Figure 6.7).

Supraglottic airway devices

In simple terms, supraglottic airway devices (SADs) consist of a cuffed tube that is inserted blindly into the pharynx and allows ventilation over the glottis. As their name implies they are not designed to be inserted beyond the vocal cords into the trachea. One attractive feature about SADs is that laryngoscopy and muscle relaxation are not necessary for insertion, making placement easier and faster than endotracheal intubation. A major disadvantage, though, is that they do not fully protect the lower airways against aspiration of gastric contents, secretions or blood. This risk must be weighed against the ease of use and potential life-saving benefits in the prehospital arena.

A number of different SADS are available (Figure 6.8) and practitioners should familiarize themselves with the type used within their service. The I-Gel® and the Proseal LMA® provide a better airway seal and allow higher airway pressures to be used than the other variants. The intubating LMA® and I-Gel® allow

Oropharyngeal Airway Sizes	
000	Neonate
00	Infant
0	Small Child
1	Child
2	Small Adult
3	Medium Adult
4	Large Adult

Figure 6.5 Oropharyngeal Airway Sizing.

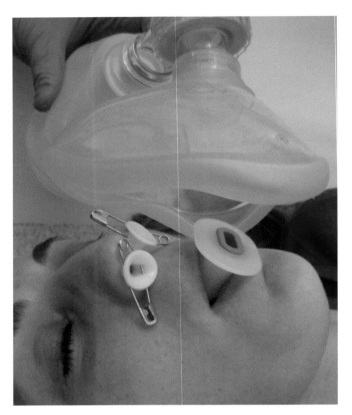

Figure 6.7 Multiple airway technique.

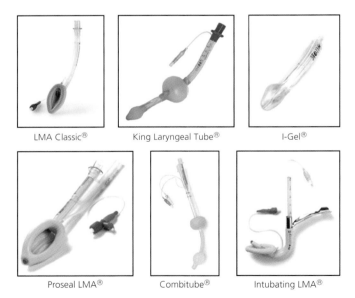

| LMA Classic® | King Laryngeal Tube® | I-Gel® |
| Proseal LMA® | Combitube® | Intubating LMA® |

Figure 6.8 Supraglottic airways.

subsequent intubation through the device if required. Most of the modern devices have an oesophageal drainage channel through which a nasogastric tube can be inserted and the stomach contents aspirated to reduce the risk of regurgitation and subsequent aspiration.

All emergency medical services providing advanced prehospital care should include at least one SAD in their standard equipment.

Which SAD to include will depend on local preference, training and availability. Such devices can provide a life-saving solution to a severe airway problem, especially when endotracheal intubation skills are not available. Disposable SADs are available in both paediatric and adult sizes.

Endotracheal intubation

Endotracheal intubation is potentially harmful in unskilled hands and undetected oesophageal intubation may be fatal for the patient. The procedure should be drug assisted (see Chapter 9) unless the patient is in cardiac arrest or deeply unconscious with an absent gag reflex.

The basic equipment required for endotracheal intubation is shown in Box 6.4. The age-appropriate size and type of laryngoscope blade and endotracheal tube are listed in Box 6.5. Cuffed endotracheal tubes are now acceptable in all age groups. Endotracheal tubes with a Parker flex-tip (e.g. GlideRite®) are preferred as they are less traumatic and less liable to catch on the laryngeal cartilages on insertion. A lubricated bougie should be used for all prehospital intubations. Laryngoscopes are notoriously unreliable and a secondary handle and blade should be available in case of failure of the primary device.

Box 6.4 **Equipment for intubation**

SAVE THE DAMSELS
Suction
Airway adjuncts
Ventilator or BVM
Emergency cricothyroidotomy kit/SAD
Tape or tie
HME filter
Endotracheal tube(s)
Drugs – if RSI required
Angle piece catheter mount
Monitoring, including ETCO$_2$
Stethoscope
Elastic bougie
Laryngoscope(s)
Syringe (10 mL)

Box 6.5 **Endotracheal tube and laryngoscope blade guide**

Age	Laryngoscope blade	ETT Length	ETT diameter
Preterm	0 Miller	8 cm	2.5 mm
Newborn		10 cm	3.0 mm
6 months	1 Miller	11 cm	3.5 mm
1 year		12 cm	4.0 mm
1–2 years		11 cm	4.5 mm
2–4 years	2 Miller	(Age/2) + 12	(Age/4) + 4 Uncuffed
4–9 years	2 Miller/Mackintosh		
9–16 years	3 Mackintosh		(Age/4) + 3.5 Cuffed
>16 years	3 or 4 Mackintosh	21 cm (Female) 23 cm (Male)	8.0 mm (Female) 9.0 mm (Male)

It is imperative to optimize intubation conditions in order to increase the rate of first pass success (Box 6.6). Where conditions are suboptimal (e.g. patient trapped sitting in a car) alternative airway devices (e.g. NPA, SAD) should be employed and intubation postponed until optimal conditions can be achieved (i.e. after extrication). A number of additional techniques (Box 6.7) may be employed should the initial laryngoscopic view be suboptimal. These form the basis of the '30-second drills' – 30 seconds being the time they should be completed in. Cricoid pressure should be released as there is limited evidence to say it is beneficial but has been shown to impair laryngoscopic view if performed poorly. External laryngeal manipulation with backward, upward and rightwards pressure (BURP) can then be attempted and has also been shown to improve the grade of view. A McCoy blade (Figure 6.9) may be used to elevate the epiglottis and improve the view at laryngoscopy in difficult intubations (e.g. anterior larynx).

Box 6.6 **Tips for optimizing intubation**

Position patient on a stretcher at optimal height
Place stretcher in shade with the sun behind the intubator
Ensure 360 degree access to the patient
Ensure stretcher, patient and intubator optimally aligned
Open the anterior part of the cervical collar (but continue MILS)
Use a pillow behind the head of medical patients to aid optimal positioning
Obese patients should be positioned so that the ear canal and sternum are in the same horizontal plane
All equipment laid out and protected in kit dump
Alternative laryngoscope and smaller ET tube available
Use largest blade from outset.

Box 6.7 **30-second drills**

Adjust operator position
Adjust patient position
Change operator
Suction
Use longer blade
Use McCoy Blade
Backward upward rightward pressure (BURP)
Release cricoid pressure
Insert blade fully and withdraw.

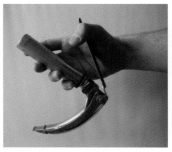 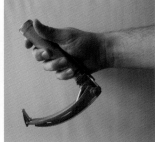

Figure 6.9 The McCoy blade.

Every system should have a written, and well rehearsed, 'failed intubation plan' for use in the event of failure of the 30-second drills. This should include supraglottic airway rescue devices and provision for performing a surgical airway.

Following intubation, confirmation of tube placement is essential. Direct visualization of the tube passing through the cords is the first step in this process. Auscultation is then performed first in the epigastric area, then in both axillae. If the tube is in the oesophagus it will bubble violently in this area in synchrony with your bag–valve–tube ventilation. If that happens, the patient must be extubated. Keep in mind that after an oesophageal intubation, sound will be transmitted from the stomach to the lungs resulting in bilateral sounds over thorax that easily can be mistaken as normal lung sounds. Therefore always auscultate the epigastric area first. Measurement of the end-tidal carbon dioxide using waveform capnography completes the final step in tube confirmation.

A number of options are available for securing the correctly placed endotracheal tube. These include adhesive tape, a tube tie (tied as a larks foot), and commercial tube holders (e.g. Thomas tube holder®).

Cricothyroidotomy

A cricothyroidotomy is indicated when a patent airway cannot be achieved by any other means, e.g. severe maxillofacial trauma, poor access to the face (e.g. in entrapment) or as part of the failed airway drill. As the name suggests access to the airway is gained through the cricothyroid membrane (Figure 6.10).

Needle cricothyroidotomy is preferred in children under the age of 12 years because there is a greater risk of subsequent subglottic stenosis with the open surgical approach. Equipment should be carried pre-assembled for immediate use (Figure 6.11).

The patient should be placed supine and if there is no risk of cervical spine injury the neck extended. The cricothyroid membrane should be identified and the larynx stabilized with the operator's left hand. With the free hand the needle is inserted at a 45-degree caudal angle through the skin over the cricothyroid membrane. The syringe should be used to aspirate as the needle is inserted, stopping when there is free aspiration of air after the cricothyroid membrane is punctured. At this point the needle tip is in the airway and the cannula may be advanced over the needle into the airway. The needle can now be withdrawn and the position confirmed with a second aspiration of air. At this point the three-way tap of the ventilation assembly can be attached to the cannula. The oxygen tubing should be connected to an oxygen supply set at a flow rate (in litres) equal to the patient's age (maximum 15 L/min).

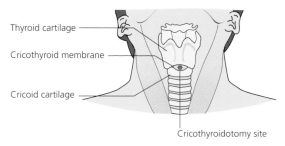

Thyroid cartilage
Cricothyroid membrane
Cricoid cartilage
Cricothyroidotomy site

Figure 6.10 Cricothyroidotomy anatomy.

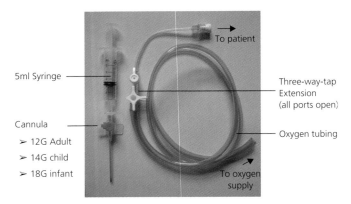

Figure 6.11 Needle cricothyroidotomy apparatus.

Occlusion of the open three-way tap port for 1 second should lead to visible chest movement. If it does not, the flow rate may be increased by increments of a litre until it does. The open port should then be released for 4 seconds to allow passive exhalation via the upper airway in a partial airway obstruction. This ratio of 1 second on to 4 seconds off should be continued while transporting the patient rapidly to definitive care. In a complete obstruction the gas flow should be reduced to 1–2 L/min to provide oxygenation without ventilation in order to prevent barotrauma.

Open surgical cricothyroidotomy is preferred in patients who are 12 years and over. It requires only minimal equipment: a scalpel (e.g. 20 blade), a 6-mm cuffed airway (endotracheal tube or tracheostomy tube), and a set of tracheal dilators (or tracheal hook). The patient should be positioned supine with the neck extended where possible. The larynx is then stabilized with the operator's left hand (which must then remain in place until the procedure is complete) and the cricothyroid membrane identified. A horizontal stab incision is made with the scalpel through the skin and underlying membrane into the airway (Figure 6.12). The scalpel should then be held in position while an assistant passes the tracheal dilators or tracheal hook into the airway alongside the blade (which can then be removed). Air or blood (or both, bubbling) may pass through the incision and the patient may cough violently if not sufficiently

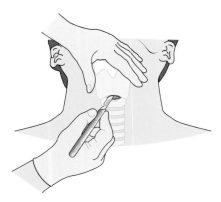

Figure 6.12 Open Surgical Cricothyroidotomy.

sedated or paralysed. The incision should be dilated and an appropriately sized endotracheal tube (internal diameter 6 mm in adults) or tracheostomy tube inserted. Once in position the cuff should be inflated and the position verified by auscultation and end-tidal carbon dioxide measurement during ventilation.

In patients with difficult neck anatomy (e.g. obesity, surgical emphysema, burns) consider performing an initial longitudinal incision to allow palpation and/or visualization of the cricothyroid membrane before incising it horizontally. A bougie can then be threaded into the incision to maintain patency and an uncut endotracheal tube railroaded into the airway.

Tips from the field

- In heavily soiled airways, suction tubing can be cut off and used directly to suction the airway in place of the narrower diameter Yankauer
- A cut-down endotracheal tube may be used as an NPA in paediatric patients
- Always lubricate a bougie prior to use
- During paediatric intubation an anterior larynx should be anticipated – look in and up
- Maintain laryngoscopy until the tube position is confirmed and the cuff inflated
- Use of a cervical collar to help reduce risk of tube displacement during transfer
- Consider performing a cricothyroidotomy under ketamine sedation in the breathing patient with an impending airway obstruction where RSI is unavailable
- Always re-check the tube position after moving an intubated patient.

Further reading

Berlac P, Hyldmo PK, Kongstad P, Kurola J, Nakstad AR, Sandberg M. Prehospital airway management: guidelines from a task force from the Scandinavian Society for Anaesthesiology and Intensive Care Medicine. *Acta Anaesthesiol Scand* 2008;**52**:897–907.

Cook TM, Hommers C. New airways for resuscitation? *Resuscitation* 2006; **69**:371–387.

Dimitriadis JC, Paoloni R. Emergency cricothyroidotomy: a randomised crossover study of four methods. *Anaesthesia* 2008;**63**:1204–1208.

Hsiao J, Pacheco-Fowler V. Videos in clinical medicine. *Cricothyroidotomy*. *N Engl J Med* 2008;**358**:e25.

Hubble MW, Brown L, Wilfong DA, *et al*. A meta-analysis of prehospital airway control techniques part I: orotracheal and nasotracheal intubation success rates. *Prehosp Emerg Care* 2010;**14**:377–401.

Kabrhel C, Thomsen TW, Setnik GS, Walls RM. Videos in clinical medicine. Orotracheal intubation. *N Engl J Med* 2007;**356**:e15.

Murphy M, Hung O, Law J. Tracheal intubation: tricks of the trade. *Emerg Med Clin North Am* 2008;**26**:1001–1014.

Nolan JD. Prehospital and resuscitative airway care: should the gold standard be reassessed? *Curr Opin Crit Care* 2001;**7**:413–421.

Santillanes G, Gausche-Hill M. Pediatric airway management. *Emerg Med Clin North Am.* 2008;**26**:961–975.

CHAPTER 7

Breathing Assessment and Management

Per Kristian Hyldmo[1], Peter Anthony Berlac[2], Anders Rostrup Nakstad[3], Mårten Sandberg[4], and Matthew Boylan[5]

[1]Sorlandet Hospital, Kristiansand, Norway
[2]University of Copenhagen, Copenhagen, Denmark
[3]Oslo University Hospital, Oslo, Norway
[4]University of Oslo, Oslo, Norway
[5]Royal Centre for Defence Medicine, University Hospitals Birmingham, Birmingham, UK

OVERVIEW

By the end of this chapter you should be able to:

- Recognize the signs of impending respiratory failure
- Understand the importance of a thorough respiratory assessment
- Identify life-threatening chest injuries
- Initiate the management of patients with life-threatening breathing disorders.

Introduction

A patent airway does not ensure adequate ventilation and oxygenation. These vital functions rely upon an intact respiratory centre, adequate pulmonary function and the coordinated movement of the diaphragm and chest wall. A number of life-threatening traumatic and medical disease processes may interfere with one or more of these essential processes and lead to respiratory failure (Box 7.1).

Box 7.1 Life-threatening breathing problems

Trauma	Medical
Tension pneumothorax	Tension pneumothorax
Open pneumothorax	Life-threatening asthma
Massive haemothorax	Acute exacerbation of COPD
Flail chest	Pulmonary oedema
Blast lung	Pulmonary embolism

Respiratory failure

Hypoxaemic (type 1) respiratory failure is characterized by a failure of blood oxygenation in the presence of adequate ventilation. Mismatch between ventilation and perfusion within the lungs is the commonest mechanism by which this occurs (e.g. pulmonary embolism, pneumonia, pulmonary oedema, pulmonary contusion). Pulmonary diffusion defects (e.g. interstitial lung disease)

and reduced inspiratory oxygen concentration (e.g. smoke inhalation) are other causative mechanisms.

Hypercarbic (type 2) respiratory failure is characterized by failure of ventilation. Hypoventilation prevents sufficient oxygen reaching the alveoli to replace that taken up by the blood, causing hypoxaemia. At the same time carbon dioxide accumulates leading to progressive hypercarbia. Causative mechanisms include depression of respiratory drive (e.g. drugs, alcohol, head injury), impaired mechanics of ventilation (neuromuscular disorders, flail chest, fatigue), and airway obstruction (epiglottitis, life-threatening asthma, severe chronic obstructive pulmonary disease (COPD)).

It is vital to recognize the early signs of respiratory failure in order to prevent further deterioration and respiratory arrest. The clinical features of hypoxia and hypercarbia are shown in Box 7.2.

Box 7.2 Symptoms of hypoxaemia and hypercarbia

Hypoxaemia	Hypercarbia
Dyspnoea	Headache
Restlessness	Peripheral vasodilatation
Agitation	Tachycardia
Confusion	Bounding pulse
Visual hallucinations	Tremor or Flap
Central cyanosis	Papilloedema
Arrhythmias	Confusion
Aggression	Drowsiness
Coma	Coma

Assessment of breathing

Assessment of breathing in the prehospital environment is often hindered by impaired access to the patient and high ambient noise. In such environments a greater reliance is placed on signs that can be seen or felt, rather than auscultatory findings. A thorough assessment of breathing is essential.

Look

Assess the patients colour, respiratory rate, respiratory effort and symmetry of chest movement. In trauma patients the chest should be examined for signs of chest injury.

ABC of Prehospital Emergency Medicine, First Edition.
Edited by Tim Nutbeam and Matthew Boylan.
© 2013 John Wiley & Sons, Ltd. Published 2013 by John Wiley & Sons, Ltd.

Colour

Assess for central cyanosis. Beware of ambient light conditions; cyanosis may not be apparent in yellow street lighting or in the bluish glow from LED headlamps. Peripheral cyanosis is common at the extremes of age but does not always indicate hypoxaemia. Infants and particularly neonates may vasoconstrict and appear pale when hypoxic.

Respiratory rate

The normal respiratory rate is age dependent (Box 7.3). Reassess regularly as changes in respiratory rate are often the first indicator of deteriorating respiratory and circulatory function. Tachypnoea indicates either hypoxia or compensation for a metabolic acidosis (e.g. diabetic ketoacidosis, shock). The inability to speak in full sentences or count to 10 in one breath are indirect indicators that tachypnoea is present. A reduced respiratory rate indicates reduced respiratory drive or fatigue induced hypoventilation.

Box 7.3 **Respiratory rate by age**

Age	Heart Rate
Newborns	40–60
Infants	30–40
Preschool children	20–30
Older children	15–25
Adults	12–20

Respiratory effort

In adults use of accessory muscles and intercostal recession indicates increased effort of breathing, usually as result of lower airway obstruction (e.g. asthma, COPD). Recession is more prominent in children due to increased chest wall compliance and may be subcostal, intercostal and even sternal in young infants. Tracheal tug, nasal flaring and grunting are further indicators of increased respiratory effort in the paediatric patient.

Respiratory symmetry

Assess for symmetrical chest movements. Asymmetry may indicate pathology on the side with reduced movement, e.g. pneumothorax, haemothorax, pleural effusion. Look for areas of paradoxical motion throughout the breathing cycle indicative of a flail segment.

Signs of injury

Are there visible signs of injury? Assess for bruising, deformity and wounds. Remember to check the neck, axilla (Figure 7.1) and back. Be thorough as small penetrating wounds can be easily overlooked.

Feel

Palpate the neck and chest wall to elicit areas of tenderness or wounds. Note crepitus from fractured ribs or subcutaneous emphysema, suggestive of an underlying pneumothorax. In low light the hands may be placed on the chest to assess for the presence of chest wall movement and symmetry. The position of the trachea should be noted.

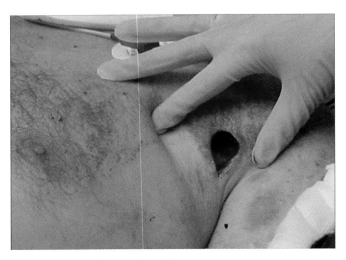

Figure 7.1 Penetrating wound to axilla.

Percussion is unreliable in a noisy environment but with practice one may 'feel' the percussion quality and enable differentiation of hyper-resonance or dullness from normal. A dull sound may indicate a haemothorax or pleural effusion. Hyper-resonance is suggestive of a pneumothorax.

Listen

Conscious patients should be asked about any pain on inspiration and difficulty breathing.

Listen to the breathing. Note any wheeze or prolonged expiratory time suggestive of lower airway obstruction. Auscultate the chest with a stethoscope. This may be difficult in the noisy prehospital environment, but should be attempted. A slight unilateral wheeze may be the only indicator of an evolving pneumothorax in a trauma patient and may be missed if auscultation is omitted. Confirm bilateral and equal breath sounds. Absent breath sounds may be due to pneumothorax, haemothorax, pleural effusion or a right main stem bronchus intubation. Assess for added sounds such as wheezes or crackles.

The mnemonics 'RISE N FALL' and 'TWELVE' can be used to remember the components of the respiratory assessment (Figure 7.2).

Monitor

A pulse oximeter should be attached and the oxygen saturation noted. In the presence of a good trace a saturation of 90% equates to a PaO_2 of 8 kPa and respiratory failure. The pulse oximeter however gives no indication of adequacy of alveolar ventilation and in the pre-oxygenated patient will not provide warning of a respiratory arrest until sometime after the event has occurred.

Non-invasive capnography (Figure 7.3) is under-used and can be extremely useful in monitoring a conscious patient's ventilatory status. It provides an accurate respiratory rate and an immediate warning of respiratory arrest. A rising end tidal carbon dioxide may be an indication of progressive hypoventilation

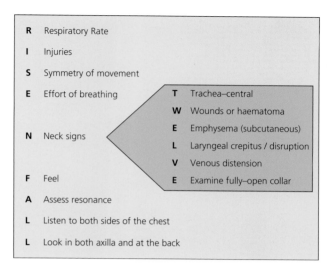

R	Respiratory Rate
I	Injuries
S	Symmetry of movement
E	Effort of breathing
N	Neck signs
F	Feel
A	Assess resonance
L	Listen to both sides of the chest
L	Look in both axilla and at the back

T	Trachea–central
W	Wounds or haematoma
E	Emphysema (subcutaneous)
L	Laryngeal crepitus / disruption
V	Venous distension
E	Examine fully–open collar

Figure 7.2 Breathing examination.

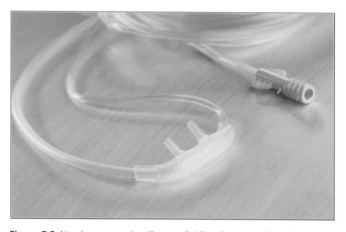

Figure 7.3 Nasal capnography. (Source: Oridion Capnography Inc).

secondary to disease or fatigue and alerts the prehospital provider to impending hypercapnic respiratory failure. The presence of a ramp-shaped capnography trace indicates bronchospasm and can be helpful in differentiating obstructive airway disease from heart failure in elderly people, and in monitoring the effectiveness of treatment of bronchospasm in obstructive airway disease. Continuous quantitative waveform capnography should be used in all ventilated patients. Simple qualitative colorimetric devices may be useful as an additional confirmatory device but should not be used alone.

Capnography has been shown to be less accurate in patients with severe chest injuries and severe shock. In these cases, hand-held arterial blood gas analysers (e.g. i-STAT) can be used to determine the true arterial blood gases and allow better titration of ventilation and oxygenation particularly in the ventilated patient during long transfers.

Focused ultrasound is also rapidly gaining popularity as a supplement to the stethoscope in the prehospital arena, where traditional auscultation may be unreliable due to ambient noise. Ultrasound may, for example, be used to detect or exclude pneumothoraces.

Management of respiratory failure

The management of respiratory failure is targeted towards optimizing oxygenation and ensuring adequate ventilation.

Oxygen administration

All critically ill medical and trauma patients requiring resuscitation should receive immediate supplemental oxygen irrespective of their oxygen saturation. Other non-critically ill patients should only receive supplemental oxygen if their SpO_2 is <94% aiming for a target saturation of 94–98%. The two exceptions to this rule are patients at risk of hypercapnic respiratory failure (Box 7.4) and patients with paraquat poisoning. These patients only require supplementation if the SpO_2 is <88% aiming for a target saturation of 88–92%.

Box 7.4 Patients at risk of hypercapnic respiratory failure

Chronic Obstructive Pulmonary Disease (COPD)
Exacerbation of cystic fibrosis
Chronic neuromuscular disorders
Chest wall disorders
Morbid obesity (BMI >40).

For most patients oxygen can be administered using a variable performance device such as a non-rebreather mask, Hudson face mask or nasal cannula set (Figure 7.4). The inspired oxygen concentration provided by these devices is determined by the patient's respiratory pattern and the flow of oxygen to the device. The flow of air that is entrained alongside the constant flow of oxygen is determined by the patient's inspiratory flow rate. As this rises more air is entrained alongside the constant oxygen flow and the overall inspired oxygen concentration may drop.

When it is important to deliver a precise concentration of oxygen (e.g. those at risk of hypercapnic respiratory failure) a fixed-performance device such as a Venturi mask (Figure 7.4) should be used. The Venturi valve increases the flow rate of oxygen and entrained air to above the patient's inspiratory flow rate, thereby providing a constant oxygen concentration whatever the respiratory pattern. A different Venturi valve is required for each different concentration of oxygen. For patients at risk of hypercapnic respiratory failure, start with a 28% Venturi mask and switch up or down to achieve the target saturation range.

Oxygen should not be delivered via a bag–valve–mask (BVM) device to the spontaneously breathing patient as the respiratory effort needed to overcome valve resistance during inspiration and expiration increases respiratory work and may hasten respiratory muscle fatigue. Anaesthetic breathing circuits such as the Mapleson C (adults) or Mapleson F (paediatric patients) are more efficient and better tolerated by patients for short-term pre-oxygenation but do require experience.

Ventilation

If a patient becomes apnoeic or their ventilation is inadequate to maintain oxygenation despite supplementation they will require ventilation. In its simplest form this may be delivered through

Nasal cannula

Flow rate: 1–4 L/min
FiO_2 increases 4% for each L/min
Well tolerated
Use: Mild or no respiratory distress or oxygenation problem

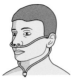

Simple face mask

Flow rate: 5–8 L/min
FiO_2: 5–6 L/min is 40%, 6–7 L/min is 50%, 7–8 L/min is 60%
Mask doesn't need tight seal
Use: Mild-moderate respiratory distress or oxygenation problem

Non-rebreather mask

Flow rate: 8–15 L/min
Proper use at 15 L/min supplies up to FiO_2 80%
Requires tight fitting mask
Should be used when >50% oxygen required
Use: Moderate-severe respiratory distress or oxygenation problem

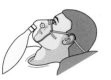

Venturi mask

Flow rate: 4–12 L/min dependant on venturi valve
FiO_2: can be set specifically with different venturi valves
Venturi valves: 24% Blue, 28% White, 35% Yellow, 40% Red, 60% Green
Use: Patients at risk of hypercapnic respiratory failure or paraquat poisoning

Figure 7.4 Oxygen delivery devices.

mouth-to-mouth or mouth-to-face mask ventilation as part of basic life support. More commonly however prehospital providers will use a BVM device. Ventilation using a BVM can be difficult and considerable practice on a regular basis is necessary for skill retention. The self-expanding bag can give the illusion of sufficient ventilation although very little air is entering the lungs. Pay close attention to the movement of the chest and abdomen and the bag compliance during ventilation. Correct mask sizing and positioning is essential (Figure 7.5).

Edentulous patients pose a significant challenge that may be overcome by altering the position of the face mask (Figure 7.6). Patients with facial hair may require the application of lubricant to the face to achieve a seal. Early use of a supraglottic airway in these patients should be considered.

Ventilation should only be delivered once the airway has been cleared and in combination with a jaw thrust and simple airway

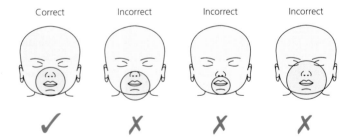

Mask Size and Position
- Should cover face from nasal bridge to alveolar ridge
- Should not press on the eyes
- Should not extend beyond chin
- Use circular masks for infants and young children

Figure 7.5 Correct mask size and position. (Source: C John Eaton, *Essentials of Immediate Medical Care 2nd Edition*, 2000).

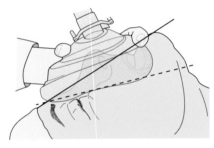

Figure 7.6 Improving the mask seal in edentulous patients: the mask is repositioned with the caudal end of the mask above the lower lip. Head extension is maintained. (Source: Racine et al. Anesthesiology 2010; 112:1190–4.)

adjuncts. A two-person technique is recommended in order to reduce the risk of gastric inflation and improve the efficacy of ventilation.

Anaesthetic breathing circuits may be used for ventilation but do rely on continuous gas flow for bag inflation and carbon dioxide clearance, which cannot always be guaranteed in the prehospital environment. A back-up BVM will therefore be required.

Transport ventilators

Where available a portable transport ventilator should be used during the transfer of ventilated patients. Ventilators provide more consistent ventilation than manual ventilation and allow better targeting of end tidal carbon dioxide. Controlled mandatory ventilation (CMV) is the most commonly used mode of ventilation in the emergency setting. The respiratory rate and tidal volume are set to determine the minute volume delivered. The peak airway pressure limiting valve should be set to alert the practitioner to the development of high airway pressures. Most ventilators allow the addition of positive end expiratory pressure (PEEP) through the addition of a PEEP valve or as an integral function of the ventilator. Complex ventilators may allow titration of oxygen concentration whereas simple ventilators are usually limited to either 100% or 45% (air mix). Suggested start values are shown in Box 7.5. It is mandatory to employ a transport ventilator with pressure alarms that will warn you if the ventilator is disconnected resulting in a non-ventilated patient.

Box 7.5 **A guide to initial portable ventilator settings**

Functions	Setting
Ventilator frequency (breaths per min)	6 month–2 yrs: 20–40 2 yrs–6 yrs: 20–30 >6 yrs: 12–20
Tidal volume (TV):	6–10 mL/kg
Peak airway pressure (P_{max})	40 cmH$_2$O
Oxygen fraction in inspired gas (FIO$_2$):	0.5–1.0
Positive end expiratory pressure (PEEP):	5 cmH$_2$O
Inspiration: Expiration ratio (I:E ratio)	1:2

- Start with a high FiO$_2$ (1.0) and titrate down
- Set the ventilator frequency to a rate suitable for the patients age
- Start with a low TV (6 mL/kg) and titrate to target ETCO$_2$
- If pressure mode is available, set inspiratory pressure to 20 cmH$_2$0 and adjust to obtain adequate T V and ETCO$_2$.

Patient positioning

A patient in respiratory distress will often not accept transport in the supine position. Elevation of the head of the stretcher or transportation in the sitting position should be considered Figure 7.7. If the patient is transported in the lateral position, most patients are better lying on the non-injured side because this results in better perfusion and therefore gas exchange in the non-injured lung. Sufficient analgesia is important in facilitating transportation. Most trauma patients are fitted with a rigid neck collar until the cervical spine is cleared. However, patients in respiratory distress are often anxious and find it extremely uncomfortable to wear a neck collar. Alternative measures (for instance manual stabilisation or sandbags) may be more acceptable for the patient and should be considered since a combative patient in respiratory distress with a potential spinal injury runs the risk of exacerbating the injury.

Life-threatening breathing problems: trauma

There are a number of traumatic chest injuries that pose an immediate threat to oxygenation and ventilation and require management in the prehospital phase.

Tension pneumothorax

A tension pneumothorax is a potentially lethal condition which occurs when air accumulates under pressure within the pleural cavity as a result of a pleural defect acting as a one-way valve (Figure 7.8). The defect is usually caused by thoracic trauma, but can occur in medical patients as a result of underlying respiratory disease (e.g. asthma, spontaneous pneumothorax). Air enters the pleural cavity on inspiration and is unable to leave on expiration. As intrapleural pressure increases there is compression and collapse of the ipsilateral lung leading to progressive hypoxia. Spontaneously breathing patients will attempt to compensate by increasing their respiratory rate and effort of breathing. Progressive respiratory distress and pleuritic chest pain are universal findings. The affected side of the chest may appear hyperexpanded, be hyper-resonant to percussion and demonstrate reduced breath sounds on auscultation. Respiratory failure leading to respiratory arrest ensues unless treatment is initiated.

The application of positive pressure ventilation, either to support the patients failing ventilation or following prehospital anaesthesia, will accelerate the build-up of intrapleural pressure exponentially. Resistance to bagging or raised ventilator peak airway pressures may be the first indicator of tension pneumothorax in the ventilated patient. Oxygen saturation will decrease rapidly. Increasing pressure leads to displacement of the mediastinal structures, including the superior and inferior vena cava, to the opposite side. This in combination with elevated intra-thoracic pressure reduces venous return to the right side of the heart, leading to hypotension and ultimately cardiovascular collapse. Progression is rapid. Deviation of the trachea and distended neck veins in the normovolaemic patient may be seen at this point and warn of imminent cardiac arrest.

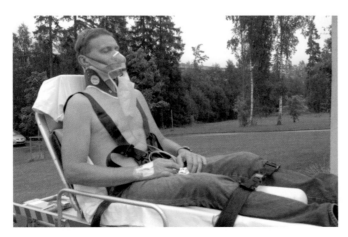

Figure 7.7 Patient positioning.

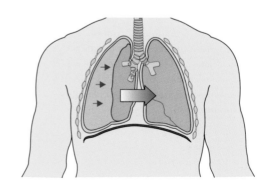

Figure 7.8 Tension pneumothorax.

Needle Decompression	
Decompression Technique	**Decompression Landmarks**

1. Prepare equipment
  • Skin prep
  • Decompression needle or wide-bore cannula
  • Syringe
2. Identify landmarks
  • Fifth Intercostal Space, Mid-Axillary Line
  • Second Intercostal Space, Mid-Clavicular Line
3. Clean the skin
4. Insert the needle above the lower rib
5. Aspirate during insertion with syringe
6. When air is aspirated advance cannula
7. Withdraw needle (→ hiss of air)
8. Stabilize cannula
9. Observe patient
	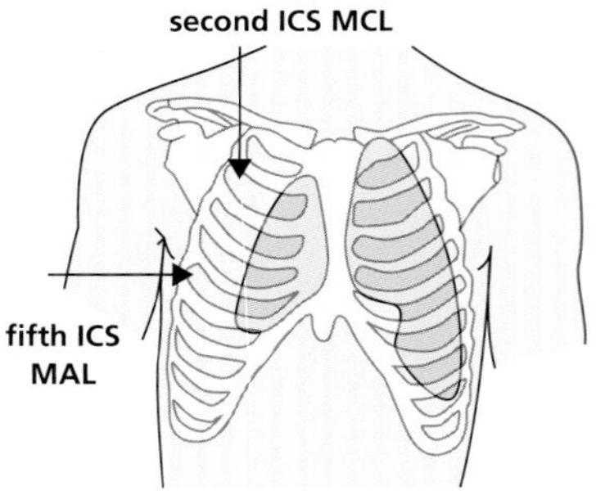 second ICS MCL
	
	fifth ICS MAL
	
	• **Neurovascular bundle runs below rib**

Figure 7.9 Needle decompression.

Simple Thoracostomy	
Thoracostomy Technique	**Landmarks**

1. Prepare equipment
  • Skin prep
  • Scalpel (22 blade)
  • Spencer Wells forceps
2. Abduct arm to 30 degrees
3. Identify landmarks
  • Fourth-fifth intercostal space, mid-axillary line
4. Clean the skin
5. Make a 5 cm skin incision along lower rib
6. Blunt dissect with forceps over lower rib
7. Penetrate the pleura under control
8. Enlarge hole in pleura to accept finger
9. Perform a finger sweep
  • Note whether any air/blood release
  • Note whether lung is up and expanded
  • Beware bone fragments
10. Observe patient
11. Re-finger if required
	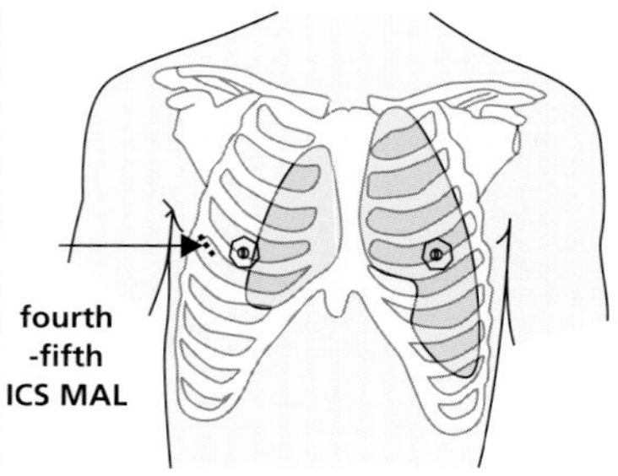 fourth -fifth ICS MAL
	
	• **In-line with male nipple**
	• **Patients hand-width below axilla**
	• **Dissect over the top of lower rib**

Figure 7.10 Simple thoracostomy.

Once recognized, tension pneumothorax is simple to treat. In the awake patient, needle decompression with a large-bore cannula is both simple and effective and aims to convert the tension pneumothorax into a simple pneumothorax. Insertion in the lateral chest is more likely to be successful than the traditional anterior approach due to reduced chest wall thickness. The procedure is summarized in Figure 7.9.

In the ventilated patient a simple thoracostomy is the preferred means of treating a tension pneumothorax (Figure 7.10). These must be monitored during transfer as they may occlude and any unexpected deterioration should prompt immediate refingering. Insertion of a chest drain may ensure patency where transfer times are prolonged (Figure 7.11). Chest drain insertion in conscious patients requires infiltration of local anaesthetic prior to incision of the chest wall. In the agitated patient ketamine sedation may be used to facilitate insertion.

Open pneumothorax

An open pneumothorax is an open chest wound that communicates with the pleural cavity (Figure 7.12). If the chest wound approximates to, or is greater in size than the tracheal diameter, air will preferentially flow through the chest wall rather than the upper airway on inspiration ('sucking chest wound'). An open pneumothorax should be obvious during inspection of the chest and immediately sealed as part of primary survey management. Purpose-made seals (e.g. Asherman, Bolin) that incorporate a one-way valve are effective and simple to apply. Alternatively an airtight, three-sided dressing may be applied. In the presence of multiple wounds one only (ideally the largest) needs to be vented and the remainder can be sealed. Resealing or clotting of the wounds or seal may occur and lead to the development of a tension pneumothorax. If this occurs the dressing should be lifted to allow venting and if this manoeuvre fails decompression with a needle or incision should be performed.

Massive haemothorax

Massive haemothorax is defined as a collection of more than 1500 ml of blood in the pleural cavity and occurs most commonly as a result of a vascular injury within the lung parenchyma, pulmonary hilum or mediastinum. Unexplained hypovolaemic shock

Chest Drain Insertion	
Technique	**Portex® Ambulatory Chest Drain Set**

1. Prepare equipment
   • Equipment as for simple thoracostomy
   • Chest drain - Adult: 28-32Fr   Paed: (Age + 16)Fr
   • Drainage bag with flutter valve (primed)
   • Syringe for priming flutter valve
   • Suture
2. Follow procedure for simple thoracostomy
3. Insert chest drain into the incision using
   the finger as a guide +/- blunt introducer
   • Guide the tube anteriorly and apically
   • Ensure all drainage holes lie within the chest
4. Attach the tube to drainage bag
5. Confirm flutter valve patency
   • Free drainage of fluid from chest into bag
   • Get patient to cough and valve leaflets should part
6. Suture drain to skin securely
7. Dress insertion site
8. Observe patient
	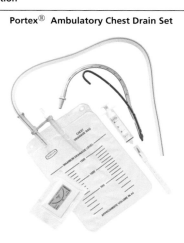

Figure 7.11 Intercostal drain insertion. (Source: Portex Ambulatory Chest Drain Set, courtesy of Smiths Medical.)

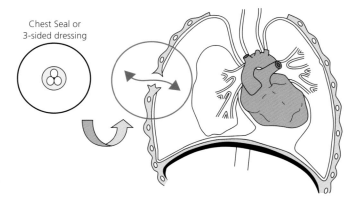

Figure 7.12 Open pneumothorax. (Source: Clinical Guideleines for Operations (CGO's) JSP-999).

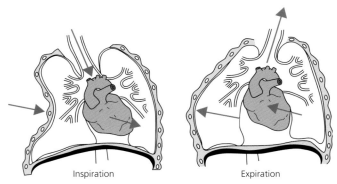

Figure 7.13 Flail chest. (Source: Clinical Guideleines for Operations (CGO's) JSP-999).

in combination with unilateral (or occasionally bilateral) chest dullness and reduced air entry suggests the diagnosis. Management of hypovolaemia takes priority. Where transfer times are short, rapid movement to a trauma centre with supplemental oxygen and carefully titrated intravenous fluids en route is required. Patients with significant respiratory compromise and those with prolonged transfer times may require chest drain insertion and/or positive pressure ventilation prior to evacuation. This is likely to be more effective at halting any ongoing bleeding than any theoretical tamponade provided by a contained haemothorax.

Flail chest

A flail chest is defined as the fracture of two or more adjacent ribs in two or more places and leads to segmental loss of continuity with the rest of the thoracic cage. A small flail segment may be difficult to identify because of local muscle spasm and splinting; however, large flail segments are usually obvious. The flail segment moves paradoxically inwards during inspiration and outwards during expiration (Figure 7.13). Tidal volume is reduced and ventilation compromised. Underlying pulmonary contusions add to the insult

on the respiratory system and cause hypoxia. Paradoxical chest movement, hypoxia and respiratory distress characterize a patient with a flail chest.

High-flow oxygen (15 L/min) and sufficient analgesia for painless spontaneous breathing is often sufficient field treatment of this condition. Large flail segments with resistant hypoxia may require urgent prehospital anaesthesia and positive pressure ventilation. Prophylactic thoracostomy with or without drain insertion should be performed on the side(s) of the injury due to the high frequency of associated haemopneumothoraces.

Other chest injuries

Several other thoracic injuries may present in the prehospital phase (Box 7.6). If suspected, continued resuscitative care should be provided and the injury communicated to the receiving trauma team.

Life-threatening breathing problems: medical

Acute breathlessness is a common medical emergency in both adults and children, and the differential diagnosis is broad (Box 7.7). Supplemental oxygenation will improve oxygenation and hypoxic

Box 7.6 Other chest injuries

Thoracic injury	Clinical features	Prehospital management
Cardiac tamponade	Penetrating chest wound Hypotension Neck vein distension	Rule out tension pneumothorax Rapid transfer to Trauma Centre Thoracotomy if cardiac arrest (See cardiac arrest chapter)
Blunt aortic injury	High-energy mechanism Chest/Back pain Differential pulses/BP	Rapid transfer to Trauma Centre Permissive hypotension
Pulmonary contusion	Hypoxia Evidence of chest wall injury Haemoptysis	Supplemental Oxygen ± Ventilation Judicious fluid resuscitation Prophylactic thoracostomy if ventilated
Tracheobron-chial injury	Subcutaneous emphysema in neck Laryngeal crepitus Haemoptysis Air leak from wound Pneumothorax (often tension)	Supplemental Oxygen If possible defer definitive airway management Careful intubation with smaller ETT if necessary Consider primary surgical airway Selective bronchial intubation if massive haemoptysis
Myocardial contusion	Blunt chest injury (e.g. sternal fracture) Dysrhythmias Cardiogenic shock	Supplemental Oxygen Arrhythmia management
Simple pneu-mothorax	Penetrating or blunt mechanism Hypoxaemia Ipsilateral ↓ air entry / ↑ resonance Non-progressive symptoms	Supplemental Oxygen Monitor for tension Prophylactic thoracostomy if ventilated

Box 7.7 Medical causes of acute breathlessness

Airway obstruction

- croup,
- epiglottitis,
- foreign body

Acute asthma
Bronchiolitis
Pneumonia
Exacerbation of COPD
Pneumothorax
Pulmonary oedema
Pulmonary embolism.

Tips from the field

- Always check the neck, axilla and back when examining the chest
- Always do a full breathing reassessment after intubation and ventilation
- Increasing respiratory rate and effort are subtle but important signs of deterioration
- BVM ventilation is not easy so should be practised regularly
- A simple pneumothorax may tension rapidly after ventilation is started
- An endotracheal tube can be used as a chest drain in an emergency with the finger of an examination glove used as a flap valve.

Further reading

Callahan JM. Pulse oximetry in emergency medicine. *Emerg Med Clin North Am* 2008: 869–279.

Donald MJ, Paterson B. End tidal carbon dioxide monitoring in prehospital and retrieval medicine: a review. *Emerg Med J* 2006;**23**:728–730.

Jørgensen H, Jensen CH, Dirks J. Does prehospital ultrasound improve treatment of the trauma patient? A systematic review. *Eur J Emerg Med* 2010;**17**:249–253.

Lee C, Revell M, Porter K, Steyn R, Faculty of Prehospital Care RCOSOE. The prehospital management of chest injuries: a consensus statement. Faculty of Prehospital Care, Royal College of Surgeons of Edinburgh. *Emerg Med J* 2007;**24**:220–224.

Waydhas C, Sauerland S. Prehospital pleural decompression and chest tube placement after blunt trauma: A systematic review. *Resuscitation.* 2007;**72**:11–25.

symptoms in most cases allowing transportation to hospital for further assessment. For further detail the reader should refer to Chapters 23 and 29.

CHAPTER 8

Circulation Assessment and Management

R. J. Dawes[1] and Matthew Boylan[2]

[1]Defence Medical Services, UK
[2]Royal Centre for Defence Medicine, University Hospitals Birmingham, Birmingham, UK

OVERVIEW

By the end of this chapter you should:

- Be able to define shock and its subtypes
- Be aware of the possible sources of bleeding in the trauma patient
- Understand the role the 'lethal triad' in the bleeding patient
- Be able to identify shock in the prehospital phase
- Be able to demonstrate a structured approach to the initial management of the shocked patient
- Understand the importance of targeting the 'lethal triad' in the management of haemorrhagic shock.

Introduction

The early identification and aggressive management of shock is an important component in the resuscitation of the seriously ill or injured patient. Shock is defined as failure of the circulatory system leading to inadequate organ perfusion and tissue oxygenation. Inadequate perfusion may result from failure of the pump (the heart), inadequate circulating blood volume (absolute or relative) or obstruction to the flow of blood through the circulatory system. Traditionally shock has been subdivided into four main subtypes (Figure 8.1). In practice there is often considerable overlap, with different types of shock co-existing in the same patient. Whatever the mechanism, inadequate perfusion leads to anaerobic metabolism, lactic acidosis and progressive cellular and organ dysfunction.

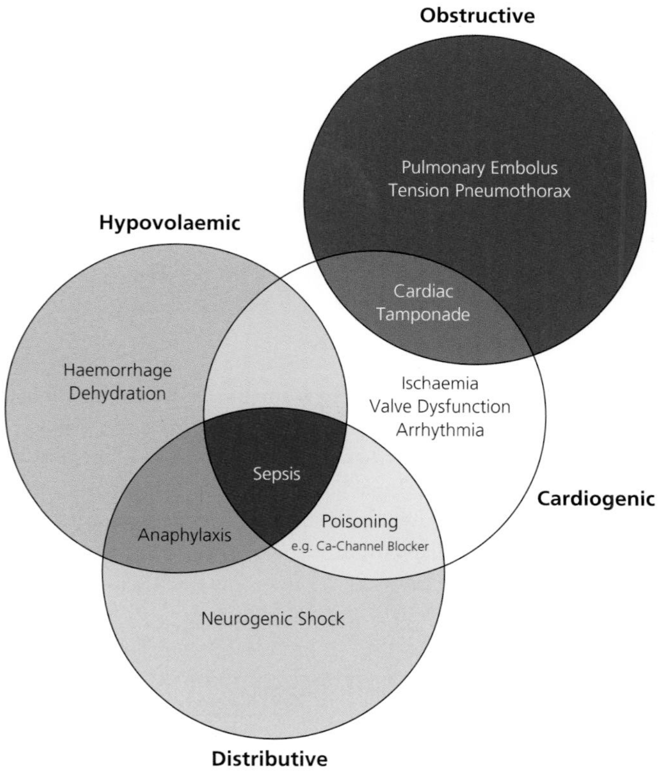

Hypovolaemic shock

Hypovolaemic shock is shock resulting from inadequate circulating blood volume. It may result from haemorrhage (e.g. trauma, gastrointestinal bleed) or excessive fluid loss from the gastrointestinal tract (e.g. cholera), urinary tract (e.g. DKA) or skin (e.g. severe burns). Fluid may also be lost into body tissues or compartments (so called 'third spacing'), particularly after significant tissue trauma or inflammation (e.g. pancreatitis), worsening volume depletion.

ABC of Prehospital Emergency Medicine, First Edition.
Edited by Tim Nutbeam and Matthew Boylan.
© 2013 John Wiley & Sons, Ltd. Published 2013 by John Wiley & Sons, Ltd.

Figure 8.1 Types of shock. (Source: Anaesthesia & Intensive Care Medicine, Causes and Investigation of Shock, *Ben Shippey*, 2010, **11**; 509–512).

Hypovolaemia in trauma

Hypovolaemic shock secondary to uncontrolled haemorrhage is by far the most common shock scenario seen in prehospital practice. Bleeding may occur from damaged blood vessels and fractured bone ends. Progressive blood loss leads to hypovolaemia and inadequate perfusion of the vital organs. In an attempt to maintain perfusion to these areas, the body's compensatory mechanisms sacrifice the perfusion of less critical areas such as the skin and gastrointestinal tract. Anaerobic metabolism in these areas causes progressive systemic lactic acidosis and limit endogenous heat production promoting hypothermia. Both acidosis and hypothermia impair the blood's ability to clot (coagulation), leading to further bleeding. These three components are known as the 'lethal triad' (Figure 8.2).

The Lethal Triad

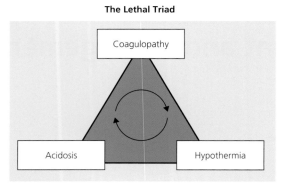

Figure 8.2 The lethal triad.

Traumatic injury to tissue and subsequent poor perfusion activates anticoagulant and fibrinolytic pathways within the coagulation cascade. The result is a primary coagulopathy termed the Acute Coagulopathy of Trauma Shock (ACoTS). ACoTS may be found in up to a quarter of patients with major trauma and is associated with a fourfold increase in mortality. Blood clot formed immediately after injury will therefore be the most stable and effective clot and should be preserved at all costs: first clot = best clot.

Cardiogenic shock

Cardiogenic shock is shock resulting from myocardial dysfunction in the presence of adequate left ventricular filling pressures. Myocardial dysfunction may be the result of arrhythmia, myocardial infarction, ischaemia, contusion or underlying cardiomyopathy. Without intervention myocardial dysfunction leads to a progressive reduction in cardiac output, reduced coronary perfusion and worsening ischaemia (Figure 8.3).

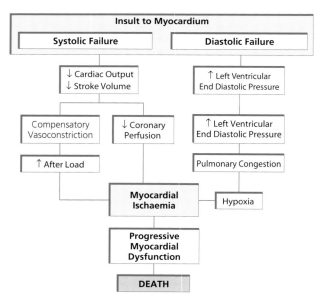

Figure 8.3 Cardiogenic shock.

Distributive shock

Distributive shock is shock resulting from a reduction in peripheral vascular resistance caused by inappropriate vasodilatation. The circulating volume is insufficient to fill the dilated vascular space resulting in a state of relative hypovolaemia and systemic hypoperfusion. Septic, anaphylactic and neurogenic shock are the most common subtypes of distributive shock. Vasodilatation in septic shock is caused by inflammatory/anti-inflammatory mediators released as part of the systemic inflammatory response syndrome (SIRS) after infection. In anaphylactic shock vasodilatation results from the antigen-induced systemic release of histamine and vasoactive mediators from mast cells. Neurogenic shock occurs when there is damage to the spinal cord above the level of T4 with subsequent loss of sympathetic outflow leading to unopposed peripheral vasodilatation.

Obstructive shock

Obstructive shock is shock resulting from extracardiac obstruction to blood flow leading to impaired diastolic filling or excessive afterload. Common causes include cardiac tamponade, tension pneumothorax and massive pulmonary embolism. Dynamic hyperinflation (gas trapping) due to excessive positive pressure ventilation in patients with severe bronchospasm may also reduce venous return (particularly in the presence of hypovolaemia) sufficient to cause an obstructive shock state.

Assessment of the circulation

Accurately assessing whether a patient is shocked is one of the most difficult skills to acquire in prehospital emergency medicine. Lack of monitoring, poor lighting, an austere environment, unknown mechanism of injury and little knowledge of premorbid state all conspire against you. The initial circulation assessment process aims to identify signs of compensated and decompensated shock (Figure 8.4).

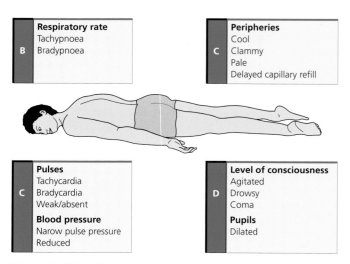

Figure 8.4 Clinical signs of shock.

Compensated shock

Hypovolaemic, cardiogenic and obstructive shock states are all characterized by a reduced cardiac output. In an attempt to maintain cardiac output the body increases the heart rate. It does this through the activation of the sympathetic nervous system (SNS). The SNS also stimulates peripheral vasoconstriction, diverting blood centrally and restoring preload. This is recognized clinically by the presence of pale, cold, clammy skin, prolonged capillary refill time and a reduced pulse pressure (palpable or measured). The SNS also induces tachypnoea. This has little effect on the actual oxygen content of the blood but does serve as an important marker of early compensation in shock. In these early stages cardiac output and blood pressure are maintained and the shock is considered *compensated*. It is important to recognize that although the systolic blood pressure is maintained, perfusion of the peripheral tissues is impaired and continued lactate formation and progressive systemic acidosis result.

Distributive shock states may not present with the classic skin changes or tachycardia described above. Pathological vasodilatation may prevent compensatory vasoconstriction, resulting in flushed and warm peripheries in the early stages. Tachycardia may also be absent in neurogenic shock due to unopposed vagal tone.

By assessing the respiratory rate, feeling the pulse rate and strength, and by looking and feeling the patient's peripheries, the prehospital practitioner can rapidly assess for signs of compensated shock (Box 8.1).

Box 8.1 **Signs of compensated shock**

Tachycardia
Tachypnoea
Delayed capillary refill
Pale / cool / clammy peripheries
Reduced pulse pressure
Poor SpO_2 trace.

Decompensated shock

A point will be reached at which the compensatory mechanisms fail to compensate for the reduction in cardiac output or systemic vascular resistance. At this point *decompensation* will occur and perfusion to the vital organs becomes compromised. The brain relies on a constant blood flow to maintain function, and as blood flow is compromised the conscious level drops. Loss of the radial pulse indicates a critical reduction in blood flow to the peripheries and correlates with impaired perfusion of the vital organs. The systolic blood pressure (SBP), having been maintained by the actions of the sympathetic nervous system, will also drop.

By assessing the patient's radial pulse and level of consciousness the practitioner can assess for signs of decompensation (Box 8.2). Non-invasive blood pressure (NIBP) measurements are

---

Box 8.2 **Signs of decompensated shock**

Altered Level of Consciousness
Loss of Radial Pulse
Drop in Systolic Blood Pressure.

---

notoriously inaccurate in low flow states and should be interpreted in combination with the other clinical signs.

The speed at which decompensation occurs will depend partly on the physiological reserve of the patient and the cause of the shock state. Patients in cardiogenic and distributive shock states have a limited ability to compensate and therefore are liable to decompensate rapidly. Certain other factors can affect the response to shock (Box 8.3). A high index of suspicion is essential in these patient groups if shock is to be identified.

Box 8.3 **Factors affecting the physiological response to shock**

Patient Group	Caution
Elderly	The elderly have less physiological reserve and will decompensate earlier
Drugs	Drugs such as Beta blockers will limit the ability for the patient to mount a compensatory tachycardia and lead to earlier decompensation
Pacemakers	A pacemaker with a fixed rate will limit the ability for the patient to mount a compensatory tachycardia and lead to earlier decompensation
The Athlete	The resting heart rate of an athlete may be in the region of 50 bpm. This should be taken into account when assessing for relative tachycardia
Pregnancy	In pregnancy the normal physiological changes of pregnancy (increased plasma and red cell volume) allow the patient to compensate for longer.
Hypothermia	Hypothermia can reduce HR, RR and BP independently hypovolaemia making fluid titration more difficult.
Penetrating trauma	A vagal response (relative bradycardia) stimulated by intra-peritoneal blood may lead to underestimation of the degree of shock.

Aids to identifying shock

A lack of plethysmography trace may reinforce suspicions of poor peripheral perfusion; however, hypothermia may have the same effect. Direct measurement of tissue oxygen saturation (StO_2) provides a more accurate indication of peripheral perfusion, with values <75% corresponding to inadequate perfusion in haemorrhagic shock. The size and weight of StO_2 monitors limits their applicability in the prehospital environment at the current time. Point of care blood gas analysis (e.g. I-Stat) will allow direct measurement of serum lactate and/or acid–base status, both of which may give an indication of impaired perfusion.

Management of the shocked trauma patient

A rapid and systematic primary survey should identify the most likely cause(s) of shock and guide treatment (Figure 8.5). Haemorrhage is the most common cause of shock following trauma and may occur in five key sites: on the floor (external) and four more

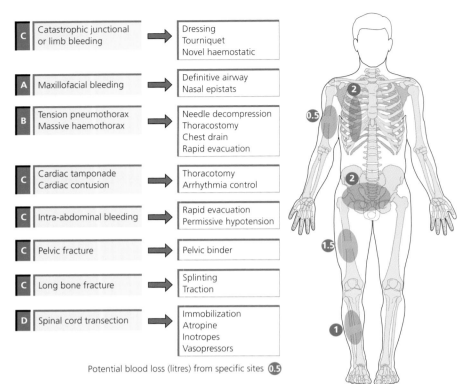

C Catastrophic junctional or limb bleeding	→	Dressing Tourniquet Novel haemostatic
A Maxillofacial bleeding	→	Definitive airway Nasal epistats
B Tension pneumothorax Massive haemothorax	→	Needle decompression Thoracostomy Chest drain Rapid evacuation
C Cardiac tamponade Cardiac contusion	→	Thoracotomy Arrhythmia control
C Intra-abdominal bleeding	→	Rapid evacuation Permissive hypotension
C Pelvic fracture	→	Pelvic binder
C Long bone fracture	→	Splinting Traction
D Spinal cord transection	→	Immobilization Atropine Inotropes Vasopressors

Potential blood loss (litres) from specific sites **0.5**

Figure 8.5 Traumatic causes of shock.

(chest, abdomen, pelvis, long bones). Evaluation of these sites forms a key part of the circulation assessment.

Prehospital ultrasound can be a useful adjunct to help localize the site of bleeding and aid management decisions. Useful findings include free fluid within the abdominal or thoracic cavity and increased pubic diastasis.

Control of external haemorrhage

In most circumstances external haemorrhage can be controlled by the stepwise application of basic haemorrhage control techniques – the haemostatic ladder (Figure 8.6). Modern dressings now come in a variety of sizes with elasticated bandages and integral pressure bars or caps to aid in the application of pressure. Where bleeding cannot be controlled by basic measures, or the environment precludes their use (e.g. military), the use of tourniquets or haemostatic dressings may be considered. These may also be used immediately in cases where haemorrhage is so severe that if not immediately controlled, would lead rapidly to death (e.g. transected carotid or femoral artery).

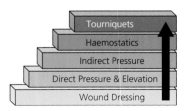

Figure 8.6 Prehospital haemostatic ladder.

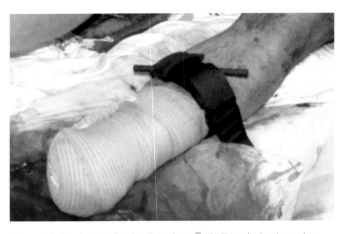

Figure 8.7 Combat Application Tourniquet® (CAT) applied to lower leg.

Tourniquets

When used tourniquets should be placed as distally as possible on the affected limb and should be tightened until all bleeding ceases (Figure 8.7). Note the time they are applied. They can often be more painful than the injury itself and judicious use of ketamine and opioids can be useful. Proximal lower limb (e.g. thigh) bleeding may require the application of more than one tourniquet to achieve control. It is vital that tourniquets are reassessed regularly during the resuscitation process as they may require adjustment.

Haemostatic dressings

Haemostatic dressings are particularly useful for controlling bleeding at junctional zones (e.g. neck, axilla, groin, perineum) where tourniquets cannot be applied. A number of impregnated

Factor concentrators	Mucoadhesive agents
• Granules absorb water • Concentrates coagulation factors • Promotes clotting	• Chitosan-based products • Anionic attraction of red cells • Adherence to wound surface
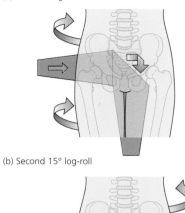	
e.g. Quickclot®	e.g. Celox™, HemCon™

Figure 8.8 Novel haemostatics. (Source: Right hand image courtesy of Z-MEDICA, LLC. Left hand image courtesy of Medtrade Ltd).

gauzes/ribbons and granules are available which work by two main mechanisms (Figure 8.8) to promote clotting. All must be used in conjunction with a standard dressing and direct pressure.

Control of non-compressible torso haemorrhage

The optimal management for uncompressible haemorrhage within the thoracic or abdominal cavity is rapid and definitive operative haemostasis. Early recognition and rapid evacuation to a major trauma centre is therefore essential. A clear appreciation of the mechanism of injury, pattern of physical injury and temporal changes in physiology will allow the prehospital practitioner to identify those patients at risk. The only exception to rapid evacuation is when a massive haemothorax compromises ventilation and oxygenation, whereupon intercostal drainage should be performed prior to transfer. Re-expansion of the lung on the affected side may also control pulmonary bleeding.

Control of skeletal haemorrhage

Following significant trauma conscious patients with pelvic pain, lower back pain or physical signs of pelvic injury should have a pelvic binder applied. Under no circumstances should the pelvis be 'sprung' to assess for stability. All obtunded patients with a significant mechanism should also undergo pelvic binding. The early application of a pelvic binder will reduce bleeding through bone end apposition and limit further movement which could disrupt established clot. Binders should be applied to skin as part of skin-to-scoop packaging. The binder should be folded into an inverted L shape and the corner inserted at the level of the greater trochanter during the first limited log-roll. During the second limited logroll the folded end is pulled through and when supine the binder is tightened to achieve anatomical reduction (Figure 8.9). It is important to ensure the feet and knees are bound to limit rotational forces at the hip joint.

Long bone fractures should be drawn out to length and splinted in position to prevent further movement of bone ends and tissue damage. Femoral fractures may require the application of traction

(a) First 15° log-roll

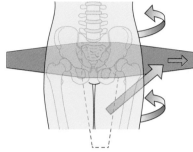

(b) Second 15° log-roll

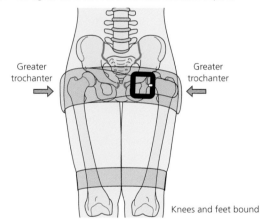

(c) Binder tightened to achieve anatomical reduction of pelvis

Greater trochanter   Greater trochanter

Knees and feet bound

Figure 8.9 Application of a pelvic binder.

to overcome the contractile forces of the thigh muscles. This should be performed as part of the primary survey.

Control of maxillofacial haemorrhage

Severe maxillofacial trauma may result in significant haemorrhage from damaged branches of carotid artery (usually maxillary artery). Airway obstruction and hypovolaemia are the main problems associated with this type of injury. After securing the airway, haemorrhage control can be achieved through a combination of facial bone splinting and intranasal balloon tamponade. A cervical collar is applied to fix the mandible before the maxillae are manually reduced and fixed using dental bite blocks (BreathSafe®). Nasal epistats (Epistat II®, Xomed) are then inserted into each nasal cavity and simultaneously inflated with saline until haemorrhage is controlled (Figure 8.10).

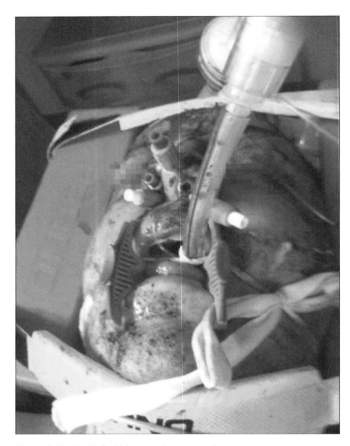

Figure 8.10 Maxillofacial haemorrhage control.

Circulatory access

Gaining access to the circulatory system is an essential part of the resuscitative process in the critically injured patient. In most cases access can be gained quickly by the insertion of an intravenous cannula into a peripheral vein. Standard access for fluid resuscitation is a large gauge cannula in the forearm. The dorsum of the hand, antecubital fossa, and medial ankle (long saphenous) are good alternative sites. Ideally two points of venous access in separate

limbs should be obtained. Injured limbs should be avoided. Prior to insertion, a venous tourniquet should be placed no more than 10 cm away from the insertion point and sufficient time allowed for it to work. When only a small vein can be cannulated, keeping the tourniquet on then infusing 50–100 mL of fluid dilates larger veins allowing larger gauge access. Care should be taken to secure cannulae and intravenous lines with dressings and tape prior to any patient movement.

There are situations where peripheral intravenous access may be difficult or even impossible (Figure 8.11). In these cases intraosseous access should be considered. Any drug, fluid or blood product that can be given intravenously can be given via the intraosseous route. In addition to the standard Cook® needle there are a number of mechanical intraosseous devices that allow needle insertion into both adult and paediatric patients, e.g. EZ-IO® intraosseous infusion system and the Bone Injection Gun™ (Figure 8.12). Specific sternal intraosseous devices (e.g. FAST Responder™ sternal intraosseous device) are also available and can be useful in

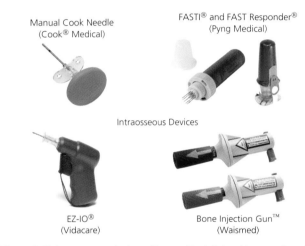

Figure 8.12 Intraosseous devices. (Source: Top left hand image – Permission for use granted by Cook Medical Incorporated, Bloomington, Indiana. Top right hand image – Permission for use granted by Pyng Medical. Bottom left hand image – Permission for use granted by Vidacare. Bottom right hand image – Permission for use granted by Waismed).

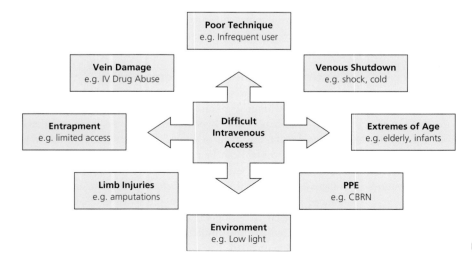

Figure 8.11 Difficult intravenous access.

Humeral Head
- Adduct arm to body and flex elbow to 90°
- Internally rotate arm so hand over umbilicus
- Greater tubercle now lies anterior on shoulder
- Insert needle perpendicular to bone
- Splint limb to side to prevent dislodgement

Proximal tibia

Adult
- One finger breadth medial to tibial tuberosity

Child
- One finger breadth below and medial to tibial tuberosity
- Two finger breadth below patella and one finger medial

Distal tibia

Adult
- Three finger-breadths above tip of medial malleolus

Child
- Two finger-breadths above tip of medial malleolus

Figure 8.13 Common intraosseous insertion sites.

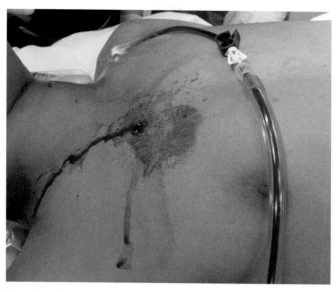

Figure 8.15 Central venous access with a large-bore subclavian line.

patients with limb polytrauma. Standard insertion sites are shown in Figure 8.13. The humeral head and sternal insertion sites permit flow rates five times higher than those in the tibia. Care should be taken to splint limbs and secure needles with commercial stabilizers or dressings to prevent dislodgement. All intraosseous needles require an initial flush prior to use. Infusion should then be performed using a bolus technique with a 50-mL syringe attached to a three-way tap and fluid bag (Figure 8.14). Monitor for extravasation particularly in infants as there is a risk of compartment syndrome if this is not recognized.

Some prehospital systems utilize large bore central venous lines (e.g. MAC™ or Swan Sheath; Arrow® international) to deliver high-flow, large-volume prehospital transfusion of blood products to patients with critical hypovolaemia (Figure 8.15). The subclavian vein offers better anatomical access than other routes and remains patent even during cardiac arrest. The femoral veins are a viable alternative but may collapse in severe shock and present a higher risk of arterial puncture, infection and thrombosis.

Fluid resuscitation

Fluid resuscitation following trauma may be indicated to replace lost blood volume and optimize haemodynamics in order to maintain oxygen delivery to the tissues and limit acidosis. There are two main classes of resuscitation fluids – crystalloids and colloids. Despite a huge amount of research, there remains no definitive answer as to which one is best. Owing to their lower cost and lower risk of adverse events (e.g. anaphylaxis, coagulopathy) crystalloids are favoured by most. Normal saline and lactated Ringers (Hartmann's) are used most commonly. More important is the amount infused and the temperature at which they are given. All fluids given to trauma patients should be warmed and the use of prehospital fluid warming devices is encouraged. Some prehospital systems administer warmed blood and plasma (Figure 8.16); however, the logistical hurdles of delivering prehospital blood products should not be underestimated.

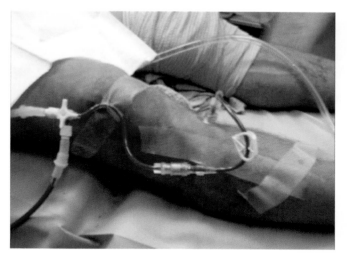

Figure 8.14 Blood administration via an intraosseous needle.

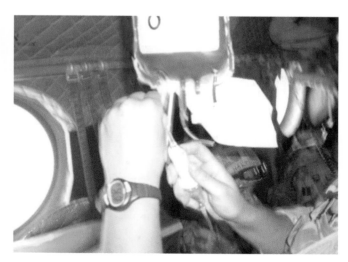

Figure 8.16 Prehospital blood administration.

Permissive hypotension

Permissive hypotension describes the technique of partial restoration of blood pressure after haemorrhage, prior to definitive haemorrhage control. It is now standard practice in most prehospital systems and is backed up by both animal and human trial data. Hypotension facilitates *in vivo* coagulation, whereas the avoidance of needless infusion of cold crystalloid fluid preserves normothermia and prevents excessive dilution of red blood cells, platelets and clotting factors. A lower than normal mean arterial pressure (MAP) of 60–70 mmHg (equivalent to a SBP of 80–90 mmHg) is taken as the target for fluid administration, unless there is an associated traumatic brain injury where a MAP of 80 mmHg (SBP >100 mg) is preferred. The presence of a palpable radial pulse is indicative of blood *flow* to the peripheries rather than any specific blood pressure. Flow is a good indicator of perfusion and so it makes sense to use this as an end point to guide fluid resuscitation in the absence of accurate blood pressure monitoring. The level of consciousness provides another easy end point against which fluid therapy can be titrated. Normal mentation indicates adequate blood supply to the brain and therefore by definition to the vital organs. Fluids are administered in 250-mL (5 mL/kg) aliquots until the desired end point is achieved. Recent research by the UK military has shown that hypotensive resuscitation should be restricted to the first hour following injury, after which normotensive resuscitation should be commenced to prevent organ damage due to hypoperfusion. This has been termed 'novel hybrid resuscitation'.

Minimal handling techniques

Excessive patient movement risks disruption of formed clot through movement of tissue and bone ends. Careful cutting of clothing to permit full exposure and the application of a scoop stretcher directly against the skin using limited (15 degree) log-rolling will lead to reduced overall movement both in the prehospital phase and in the emergency department (Figure 8.17). Care should be taken to protect the patient against hypothermia at all times during this process.

Tranexamic acid

Tranexamic acid acts to limit the hyperfibrinolysis seen in the acute coagulopathy of trauma. The CRASH 2 trial showed that the administration of tranexamic acid within 3 hours of injury to trauma patients with, or at risk of, significant bleeding reduced the risk of death from haemorrhage, with no apparent increase in fatal or non-fatal vascular occlusive events. The most benefit is seen if given within 1 hour of injury. Tranexamic acid is given as an initial intravenous bolus of 1 gram over 10 minutes, followed by a further 1 gram infused over 8 hours. The paediatric dose is 15 mg/kg (max 1 g) followed by 2 mg/kg/hr. Hypotension may occur if administered too quickly.

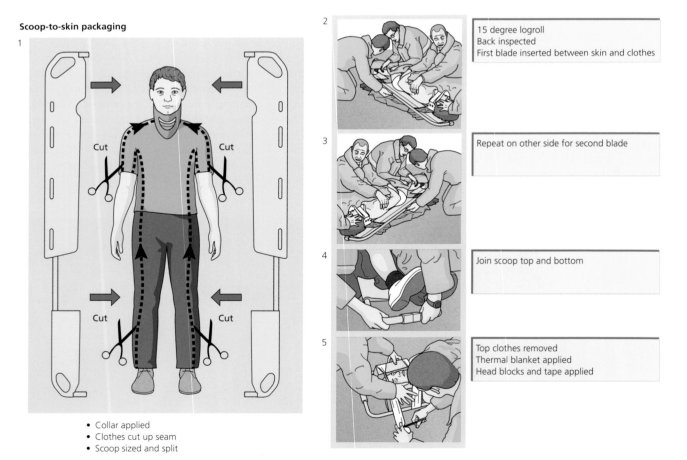

Scoop-to-skin packaging

1
- Collar applied
- Clothes cut up seam
- Scoop sized and split

2 — 15 degree logroll / Back inspected / First blade inserted between skin and clothes

3 — Repeat on other side for second blade

4 — Join scoop top and bottom

5 — Top clothes removed / Thermal blanket applied / Head blocks and tape applied

Figure 8.17 Scoop-to-skin packaging.

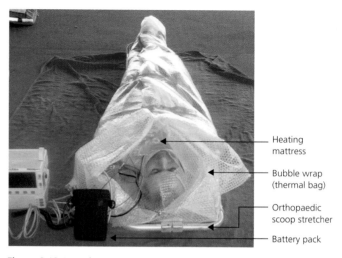

Heating
mattress

Bubble wrap
(thermal bag)

Orthopaedic
scoop stretcher

Battery pack

Figure 8.18 Hypothermia mitigation (Courtesy of London HEMS).

Hypothermia mitigation

Hypothermia forms part of the lethal triad and will exacerbate acidosis, coagulopathy and cause further bleeding if ignored. It is essential that the patient is protected from the environment at all times with exposure for critical interventions only. Various thermal blankets and wraps are available (Figure 8.18) some with integral warming pads and access ports. Intravenous fluids should all be warmed and vehicle heaters should be turned on during transfer.

Triage

All shocked trauma patients should be triaged to a major trauma centre with an ability to deliver massive transfusion and rapid transfer to theatre. Some systems allow prehospital alerting for massive transfusion in order to minimize delays to receiving blood products.

Management of the shocked medical patient

Figure 8.19 summarizes possible causes of shock in the medical patient and highlights the key interventions. The presence of jugular venous distension is suggestive of either cardiogenic or obstructive shock. The lung fields will be clear in obstructive shock and wet in cardiogenic shock due to left ventricular failure. Absence of jugular venous distension is suggestive of either hypovolaemia or distributive shock. The history and examination will be key in determining the likely cause. Medical causes of shock will be dealt with in more detail in Chapter 22 on medical emergencies.

Tips from the field

- Patients who are tachycardic, tachypnoeic, with cold clammy skin are in compensated shock until proven otherwise
- Loss of the radial pulse and/or reduced level of consciousness indicates decompensation
- Non-invasive blood pressure readings can be unreliable and provide false reassurance
- The humeral and sternal intraosseous sites allow the best flow rates
- The application of a pelvic binder and splinting of long bone fractures should be undertaken as part of the primary survey
- Always secure intravenous/intraosseus access sites and lines securely prior to patient movement.

Further reading

Brohi K, *et al.* Acute coagulopathy of trauma: mechanism, identification and effect. *Curr Opin Crit Care* 2007;**13**:680–5.

Dawes R, Thomas R. Battlefield resuscitation. *Curr Opin Crit Care* 2009; **15**:527–535.

Rossaint *et al.* Management of bleeding following major trauma: an updated European guideline. *Crit Care* 2010;**14**:R52.

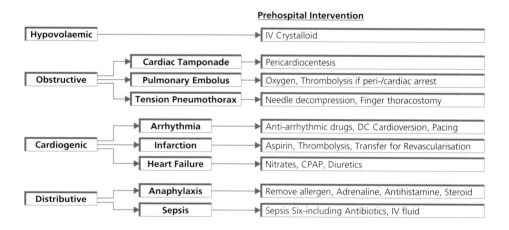

Figure 8.19 Medical causes of shock.

CHAPTER 9

Prehospital Anaesthesia

Tim Hooper[1] and David Lockey[2]

[1]London HEMS & Defence Medical Services, London, UK
[2]University of Bristol, Bristol, UK

OVERVIEW

By the end of this chapter you should know:

- Indications for prehospital anaesthesia
- Evidence base for prehospital RSI
- Equipment, training and skills necessary
- Safe practice for delivery of prehospital anaesthesia.

Box 9.1 **Indications for prehospital anaesthesia**

- Actual or impending airway compromise
- Ventilatory failure
- Unconsciousness
- Injured patients who are unmanageable or severely agitated after head injury
- Humanitarian indications
- Anticipated clinical course.

Introduction

In this chapter the indications for prehospital emergency anaesthesia and the current evidence base behind the practice will be described. The importance of training, technical skill levels and equipment and the requirement for a robust clinical governance infrastructure will be highlighted. An overview of how prehospital anaesthesia can be performed will follow.

Prehospital emergency anaesthesia is the term used to describe the administration of drugs to a patient, in the prehospital setting, to facilitate tracheal intubation (TI) and post-induction transfer to hospital. Other terms commonly used include drug-assisted intubation (DAI) and rapid sequence intubation (RSI). RSI differs from DAI in that neuromuscular blocking agents (NMBs) are always used to facilitate TI.

Prehospital emergency anaesthesia is carried out in many EMS organizations worldwide. In Europe it is predominantly physician led, while in the USA RSI is usually carried out by paramedics or nurses. Only a minority of US paramedics perform RSI. There are wide variations in practice and complication rates.

The indications for RSI in the prehospital setting are the same as for those in the in-hospital setting and are shown in Box 9.1.

Whatever the indication, the practice of prehospital RSI should achieve the same standards as in the emergency department.

Evidence base

Tracheal intubation is the standard of care for protection of the trauma airway from aspiration of gastric contents and blood while also allowing control of ventilation. It is the standard of care in the

emergency department and has therefore been extended into the prehospital phase of care. However, in the practice of prehospital care, good evidence for interventions is rare and prehospital RSI is no exception. The published evidence is difficult to interpret because RSI is often mixed with non-drug-assisted intubation and different levels of operator and varied patient case-mix mean that studies are rarely comparable.

Papers often have conflicting conclusions about the benefit of prehospital RSI. The well-reported San Diego Paramedic RSI Trial demonstrated increased mortality in RSI performed by paramedics when compared with non-intubated controls. This has been attributed to poor training and a high incidence of oxygen desaturation and subsequent hyperventilation. Other studies including a recent Scandinavian paper reported a decrease in mortality when prehospital RSI was performed by physicians in patients with severe traumatic brain injury. In the UK there is now less emphasis on training paramedics to perform intubation without drugs, and there is certainly no evidence base to support training them to perform drug-assisted intubation.

Guidelines for the safe practice of prehospital anaesthesia have been produced in the UK, Scandinavia and the USS. They have all come to similar conclusions:

- RSI may be beneficial in a relatively small proportion of prehospital patients. However, if poorly performed, it can result in unnecessary morbidity and mortality.
- It should only be performed by well-trained and competent practitioners, using appropriate equipment. This includes mandatory failed intubation plans.
- The need for a well-governed prehospital infrastructure including standard operating procedures and algorithms. High level medical direction and supervision is also needed.

ABC of Prehospital Emergency Medicine, First Edition.
Edited by Tim Nutbeam and Matthew Boylan.
© 2013 John Wiley & Sons, Ltd. Published 2013 by John Wiley & Sons, Ltd.

- Standards of practice and monitoring should be the same as those used in the in-hospital setting.

The team approach

Prehospital RSI should not usually be carried out without an operator and a trained assistant. The exact make-up of the team will vary between systems. In many European countries the operator is a physician who may come from a range of backgrounds but must have up-to-date anaesthetic and prehospital experience. The assistant is usually a health-care professional who has been specifically trained for the role (e.g. a critical-care paramedic).

It should be noted that practitioners without RSI competence can still make significant contributions to the airway management of a patient in the prehospital setting and should not be pressurized into intubating a patient without adequate support and training. Simple airway manoeuvres and airway devices can be used to provide adequate oxygenation for most patients.

The team is not just made up of an operator and assistant but also includes the senior clinical lead for the particular system and those involved with training and case review. They are particularly important in maintaining clinical quality assurance and implementing standard operating procedures and protocols.

Training and skills required

Poorly practised advanced airway procedures or inadequately trained operators are potentially harmful. Indeed the Scandinavian task force (SSAI) recommends that RSI be restricted to doctors who do drug-assisted TI in their routine practice. The precise training required to perform prehospital RSI is not clearly defined. For safe practice anaesthesia and prehospital care skills are required. Competence should be defined by these skills rather than by a physician's primary specialty.

The decision making and technical skills associated with prehospital RSI on a critically ill patient should not be underestimated. In addition to performing the procedure, the ability to manage the physiological effects of drugs administered, anticipation and management of the difficult or failed airway and the ongoing scene management are all required.

It is recognized that there is a baseline competence needed to perform RSI (in the UK it has been suggested that the ACCS programme – 2 years of training including anaesthesia, intensive care and emergency medicine – or equivalent in addition to prehospital anaesthesia training should be an absolute minimum). Regular practice of the skill and continued training are necessary to prevent skill fade. The use of simulation training may be of value but does not replace the need for clinical experience. In addition, because of the characteristics of the prehospital environment, many believe that the frequent presence of a practising senior physician on scene for direct observation and supervision is an essential governance requirement.

Each EMS system should have in place a clinical governance structure to ensure competence of team members and allow regular review of cases for personal and system development.

Minimum monitoring standards

Clinical assessment in combination with physiological monitoring should be performed throughout the prehospital anaesthetic, including preparation, induction, maintenance and transfer. Clinical assessment is vitally important and may detect changes in the patient condition prior to alteration of physiological measurements. Box 9.2 illustrates key clinical observations and Box 9.3 highlights the AAGBI and NAEMSP recommended minimum monitoring standards.

Box 9.2 **Clinical assessment of the anaesthetised patient**

- Pulse rate and strength
- Colour and coolness of peripheries
- Respiratory rate
- Pupil size and reactivity
- Lacrimation
- Evidence of muscle activity and limb movements.

Box 9.3 **Minimum standards of monitoring for the anaesthetised patient**

- **Heart rate and rhythm** (including ECG) – desaturation at induction is associated with bradycardia and dysrhythmias Tachycardia may be due to inadequate sedation or hypovolaemia
- **Non-invasive blood pressure** – Hypertension may suggest inadequate sedation or Cushing's response (significantly raised intracranial pressure with coning). Hypotension may be due to over-sedation, hypovolaemia or decreased venous return
- **Oxygen saturation** (SpO2) – Assesses adequate oxygen delivery and may give an indication of tissue perfusion
- **End Tidal Carbon Dioxide** (ETCO2) – ideally capnography Confirms correct placement of the tracheal tube (TT) and enables accurate control of ventilation, important in the management of head injuries.

Measurements should be made at least every 3 minutes and appropriate alarm limits set on the monitoring equipment. Alarms should be loud enough to be heard in the prehospital environment.

Current recommended minimum standards for practice

As discussed previously the prehospital care team intending to perform anaesthesia should be made up of a competent physician and trained assistant.

Equipment should be fit for task as well as being robust, weatherproof and portable. It should be adequately maintained and serviced with electrical equipment having appropriate battery life. The team must be familiar and have in depth knowledge of all equipment. Box 9.4 lists the necessary equipment.

Drugs

The primary goal of RSI is to achieve rapid anaesthesia with muscle relaxation while minimizing physiological derangement

Table 9.1 Drugs used in prehospital anaesthesia

Drug	Drug type/ Mode of Action	Indication	Dosage	Advantages	Disadvantages
Etomidate	Imidazole derivative GABA receptor agonist	Induction	0.3 mg/kg IV	Haemodynamic stability	Adrenal suppression Antiplatelet activity
Ketamine	Phencyclidine derivative NMDA receptor antagonist	Induction (maintenance) Analgesia	1–2 mg/kg IV (10 mg/kg IM) (titrated to effect) 0.1 mg/kg IV (1 mg/kg IM)	Haemodynamic stability Bronchodilatation Airway reflexes maintained	Tachycardia, hypertension and raised ICP Increased salivation Emergence delirium Antiplatelet activity
Thiopentone Propofol	Rarely used in the prehospital setting due to negative effects on the cardiovascular system – reduced cardiac output and hypotension. However titrated boluses or infusions of propofol are used by some for maintenance of anaesthesia				
Suxamethonium	Dicholine ester of succinic acid Depolarizing Muscle relaxant	Paralysis for RSI	1–2 mg/kg IV (2.5 mg/kg IM)	Rapid and profound neuromuscular blockade Brief duration of action	Bradycardia and dysrhythmias Hyperkalaemia Raised IOP and ICP Malignant hyperthermia Sux. Apnoea
Atracurium	Benzyl- isoquinolinium or aminosteriod	Maintenance of Paralysis	0.3–0.6 mg/kg IV	Medium acting	Histamine release
Rocuronium	Non-depolarizing muscle relaxant		0.6 mg/kg IV (Or 1 mg/kg for intubation)	Medium acting Haemodynamic stability Rapid reversal with sugammadex	Anaphylactoid reactions
Pancuronium			0.1 mg/kg IV	Long acting Sympathomimetic	
Midazolam	Benzodiazepine (BDZ) GABA receptor activator	Hypnotic Maintenance of sedation Anxiolysis	0.5–2 mg IV Boluses titrated to effect (2.5–5 mg IM)	Short acting Can be used to control agitated patients pre-RSI	Hypotension Respiratory depression
Morphine	Opioid Opioid receptor agonist	Analgesia Maintenance of sedation (used with BDZ)	1–2 mg IV Boluses titrated to effect (5–10 mg IM)	Potent analgesic	Respiratory depression Hypotension Histamine release Nausea and vomiting
Fentanyl	Opioid Opioid receptor agonist	Analgesia	1-5 µg/kg IV	Potent analgesic Rapid onset Obtunds cardiovascular response to laryngoscopy	Bradycardia Respiratory depression Rarely muscle rigidity

either from the drugs administered or laryngoscopy. The drugs used are usually selected for their haemodynamic stability, although it should be noted that there is no ideal drug – all have advantages and disadvantages.

The RSI team must have an in-depth knowledge of all drugs used and be alert to the side effects, contraindications and physiological derangement they may cause. Emergency drugs (adrenaline, atropine, naloxone, etc.) must be carried to deal with adverse drug reactions.

In systems with frequent RSI it may be appropriate to check, pre-draw and carefully label drugs so that they are ready for immediate use. This may save time and reduce the risk of drawing up errors.

Table 9.1 illustrates the common drugs used in the prehospital setting.

Procedural summary

General principles

The general principles of prehospital anaesthesia are the same as those for emergency in-hospital anaesthesia. However, the variable

prehospital environment makes it imperative that standard operating procedures are in place, well rehearsed and understood by all team members.

The choice of drugs and equipment are dependent on the system, standard operating procedures, physician preference and the patients' physiological state.

Preparation

This is essential to successful prehospital anaesthetic delivery and reduction of complications. The patient should be placed in as controlled an environment as possible, ensuring adequate light/shade and, if possible, shelter from the elements. Where possible the sun should be behind the operator so as not to affect the laryngoscopic view: 360 degree access to the patient should be sought to allow interventions to be carried out more easily. The ideal position to perform intubation is with the patient supine (or slightly tilted head up) on an ambulance trolley at thigh height allowing the operator to intubate easily while kneeling (Figure 9.1).

Box 9.4 **Equipment for prehospital anaesthesia**

Monitoring	See Box 9.2. To be attached to the patient as soon as is practical May need to be temporarily removed for extrication, etc.
Oxygen	Adequate supplies for on scene period and transfer (with redundancy)
Simple airway adjuncts	Oropharyngeal and nasopharyngeal airways
Vascular access equipment	Intravenous and intraosseous
Drugs	Limited selection to reduce drug errors. Labelled. See Table 9.1.
Intubating equipment	Laryngoscope with different sized blades, varied sized endotracheal tubes, bougie
Suction	Hand or battery operated
Ventilating system	To include circuit (catheter mount, heat and moisture exchange filter – HME, capnography device), self inflating bag (bag, valve, mask – BVM) and mechanical ventilator (if appropriate)
Airway rescue devices	Including supraglottic airways (e.g. Laryngeal Mask Airway™) and surgical airway equipment
Lighting	As appropriate
Procedural check lists	May be of benefit

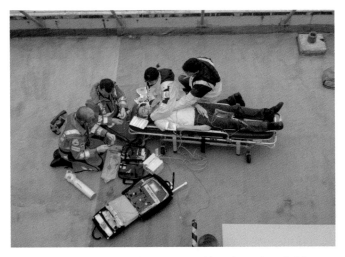

Figure 9.1 Preparation: 360-degree access with patient at knee height.

A standard 'kit dump' should be prepared. This will vary with each EMS system but should include all necessary equipment and drugs needed for the RSI, including monitoring, oxygen, intubating and ventilation equipment, suction and rescue airway devices. The use of a yellow clinical waste bag and standard equipment lay-out will aid in the checking and location of equipment in emergencies (Figure 9.2). Monitoring should be applied to the patient as soon as practically possible and two points of circulatory access gained).

Assistants should be fully briefed to ensure everyone knows their role and what is going to happen. Ideally four people are required: operator, operator's assistant, provider of manual, in-line

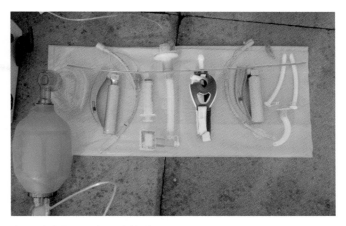

Figure 9.2 Preparation: RSI kit dump.

immobilization of the cervical spine and a person to perform cricoid pressure and manipulation (Figure 9.1).

Pre-induction

Pre-oxygenation is essential to prevent hypoxaemia during the procedure. This can be achieved using a non-rebreathing oxygen face mask with reservoir attached or a bag and mask. In a patient with respiratory compromise gentle assisted ventilation may be required.

In agitated patients it may be necessary to use small amounts of sedation (e.g. ketamine or midazolam) to facilitate pre-oxygenation and pre-optimization.

The use of an equipment check list (Figure 9.3) may be helpful to ensure all equipment is present and allow time for adequate pre-oxygenation. Decisions on laryngeal blade and tube size should be made during this time.

Once manual in-line immobilization of the cervical spine is established, the cervical collar and head blocks can be removed until intubation is completed.

Induction and intubation

Induction should be straightforward but modified to the patient's individual needs (e.g. reduced drug dosages in the profoundly

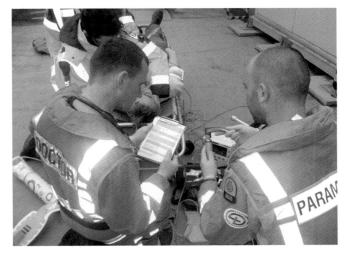

Figure 9.3 Use of a checklist during pre-oxygenation.

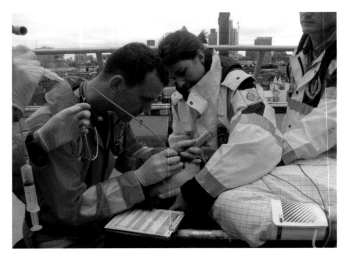

Figure 9.4 Routine use of a bougie.

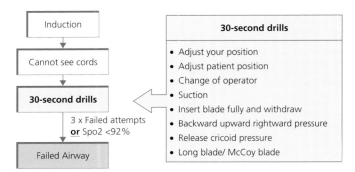

Figure 9.5 Thirty-second drills.

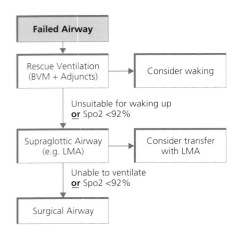

Figure 9.6 Failed intubation plan.

shocked patient). Although prehospital airways are often considered challenging well-rehearsed simple techniques produce good results. Poorly applied cricoid pressure often distorts anatomy and may need to be repositioned, or released, to aid intubation. An intubating bougie should be used routinely (Figure 9.4) and suction should be immediately available. If intubation is unsuccessful at the first attempt, patient, operator and equipment should be optimized for success on the subsequent attempt. Figure 9.5 shows the elements that can be optimized during this period. Collectively these are known as the '30-second drills', as they should be addressed within this time frame. Repeated intubation attempts should be avoided once these aspects have been optimized. If the patient desaturates during attempted intubation they should be gently ventilated using a BVM until saturation improves.

Failed intubation should be anticipated early. Every system should have a written, and well-rehearsed, 'failed intubation plan'. This should include supraglottic airway rescue devices and provision for performing a surgical airway. Figure 9.6 shows an example of a failed intubation plan.

The breathing circuit should be connected and correct placement of the tracheal tube should be confirmed as soon as possible using conventional methods (seeing the tube pass between the vocal cords, viewing chest wall rise and fall, auscultation in the axillae and stomach) and end tidal end tidal CO_2 detection devices (preferably waveform capnography). Once confirmed the endotracheal tube should secured in place using ties, adhesive tape or tube holders. Care should be taken not to obstruct venous drainage from the head by securing the endotracheal tube too tightly, especially in the head injured patient. When secured the cervical collar and head blocks can be replaced.

Post intubation

All anticipated practical procedures should be completed prior to packaging for transfer to hospital as they may be difficult to perform adequately once transfer begins. Patients should be carefully packaged with particular attention to temperature control, spinal immobilization and accessibility of intravenous access.

There should be sufficient supplies of oxygen for the whole journey, with redundancy, to ensure the patient receives optimal oxygenation. Ventilation, either by hand using a BVM or preferably a mechanical ventilator, should be adjusted to maintain normocapnia (ETCO$_2$ 4.0–4.5 kPa).

Anaesthesia should be carefully maintained to prevent hypertension and reduce the chances of awareness. Awareness is more likely where the patient was conscious prior to RSI and has received muscle relaxant drugs. Monitor for tachycardia, hypertension, pupillary dilatation and lacrimation. Aliquots of a hypnotic agent such as midazolam and an analgesic, titrated to the patients' physiological response are usually sufficient. Some EMS systems use drug infusions for maintenance of anaesthesia.

Transfer

Transfer is covered in detail in Chapter 32. Maintenance of anaesthesia, ongoing monitoring and continual assessment of the patient must take place during transfer and should be overseen by a clinician skilled in managing the anaesthetised patient. Supporting equipment (suction, intubating equipment, resuscitative fluids) must be available and a contemporaneous record of vital signs and interventions generated.

Figure 9.7 gives an overview of the steps in prehospital RSI.

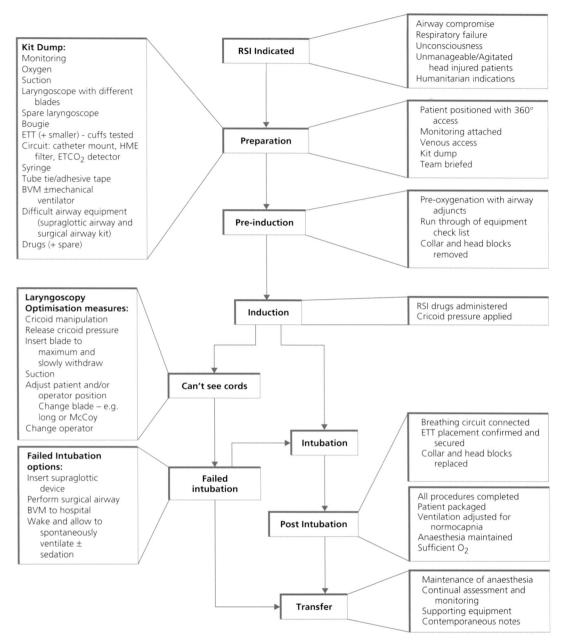

Figure 9.7 Prehospital anaesthesia: overview.

Paediatrics

Prehospital anaesthesia of small children is only rarely required. For most children the risks outweigh the benefits. Where actual airway compromise cannot be overcome with simple airway manoeuvres the risk to benefit ratio may change and drug-assisted intubation may become appropriate.

Tips from the field

- Move the patient to an area with 360-degree access early – even if peri-arrest

- Optimize pre-oxygenation by utilizing airway adjuncts, airway toilet and titrated sedation if required
- Consider the pre-oxygenation and induction of obese patients in a head-up position (with cervical spine protection maintained) or in the sitting position
- Pre-oxygenate and induce patients with severe facial injuries in the position where they are most comfortable and can maintain their own airway
- Anaesthetic agents can, if absolutely necessary, be given via the intraosseous route
- Consider reducing induction sedative dose or omitting altogether in severe shock states.

Further reading

Association of Anaesthetists of Great Britain & Ireland: Safety Guideline 'Prehospital Anaesthesia'. Feb 2009

NAEMSP Drug Assisted Intubation in the Prehospital Setting Position Statement of the National Association of Emergency Physicians. Jan 2005

Drug-Assisted Intubation in the Prehospital Setting (Resource Document to NAEMSP Position Statement). Prehospital Emergency Care. Apr-Jun 2006;10(2):261–171

Prehospital Airway Management – Time to Provide the Same Standard of Care as in the Hospital. ACTA Anaesthesiol Scand. 2008;52:877–878

Prehospital Airway Management: Guidelines from a Task Force from the Scandinavian Society for Anaesthesiology and Intensive Care Medicine. 2008;52:897–907

CHAPTER 10

Prehospital Analgesia and Sedation

Jonathan Hulme

Sandwell and West Birmingham Hospitals NHS Trust, City Hospital, Birmingham, UK

OVERVIEW

By the end of this chapter you will understand:

- The importance of effective analgesia
- The various methods of achieving effective analgesia
- The technique and monitoring required for safe sedation
- The importance of adequate training and skills prior to commencing sedation.

Analgesia

The problem with pain

Pain is common in prehospital medicine and is defined in Box 10.1.

Box 10.1 **Definitions**

Pain: An unpleasant sensory and emotional experience associated with actual or potential tissue damage, or described in terms of such damage. Pain is an individual, multifactorial experience influenced by culture, previous pain events, beliefs, mood and ability to cope

Analgesia: Relief of pain through administration of drugs or other methods

Procedural sedation: A drug-induced depression of consciousness during which patients respond purposefully to verbal commands, either alone or accompanied by light tactile stimulation. No interventions are required to maintain a patent airway, and spontaneous ventilation is adequate. Cardiovascular function is usually maintained.

Acute pain has adverse psychological and physiological consequences; both are important.

Poor analgesia worsens patients' perception of pain, both around the time of injury and long after the initial insult. The psychological consequences make effective analgesia more difficult to achieve: consider the scared patient who recoils from minor interventions such as cannulation. Psychological responses to acute pain are risk factors for the development of chronic pain states.

ABC of Prehospital Emergency Medicine, First Edition.
Edited by Tim Nutbeam and Matthew Boylan.
© 2013 John Wiley & Sons, Ltd. Published 2013 by John Wiley & Sons, Ltd.

Physiological responses include sympathetic stimulation that can potentially lead to myocardial ischaemia. Acute pain is a trigger of the 'injury response', causing activation of complex neurohumoral and immune responses (e.g. hyperglycaemia, fat and protein catabolism, blood vessel permeability, etc.), which is necessary for healing and recovery. The size of the 'injury response' is related to the extent of the painful stimulus: prolonged stimuli, without effective analgesia, can lead to counterproductive responses and worsen patient outcome.

Effective analgesia can achieve a number of aims (Box 10.2).

Box 10.2 **Objectives of effective analgesia**

To relieve suffering
To improve assessment of a patient who is no longer distressed and agitated
To reduce physiological stress and prevent avoidable deterioration
To facilitate treatment that would otherwise cause significant distress to the patient.

Physiology of pain

The body's ability to detect injury is an important protective mechanism. The individual is alerted to tissue damage by acute pain. Receptors ('nociceptors') detect a range of noxious stimuli (heat, cold, pressure, chemical). The initial response is modulated peripherally by altered conditions in damaged areas including increased concentrations of proinflammatory cytokines, substance P and prostaglandins.

Stimuli are transduced to action potentials and transmitted to the central nervous system via fast (myelinated and medium diameter) Aδ-fibres and the more numerous slow (unmyelinated and small diameter) C-fibres.

In the spinal cord, there is fast transmission to higher centres. Central sensitization can occur, typically due to repeated stimulation. Phenomena such as 'wind-up' result in heightened responses after similar noxious inputs and pain after what would previously have been interpreted as non-painful stimuli.

Interpretation in the cortex is a summation of the effects of the initial stimulus, modified peripherally and centrally, and influenced by culture, previous pain events, beliefs, mood and ability to cope.

Principles of management of acute pain

Although pain is commonly encountered, adequate treatment is often lacking.

Recommendations for prehospital pain management are internationally agreed, by civilian and military representatives, and are appropriate aims for us all (Box 10.3).

Box 10.3 **Practice recommendations on prehospital pain management from the National Association of EMS Physicians and endorsed by the UK military**

Mandatory assessment of both presence and severity of pain
Use of reliable tools for the assessment of pain
Indications and contraindications for prehospital pain therapy
Non-pharmacological interventions for pain management
Pharmacological interventions for pain management
Mandatory patient monitoring and documentation before and after analgesic administration
Appropriate handover and transfer of care to hospital
Quality improvement and management structure to ensure appropriate use of prehospital analgesia.

Some aspects are beyond the scope of this chapter but remain integral to the delivery of safe and effective analgesia to patients in the prehospital arena.

Assessment of pain

Poor analgesia provision is frequently due to under-appreciation of a patient's needs. Although a difficult concept to practice at all times, pain is whatever the experiencing person says it is, existing whenever they say it does.

Appropriate assessment is the key. There are reliable tools for scoring pain that are rapid and objective both before and after analgesia.

Visual analogue scales and simple scoring systems are the most appropriate in the majority of prehospital situations for adult patients. The Wong–Baker FACES pain scale is better for children.

For all patients, the trend in pain scores is more important than a one-off or absolute value, i.e. the practitioner should expect that after appropriate, adequate analgesia, the patient reports an improvement in the pain score.

Assessment is not possible in patients with impaired cognition, e.g. depressed consciousness. It must not be assumed that this equates to an inability to be in pain.

Treatment of pain

There are no contraindications for prehospital analgesia although some methods may be (relatively) contraindicated in some patients, e.g. opioids in brain injury may be problematic if they lead to hypercapnia.

Patients typically need a combination of non-pharmacological and pharmacological methods for effective analgesia.

Non-pharmacological interventions

Reassurance through effective therapeutic communication significantly alleviates distress; a professional, empathic approach distracts from the painful stimulus. For children, parental presence reduces distress for both child and parent.

Immobilizing fractures or dislocations reduces pain and bleeding. Traction splints are particularly good for femoral fractures, as a significant amount of pain is due to unopposed contraction of the thigh muscles.

Cold water reduces the pain of superficial burns immediately after injury. Dressings preventing airflow across the burn (e.g. cellophane wrap) and provide additional analgesia. Burns can be cooled for up to 20 minutes; the risk of causing hypothermia should be anticipated.

Pharmacological interventions

Drugs affect the pain pathway at specific points.

There are a variety of routes of administration (Table 10.1).

The use of synergistic analgesic agents is considered to be good practice if it reduces the dose required of an agent that has the potential to cause harm.

For example, co-administration of paracetamol (acetaminophen), codeine and non-steroidal anti-inflammatory drugs can reduce the amount of morphine required over several hours. Within the timeframe of the prehospital practitioner, these benefits are unlikely to be seen. So, for short-term analgesia, many avoid polypharmacy, leaving the multimodal drug approach for the hospital prescription chart.

Some specific drugs are considered further:

Paracetamol (acetaminophen) and non-steroidal anti-inflammatory drugs

These good analgesics are infrequently used in the prehospital phase. Use is mainly confined to self-administration in patients seen and discharged from scene.

Intravenous paracetamol is available, has an opiate-sparing effect, but is supplied in 100-mL glass bottles, adding significant weight to kit bags. It is better suited to early administration in the Emergency Department (ED).

Nitrous oxide: oxygen (50/50 mix): Entonox®

Rapid onset and offset of analgesia. It is used while other means of longer lasting analgesia are established or as brief additional analgesia during painful episodes, e.g. movement of an injured limb into a splint.

There are no significant side effects except sedation and nausea but it is contraindicated in patients with an air-containing closed spaces since N_2O diffuses into them with a resulting increase in pressure. This is dangerous in pneumothorax, intracranial air after head injury and decompression sickness.

Entonox® (Figure 10.1) separates into its component gases at approximately $-6°C$, risking delivery of a hypoxic mixture. Cylinders should be stored horizontally and repeated inversion of

Table 10.1 Pharmacological interventions: routes of administration

Route	Example	Pros	Cons
Oral	Paracetamol, NSAIDS,	Cost and ease Widely acceptable	Conscious and able to swallow (nausea) Slow onset Poor titration Poor for severe pain Variable absorption (gastric stasis / first pass)
Inhalational	Entonox, methoxyflurane	Rapid Self administration (titrated by patient) Short lasting Adjunct to other agents	Inability to understand / coordinate needs Short lived Nausea and vomiting Cumbersome equipment Cough, mucosal irritation
Intravenous	NSAIDS, Opioids, ketamine, paracetamol	Rapid No first pass Titratable	IV access – difficult in some and needs training
Nasal	Opioids, ketamine	Rapid Easy No needles Titratable	Absorption may be affected by mucosal conditions, blood, etc. Legislation
Topical	Local anaesthetic cream Slow release opioids	Painless	Poor titration Limited range of drugs for most patients Slow
Intramuscular	Opioids	No IV access needed	Slow and variable onset Potential for delayed overdose Damage to nerve Inadvertent IV/IA injection
Buccal	Opioids	Rapid Painless Avoids first pass Spit / swallow when finished	Limited range of drugs
Rectal	Paracetamol, NSAIDS	Rapid Avoids first pass Easily self administered	Acceptance
Intraosseous	NSAIDS, Opioids, ketamine, paracetamol	Rapid No first pass Titratable Easier than IV	Small risk of bone infection Training / legislation to be able to do it

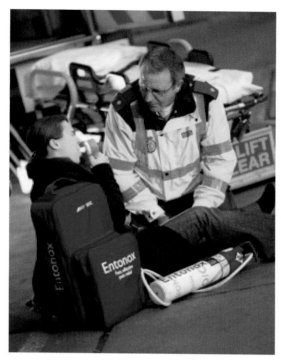

Figure 10.1 Entonox.

the cylinder prior to use at low temperatures is recommended to mix the gases.

The main limitations in the prehospital setting are not pharmacological. The cylinder and delivery system are heavy and can mean that a very useful analgesic is left in the emergency vehicle if other equipment needs to be carried to the patient.

Opioids

Opioids are widely used. Morphine and fentanyl are common and equally effective.

Fentanyl is faster acting, shorter lasting and more lipid soluble than morphine. This last property enables it to be delivered via alternative routes (nasal and buccal) while longer lasting analgesia is

arranged. The 'fentanyl lollipop' is, however, not currently licensed for acute pain.

Shortcomings with morphine include significant interpatient differences in dose requirements and a typical time to maximal effect of 20 minutes. Titration to best effect is essential but can take a long time to achieve. This is completely impractical when trying to provide good pain relief during dynamic situations such as patient transport, e.g. analgesia for a fractured neck of femur when moving downstairs or extricating an injured patient from a vehicle.

Respiratory depression is uncommon with careful titration. The incidence of nausea is small, but 10 mg metoclopramide is often co-administered. Studies have failed to show any clinically significant antiemetic effect of metoclopramide. Alternatives such as cyclizine or ondansetron are more efficacious.

Ketamine

Ketamine is a dissociative anaesthetic that is similar to phencyclidine (PCP/'angel dust', Figure 10.2).

The drug datasheet advises that ketamine should be used by, or under the direction of medical practitioners, experienced in administering general anaesthetics and in maintenance of an airway and in the control of respiratory support. It is, though, used widely and safely in prehospital care by a range of immediate care professionals. Absolute contraindications to its use are few.

For many prehospital professionals, it is the agent of choice for musculoskeletal injuries requiring strong analgesia or procedural analgesia and sedation (see later).

Most often administered intravenously, it is effective intraosseously and intramuscularly for moderate and severe pain.

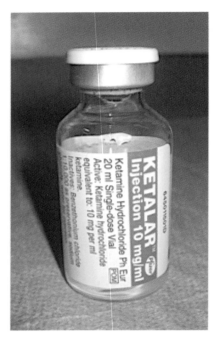

Figure 10.2 Ketamine vial (10 mg/mL).

At subanaesthetic doses (i.e. 0.25–0.5 mg/kg IV/IO) it provides excellent short-lasting analgesia, sedation and amnesia ('analgosedation'). It has a rapid onset (about 1 minute) and is easily and rapidly titrated to effect. This lasts approximately 10–15 minutes: repeated small doses are often needed, i.e. during extrication of the trapped patient.

Ketamine has a large therapeutic index: the difference between the effective dose and amount needed in overdose to cause significant harm is large.

It suppresses breathing less than other potent analgesics; apnoea is unusual unless an intravenous dose is administered too rapidly.

Airway patency and reflexes are *usually* preserved with obvious advantages in the sedated patient, although this makes tolerance of supraglottic airway devices less satisfactory than with other agents.

Hypersalivation is rarely a practical problem and co-administration of atropine is seldom used.

Increased muscular tone after ketamine can make extrication more difficult as the limbs become more difficult to bend. Reducing dislocations is more difficult.

Nausea and vomiting are uncommon.

Ketamine can cause hypertension and tachycardia: undesirable in the patient with an at-risk myocardium. The increase in blood pressure, although usually slight, may necessitate increasing tourniquet or direct pressure to maintain haemorrhage control. It is important not to assume that all tachycardia in the patient who has received ketamine is a drug effect: it may be due to shock.

Ketamine may increase cerebral perfusion pressure, which, contrary to older data from underpowered studies in non-traumatic brain injury patients, is now considered safe and a potential advantage.

Most preparations can cause psychological disturbances; up to 20% of patients experience emergence phenomenon (disorientation ± agitation ± psychological distress) as the drug wears off. Short-term hallucinations are frequent; long-term nightmares and hallucinations are reported but rare. The incidence and severity of these side effects can be reduced by co-administration of benzodiazepine and/or morphine.

Local anaesthesia
The roles for this include:

- *Topical application:* for venepuncture in non-time critical situations, for children and needle phobic adults.
- *Peripheral nerve blocks:* popular with some prehospital providers due to profound analgesia without sedation, e.g. femoral nerve blocks. However, in many settings, splinting and ketamine/morphine obviate the need for regional anaesthesia performed in difficult practical circumstances and where analgosedation is desirable.

Procedural sedation

What is it?

Some interventions are distressing for patients because they increase pain (e.g. extricating the injured, trapped patient) or are invasive (e.g. insertion of intercostal drain).

Administration of short-acting sedatives and analgesics ameliorate this problem and facilitate treatment. Previously called 'conscious sedation', the name has changed as effective sedation often alters consciousness.

How much is the patient sedated?

Sedation is a continuum, although discrete definitions are proposed (Table 10.2).

Table 10.2 Sedation

	Minimal sedation/ anxiolysis	Procedural sedation		General anaesthesia
		Moderate sedation	Deep sedation	
Responsive-ness	Normal response to verbal stimulation	Purposeful response to verbal or tactile stimulation	Purposeful response following repeated or painful stimulation	Unarousable even with painful stimulus
Airway	Unaffected	No intervention required	Intervention may be required	Intervention often required
Spontaneous ventilation	Unaffected	Adequate	May be inadequate	Frequently inadequate
Cardiovascular function	Unaffected	Usually maintained	Usually maintained	May be impaired

(Source: Continuum of depth of sedation: Definition of general anaesthesia and levels of sedation/analgesia Committee of Origin: Quality Management and Departmental Administration (2009) is reprinted with permission of the American Society of Anesthesiologists, 520 N. Northwest Highway, Park Ridge, Illinois 60068-2573).
Note: In practice there is minimal distinction between deep sedation and general anaesthesia.

Ketamine does not fit neatly into these definitions: it produces dissociative sedation, which is a trance-like state during which airway reflexes, spontaneous respiration and cardiovascular stability are typically but, importantly, *not always* maintained.

Prehospital procedural sedation should aim to be 'moderate' avoiding the potential complications with airway, breathing and circulation.

What is required for procedural sedation?
Monitoring
In accordance with minimum standards used during anaesthesia:

- ECG (three lead)
- pulse oximetry
- non-invasive blood pressure (auto cycle for every few minutes)
- visual monitoring (respiratory rate, alertness, response to painful stimuli, etc.).

Capnography is helpful to monitor respiratory rate even in the non-intubated patient (end tidal CO_2 value is not accurate but presence of a trace reassuring).

Equipment
In short, kit and drugs that would be required for emergency anaesthesia (i.e. rapid sequence induction (RSI)) and cardiovascular collapse. These are described in Chapter 9.

Drugs
Numerous drug combinations have been used.

Polypharmacy should be avoided. Successful prehospital analgesia with or without sedation can be readily achieved for most patients with the use of one or two drugs: ketamine is usually one of these. In difficult situations what is usually needed is more patience to correctly titrate the therapeutic agent, additional non-pharmacological methods (i.e. splinting) and better teamwork, not an extra drug.

A popular prehospital choice is ketamine and midazolam. Ketamine's excellent analgesic effect (that lasts beyond the period of procedural sedation) and dissociative state with fewer physiological adverse effects combined with midazolam's limitation of the psychological side effects make it an ideal combination.

A dose of 1–2 mg/kg (IV/IO) of ketamine in titrated aliquots and 1–2 mg (IV/IO) midazolam is the norm in adult patients, aiming to 'go to sleep with ketamine and wake up on midazolam'.

Supplemental oxygen is typically administered.

Training
Procedural sedation can, during 'deep' sedation and without intention by becoming general anaesthesia, precipitate physiological decompensation. This typically results in the need for emergency anaesthesia. Illness, acute or pre-existing, and injury increase the likelihood of adverse events even with small amounts of sedation.

In-hospital sedation by practitioners without anaesthetic training has been cause for concern. The less controlled prehospital arena,

without access to experienced support, means that recommendations endorsed internationally and, in the UK, by all major bodies involved in prehospital care, are that procedural sedation should only be undertaken by 'practitioners ... competent to undertake RSI and tracheal intubation'.

Handover to hospital
A verbal and written explanation of drugs administered for analgesia with or without sedation must be given to the clinician receiving the patient at hospital.

This helps clinical decision-making and planning. For example:

- The agitated and combative patient who has been sedated to facilitate safe transfer to secondary care may need RSI within the ED.
- Confusion and sedation may be due to analgosedative agents. This may be confused with organic illness if the ED physician has not received a clear handover.

Tips from the field

- In emergencies, it is easy to concentrate on other aspects of treatment and extrication and overlook pain; make it a routine part of assessment
- Ask the patient how bad their pain is. Treat it then ask them again to see if you have made it better. If not, they need more analgesia!
- A distressed patient in pain is upsetting for everyone. Effective pain relief is good for the patient, satisfying for you and calms the whole emergency team making the rest of the rescue less stressful
- Non-pharmacological methods of pain relief are very effective and can avoid or reduce drug requirements. Not always perceived as 'high-tech' they may be poorly done or missed out
- If you are going to the trouble of drawing up and administering an anti-emetic, use an effective one, such as cyclizine or a 5-HT$_3$ antagonist
- Do not administer ketamine as a fast bolus: it stops patients breathing
- Deep sedation is, in practice, general anaesthesia. If you wouldn't give your patient a general anaesthetic, don't be tempted to deepen 'sedation' to similar levels
- Attaching and maintaining monitoring (ECG, SpO$_2$, BP ± ETCO$_2$) can be difficult but the benefits of struggling occasionally far out way the problems of missing deterioration
- Avoid polypharmacy. Have a small selection of drugs you use regularly and get very used to what they do.

Further reading

AAGI. *Prehospital Anaesthesia*. London: The Association of Anaesthetists of Great Britain and Ireland, 2009.

Allison K, Porter K. Consensus on the prehospital approach to burns patient management. *Emerg Med J* 2004;**21**:112–114.

Alonso-Serra HM, Wesley K. Prehospital pain management. *Prehosp Emerg Care* 2003;**7**:482–488.

ASA Standards, Guidelines and Statements. Continuum of depth of sedation: Definition of general anaesthesia and levels of sedation/analgesia. 2009.

Cordell W. The high prevalence of pain in emergency medical care. *Am J Emerg Med* 2002;**20**:165–169.

Fisher J. UK Ambulance Service Clinical Practice Guidelines (2006). 2008.

Henzi I, Walder B, Tramèr MR. Metoclopramide in the prevention of postoperative nausea and vomiting: a quantitative systematic review of randomized, placebo-controlled studies. *Br J Anaesth* 1999;**83**:761–771.

Migita RT, Klein EJ, Garrison MM. Sedation and analgesia for pediatric fracture reduction in the emergency department: a systematic review. *Arch Pediatr Adolesc Med* 2006;**160**:46–51.

Morris C, Perris A, Klein J, Mahoney P. Anaesthesia in haemodynamically compromised emergency patients: does ketamine represent the best choice of induction agent? *Anaesthesia* 2009;**64**:532–539.

Sehdev RS, Symmons DAD, Kindl K. Ketamine for rapid sequence induction in patients with head injury in the emergency department. *Emerg Med Australas* 2006;**18**:37–44.

Sibley A, Mackenzie M, Bawden J, *et al*. A prospective review of the use of ketamine to facilitate endotracheal intubation in the helicopter emergency medical services (HEMS) setting. *Emerg Med J* 2010.

Svenson JE, Abernathy MK. Ketamine for prehospital use: new look at an old drug. *Am J Emerg Med* 2007;**25**:977–980.

CHAPTER 11

Prehospital Monitoring

Tim Harris and Peter Shirley

Royal London Hospital, London, UK

OVERVIEW

By the end of this chapter you should:

- Develop an understanding of the common monitoring modalities used in prehospital care
- Develop an awareness of the limitations of common monitoring modalities
- Understand how the prehospital environment and mode of transport may affect monitoring.

Introduction

The role of monitoring is to provide a real-time visual display of the patients' physiology and to alert the clinician when this falls outside predetermined limits. The prehospital environment presents a challenge when assessing, treating and monitoring patients. This and need for rapid assessment often lead to compromise between what is desirable and what is practical. Indeed there are situations where the time taken to place monitoring is of greater risk than benefit to a patient – for example if a patient with a penetrating chest injury is conversant and close to definitive care then the requirement for rapid transfer overrides the desire for full accurate physiological measures.

Prehospital monitoring

The same physiological variables should be monitored as in the resuscitation room – pulse, ECG, blood pressure, respiratory rate, Glasgow Coma Scale (GCS), temperature and end-tidal carbon dioxide. In patients transferred between intensive care areas, invasive blood pressure, central venous pressures and urine output may also be monitored in transit. The clinician needs to make an active choice of which variables to monitor and what alarm limits to set (Figure 11.1). A written record should be maintained in longer transfers, both to assist in detecting trends and to monitor changes to treatment.

It is important for the prehospital practitioner to recognize how these physiological variables can be affected by the prehospital environment and/or transportation. Significant fluid shifts may occur during take-off and landing on retrieval flights altering

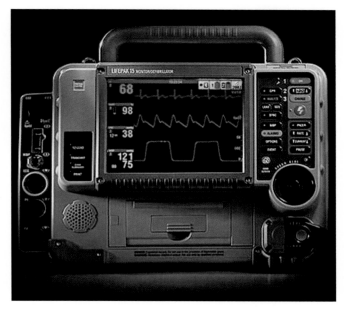

Figure 11.1 Modern multimodality monitors allow different physiological variables to be displayed simultaneously on a single screen. Assigning different colours to different physiological variables aids clarity and safety.

invasive vascular monitoring. The vibration/motion in moving ambulances or helicopters may render non-invasive blood pressure virtually redundant. Movement during patient positioning and transportation may stimulate catecholamine surges leading to rises in pulse and heart rate by over 10%. Physical characteristics such as ambient light, temperature, body fluids, mechanical fluids, aircraft safety and movement may all affect the use of monitoring. Back-up equipment, familiarity with the limits of the kit and rapid maintenance skills are therefore essential.

The human–equipment interface

Medical practitioners routinely respond to clinical cues, alarms and alerts that occur during patient care. They appraise the situation, assess the significance of these warnings and make a decision to either intervene or continue monitoring the situation. They are also aware of the subtle indicators of normal function that are in the background. With experience these become familiar and can

ABC of Prehospital Emergency Medicine, First Edition.
Edited by Tim Nutbeam and Matthew Boylan.
© 2013 John Wiley & Sons, Ltd. Published 2013 by John Wiley & Sons, Ltd.

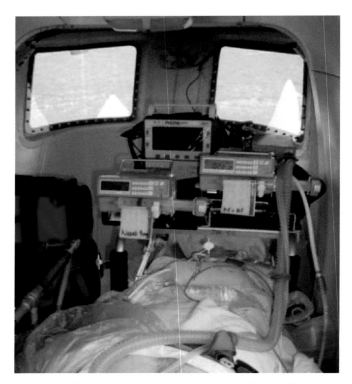

Figure 11.2 All monitoring equipment needs to be easily accessible and visible.

be a significant adjunct to monitoring. Trained and experienced practitioners are alerted to potential problems before alarms trigger and will be able to act accordingly. Noticing the change in sound as a ventilator becomes disconnected, the experienced practitioner would respond before disconnection alarms were triggered and well before a change in the patient's vital signs.

All monitoring equipment needs to be easily accessible and visible (Figure 11.2).

Box 11.1 summarizes the ideal characteristics of out of hospital monitoring equipment

The structured approach to monitoring

A structured approach to assessment allows for a rapid accurate response and minimal error under pressure. The best monitor remains the clinician. The initial clinical assessment may occur when the patient is trapped or only partially visible to the clinician and needs to be regarded as baseline monitoring. As the environment becomes more permissive and access to the patient improves, so too will the level of monitoring that may be employed.

The application of monitoring should follow and be an integral part of the <C> ABCDE primary assessment.

Airway

Clinical assessment is made for the adequacy of ventilation, airway obstruction and risk of aspiration. If the airway protected with a cuffed endotracheal tube its position at the lips and cuff pressure are noted.

Box 11.1 Ideal characteristics of prehospital monitoring equipment

1 Loud and visible alarms
  ○ Alarms should be visible and audible against background noise levels
2 Large and clear illuminated display
  ○ The display should be visible at distance, in sunlight and be capable of displaying ECG, arterial oxygen saturation, non-invasive blood pressure, two invasive pressures, capnography and temperature
3 Simplicity of operation
  ○ Easily manipulated, intuitive controls
  ○ Recognized modes and settings
  ○ Immediately available consumables
  ○ User-friendly, interchangeable with universal connections
4 Equipment characteristics
  ○ Complies with relevant regulations and standards (aviation and medical)
  ○ Lightweight, tough, portable with low centre of gravity, easily fixed, held and moved
  ○ Ability to store data and print out to highlight trends and provide a medico legal record
5 Power supplies
  ○ Multiple and independent
  ○ Mains power supply: worldwide voltage and frequency
  ○ Aircraft power supply: able to use aircraft auxiliary power supply
  ○ Battery power supply: exchangeable internal battery and external connection
  ○ Back-up battery: internal battery covering external power failure
  ○ No change in function while power supply changed
6 Function indication
  ○ Normal function indicated
  ○ Abnormal function identified promptly both visually and audibly
  ○ Fail-safe loss of function reverts to least hazardous condition
  ○ Maintain all functions in all environments
7 Reliability
  ○ High reliability, low failure risk
8 Training programme
  ○ Supplied with complete training package.

Breathing
Monitoring begins with noting the misting of the oxygen mask or tracheal tube and chest movement.

Respiratory rate
This is arguably the most sensitive detector of cardiovascular disease and its value is often minimized by inaccurate measurements. If counted manually at least 15 seconds should be used to calculate

the minute rate. There remains no agreement on what constitutes a normal respiratory rate; however, most studies suggest a range of 14–24 breaths per minute. It is measured on most monitors by the delivery of a small AC current via ECG leads I (adults) or II (neonates, infants). The changing thoracic impedance with respiration is then used to calculate the rate. This system requires 30 seconds to 'learn' a rate.

Pulse oximetry

This provides a non-invasive, continuous read out of oxygen saturation. This technology measures the absorption of red (660 nm) and infrared light (940 nm) (Figure 11.3). Oxy- and deoxyhaemoglobin have different absorptions and the proportion of each is measured around 50 times per second. The system requires pulsatile blood flow to obtain reliable readings and loses accuracy at readings below 70%. Values are affected by vibration, patient movement, poor peripheral perfusion, external light sources, severe anaemia (below 5 g/dL) and false fingernails. Falsely high values are obtained if carboxy, met- or suphaemoglobin are present. Several probe types are available for different body sites. The ear is most dependent on mean perfusion pressure and the finger on sympathetic tone. Reflectance oximetry using three LEDs and two photodetector rings is able to offer more reliable information in low signal-to-noise environments.

It is essential to remember that there is a time lag (15–30 seconds) between blood being oxygenated at the lungs and its arrival at the monitored site (pulse oximetry lag). The pulse oximetry reading therefore represents the state of lung oxygenation 15–30 seconds in the past. Vasoconstriction in shock or hypothermia will increase this time lag significantly (up to 2–3 mins). Action must be taken to improve oxygenation as soon as saturations are seen to drop and before the steep part of the oxygen dissociation curve is reached (i.e. before SpO_2 92%). An initial deterioration in saturation and a delay in improvement following intervention should be expected due to lag time. Centrally placed probes (e.g. ear lobe, forehead) will reduce pulse oximetry lag time.

Remember that saturations are a late measure of hypoxia due to the shape of the oxygen desaturation curve.

Capnography

Qualitative and quantitative measures are widely used. The latter is arguably the single most useful piece of monitoring available in prehospital care (PHC), as waveform analysis provides information on respiratory rate, airways/endotracheal tube obstruction, ventilator disconnection, muscle relaxation, cellular function and cardiac output (Figures 11.4 and 11.5). It works by spectrophotometric analysis of carbon dioxide at 4.3 nm. It should be used on all intubated and ideally non-intubated patients.

Mainstream sensors are more rapidly responsive, less susceptible to blockage (usually by water in the sample tubing) or changes in humidity or temperature than side stream but are more bulky and use more power. Side stream is designed for short-term use. Qualitative devices offer a colour change in response to the presence of carbon dioxide and are useful to confirm intubation but not as monitors.

The end-tidal carbon dioxide is lower than the arterial partial pressure and paired measures should be performed prior to departure for interhospital transfers. In health the gap is around 5 mmHg (0.7 kPa) but widens with shock and pulmonary disease.

Circulation
Pulse

This is best taken using the pulp of the first and second digits to minimize the clinician detecting their own pulse. Crude estimations of blood pressure are derived from the presence of carotid, femoral or peripheral pulses. These correlate poorly with measured pressures but are rapidly obtained and are suggested as initial guides to the administration of intravenous fluids in trauma patients, where rapid transport to hospital is paramount. The presence of a peripheral

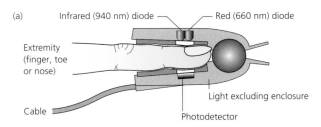

(a) Infrared (940 nm) diode — Red (660 nm) diode
Extremity (finger, toe or nose)
Cable
Light excluding enclosure
Photodetector

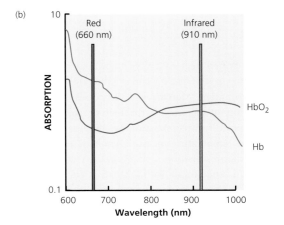

(b)

Figure 11.3 Pulse oximetry.

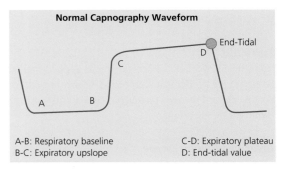

Normal Capnography Waveform

End-Tidal
A
B
C
D

A-B: Respiratory baseline
B-C: Expiratory upslope
C-D: Expiratory plateau
D: End-tidal value

Figure 11.4 Normal capnography waveform.

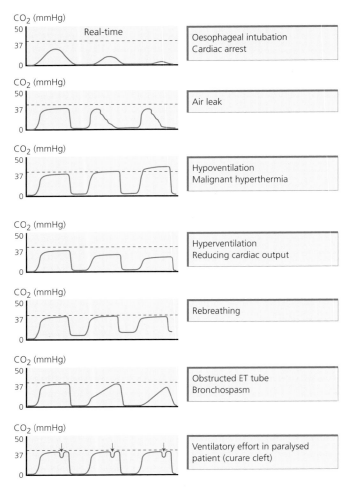

Figure 11.5 Abnormal capnography waveforms.

pulse may give a better indication of peripheral blood flow than the non-invasive blood pressure.

Electrocardiogram

ECG monitoring (three or five lead) provides a constant reading for pulse rate, cardiac rhythm and ischaemia. V4 or V5 are best leads to show ischaemia and lead II for rhythm.

Figure 11.6 shows the electrode placements for the standard 12-lead ECG. Right-sided and posterior lead ECGs should be taken in all cases of suspected acute myocardial infarction in order to rule out right ventricular and posterior infarct.

Capillary refill

Pressure sufficient to blanch a central area is applied then released with the time taken for normal colour to return measured with a normal value being 2 seconds or under. It is a useful test in children but of limited value in adults.

Non-invasive blood pressure

The cuff should be 12.5 cm wide for an average arm (40% of the mid-arm circumference) and the arm placed at the same level as the heart. If the cuff is too small blood pressure will be overestimated. Automatic machines use oscillometric methods and are more accurate than manual values, but overestimate low and underestimate high pressure. They lose accuracy with irregular rhythm and systolic pressures below 80 mmHg. In the critically ill with volume depletion, systolic pressures may be underestimated. Non-invasive blood pressure (NIBP) should me measured every 3 minutes and is inaccurate during motion.

Invasive blood pressure

The noise and vibration of all transport interfere with NIBP and makes IBP attractive for patients transferred between hospitals or over long distances. It is rarely practical for primary work but essential for interhospital transfers of unstable patients or those on vasoactive medication. The equipment is zeroed at the level of the heart and infused at 3 mL/hour with saline (Figure 11.7). Invasive systolic pressures increase as measured more peripherally but means are similar wherever measurements are taken. Since means are the true driving pressure for peripheral flow, less affected by damping and less affected by measurement site it is mean values that are the preferred physiological target. Values are affected by limb position, movement artefact and damping. Damping is reduced by minimizing the length of connector tubing from catheter to transducer, ensuring no air bubbles are present and the pressure bag is maintained at least 100 mmHg above peak systolic pressures. Damping is recognized by a narrow pulse pressure, attenuated systolic pressures, gradual pressure wave up/down slopes and is usually corrected by a flush.

Changes in blood pressure with respiration may also help assess circulating volume, with changes of over 10–15% suggesting intravascular depletion.

Disability

Clinical assessment is with either AVPU (alert, voice, pain, unresponsive) score or GCS and monitoring pupil size/reactivity. The presence of limb movement needs to be clearly recorded before moving the patient or performing procedures such as intubation. Glucose is always checked. Pain should be assessed, treated and the response monitored by either questioning or observing for physical evidence such as tachycardia or lacrimation.

Environment
Temperature

Temperature is an often-neglected physiological variable that has a profound effect on enzyme systems and is vulnerable to fluctuation in the PHC environment. Mercury is a hazardous aviation material and the fragility of mercury thermometers makes them poor choices for transport. Infrared emission detection is unreliable for field use. Invasive temperature measurements are easily obtained using electronic thermistor probes placed in the rectum, oesophagus or central vein. Anaesthesia with intubation and ventilation is associated with a temperature drop compared with spontaneously ventilating patients prehospital, and since cooling is associated with poor outcome in many disease processes, such as trauma but is a therapeutic end point in others, such as cooling post arrest, temperature recording prehospital should be utilized more widely than it is.

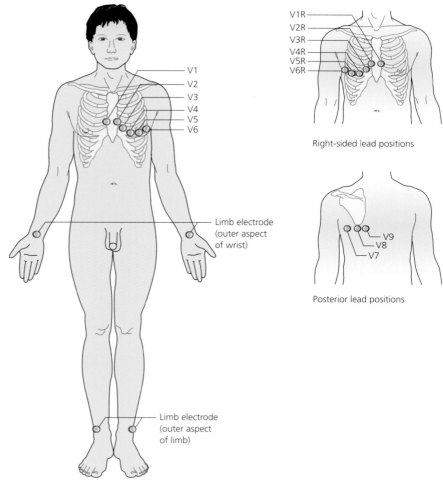

Figure 11.6 ECG electrode placement.

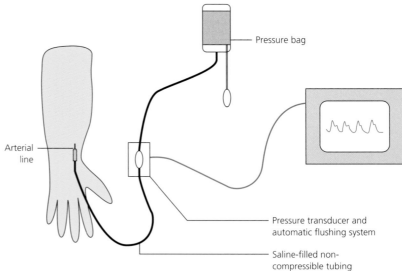

Figure 11.7 Invasive blood pressure measurement. (Source: http://www.aic.cuhk.edu.hk/web8/haemodynamic%20monitoring%20intro.htm).

Monitoring in aircraft

The functions of medical equipment as well as logistic considerations are of great importance when delivering medical care in aircraft.

At altitude the main in-flight stressors are hypoxia and gas expansion caused by decreased barometric pressure. Hypoxia should be monitored for using continuous oxygen saturation monitoring in flight and managed with oxygen supplementation. Thoracic ultrasound may be used to detect pneumothoraces prior to transfer and allow prophylactic drainage before ascending to altitude. Gas expansion may be better prevented by postponing the trip until resolution or seeking an aircraft capable of being fully pressurized.

Unlike oxygen saturation monitors, end-tidal CO_2 monitors are unaffected by altitude in the ventilated patient. If the patient's CO_2 production is constant the end-tidal partial pressure remains the same. All end-tidal devices (even those that display percentages and not partial pressure) actually measure partial pressure and as this is constant for CO_2 they will read virtually the same at altitude as they do at sea level. We note that in many patients the observed end-tidal CO_2 falls, perhaps consequent upon the increased tidal volume with decreasing pressure. The end-tidal partial pressure of oxygen and nitrogen, however, fall with altitude and therefore the actual percentage of CO_2 rises despite this. In the spontaneously breathing patient, who is compensating for hypoxia at higher altitudes, end-tidal CO_2 will decrease as a result of hyperventilation, but this is not an issue at normal cabin altitude unless lung function is abnormal to begin with, and is negated by adding inspired oxygen. It is first noticeable in the healthy at 5000 feet (1524 metres).

Change in pressure affects equipment and components that contain air. As ambient pressure is reduced bubbles may expand in fluids within monitoring transducers and cause dampening of arterial or venous pressure waves leading to inaccurate readings. Meticulous removal of air will avoid this. Most fluids contain a small amount of dissolved gas, which comes out of solution at altitude and forms bubbles, which may coalesce and present further hazard. In this situation the use of air detection monitoring in fluid delivery systems and the use of air traps is of value. Air traps have to be watched closely as their volume may increase and allow air into lines if not adjusted correctly.

Future monitoring techniques

Technology is providing an ever-increasing array of monitors and new applications of current technology. Non- or minimally invasive measurement devices are in development which have the potential to offer us a vast array of information currently requiring invasive monitoring or repeated measures. Specific examples include continuously reading micro-dialysis catheters offering glucose/acid base balance, continuously reading haemoglobin oximeters and NIRS (near infrared tissue spectroscopy). The latter provides a non-invasive measure of the tissue haemoglobin oxygen saturation in various capillary beds, for example the thenar eminence or brain, providing evidence of any ongoing tissue hypoxia and the potential requirement for further resuscitation. Other technology offers non-invasive cardiac output monitoring using thoracic bioimpedance or Doppler ultrasound.

Non-invasive tools to assess brain injury are also undergoing clinical assessment, based on ultrasound or EEG recordings. Focused ultrasound is already moving from the hospital to prehospital arena and has the potential to offer assessments of cardiac performance, intravascular volume, tracheal tube location and intracerebral pressure. This is more fully discussed in the chapter on ultrasound.

Summary

All new staff involved in prehospital care should undergo appropriate training in all aspects of prehospital patient monitoring and have experience of using the equipment in that environment. The use of monitoring should be undertaken by a healthcare professional able to interpret and act upon abnormal results. Used correctly, they provide early warnings of deterioration, record physiological trends, add to clinical assessments and provide both diagnostic and prognostic information. Used poorly, monitors increase time to definitive intervention and provide inaccurate measurements. Unless findings are likely to alter patient care, the clinician should question the value of a monitored variable. In the future, we are likely to see smaller, more accurate, combined monitors.

Tips from the field

- Your clinical skills are your best monitor – learn to trust them. High-end monitors build on clinical assessment but never replace it
- Monitoring may not always be required. Like any intervention in medicine it comes with risk (usually a delay in transfer) and benefit (more physiological detail). A patient 5 minutes from a trauma centre with a knife in the chest who can talk just needs to be there!
- Monitors prehospital have the added complexity of considerable artefact and interference. Look at the whole picture emerging before you
- Never ignore an abnormality – explain it. There is emerging evidence that even a single reading of low blood pressure is associated with increased risk. Single abnormal readings may easily be dismissed as erroneous
- Know your monitor and check the alarms before you leave!

Further reading

AAGBI Safety Guideline. Checking anaesthetic equipment (2004) The Association of Anaesthetists of Great Britain and Ireland, http://www.aagbi.org.

AAGBI Safety Guideline. Interhospital Transfer (2009) http://www.aagbi.org.

Australian and New Zealand College of Anaesthetists, Joint Faculty of Intensive Care Medicine, Australasian College for Emergency Medicine. Minimum standards for intrahospital transport of critically ill patients. 2003.

Donald MJ, B Paterson B. End tidal carbon dioxide monitoring in prehospital and retrieval medicine: a review. *Emerg Med J* 2006;**23**:728–730.

Hulme J. Monitoring the injured patient. *Trauma* 2006;**8**:85–93.

McGuire NM. Monitoring in the field. *Br J Anaesth* 2006;**97**:46–56.

Warren J, From RE, Orr RA, *et al.* Guidelines for the inter and intrahospital transport of critically ill patients. *Crit Care Med* 2004;**32**:256–262.

CHAPTER 12

Prehospital Ultrasound

Tim Harris¹, Adam Bystrzycki², and Stefan Mazur³

¹Royal London Hospital, London, UK
²Alfred Hospital, Melbourne, VIC, Australia
³MedSTAR South Australian Emergency Medical Retrieval Service, QLD, Australia

OVERVIEW

By the end of this chapter you should:
- Understand the basic principles of focused ultrasound
- Understand how focused ultrasound can be used in prehospital care to aid diagnosis and reduce adverse events
- Understand where ultrasound may be used within the primary and secondary survey.

Introduction

Focused ultrasound is an emerging tool that non-imaging specialists are increasingly using in hospital to assess and monitor patients. The use of ultrasound under these circumstances is directed towards answering a specific clinical question, or improving the safety of a specific clinical procedure. Ultrasound provides real-time imaging of many structures otherwise 'invisible' to the practitioner and is not limited by environmental noise.

The development of lighter, stronger, cheaper and more portable ultrasound devices means that focused ultrasound may now be employed in the prehospital environment (Figure 12.1).

What is ultrasound?

Ultrasound involves the use of high-frequency sound waves, typically between 2.5 and 12 MHz, to form two-dimensional real-time motion images. Equipment consists of a transducer or probe which produces and then detects reflected sound waves, a computer to process the images and a screen to display them. Higher frequencies are used for higher resolution and lower frequencies for increased penetration to display deeper structures. Transducers may be linear, curvilinear or phased array. Linear probes are used for imaging more superficial structures – blood vessels, nerves, bone and pleura – and produce images equal in width to the transducer size (footprint). Curvilinear transducers produce images larger than their footprint and are used for imaging

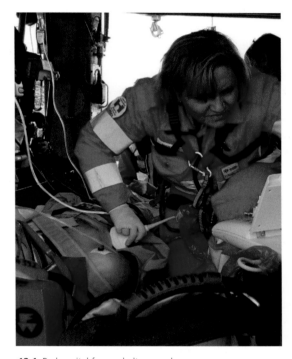

Figure 12.1 Prehospital focused ultrasound.

larger and deeper structures, such as the abdomen. Phased-array transducers have smaller footprints, which fit between the intercostal spaces image a wide area and are used for cardiac imaging.

In prehospital care (PHC) where space and weight are an issue a mini curvilinear probe will give reasonable cardiac, vascular and abdominal images. Alternatively, a selection of interchangeable probes may be carried. Gel will be required to ensure that sound is transmitted efficiently to the subject as air transmits ultrasound poorly.

The depth, focus (point of best resolution) and gain (amplitude) of the sound waves can be adjusted to maximize picture quality. The reflected signal may also be modified – for example to magnify or diminish the intensity of recorded sound from a particular depth so altering the grey scale at a particular depth (the time gain compensation).

ABC of Prehospital Emergency Medicine, First Edition.
Edited by Tim Nutbeam and Matthew Boylan.
© 2013 John Wiley & Sons, Ltd. Published 2013 by John Wiley & Sons, Ltd.

Prehospital uses of ultrasound

A – the role of ultrasound in airway management
Ultrasound and endotracheal Intubation
Intubation is a commonly performed prehospital procedure which should be performed to the same standard as in hospital. Unrecognized oesophageal intubation will result in potentially fatal hypoxia and gastric insufflation. Ultrasound scan (USS) can be used in real time to watch the endotracheal tube being placed prior to any ventilation. Studies suggest that laryngeal USS can identify tracheal placement of the endotracheal tube with 95.7–100% sensitivity and 98.2–100% specificity.

Method
A 5–10 MHz linear transducer is placed horizontally over the anterior larynx just above the suprasternal notch. If the endotracheal tube is placed in the trachea a highly echogenic image with reverberation artefact results (Figure 12.2a). In cases of oesophageal intubation the oesophagus is displaced laterally (usually to the left) in relation to the trachea and two anechoic circular structures are displayed (Figure 12.2b).

USS can also be used to help identify right main stem intubation. Reduced pleural sliding (see Pneumothorax section) and diaphragmatic movement in the left hemithorax will be present when the right main stem is intubated.

Ultrasound and cricothyroidotomy
USS can be used to identify the cricoid membrane in the bariatric patient where landmarks are difficult to palpate.

Method
A 5–10 MHz linear transducer is placed longitudinally over the anterior larynx just above the suprasternal notch. The cricothyroid membrane is easily identified.

B – The role of ultrasound in the assessment of breathing
USS can be used as an adjunct to breathing assessment to rule in life-threatening 'B' problems. These include pneumothorax, pleural effusion (e.g. haemothorax), lung consolidation and pulmonary oedema.

Pneumothorax
The parietal and visceral pleura are reflective, generating a bright pleural line with poorly defined lightly echogenic lung parenchyma beneath. The movement of the lung with respiration creates artefacts. These are:

1 Pleural or lung sliding: the two pleural layers slide on one another, appearing to shimmer
2 Baubles or walking ants: bright dots moving within the pleura with respiration
3 B lines or 'comet tails': artefactual vertical lines arising from the pleura. The appearance is that of well-defined beams arising from the pleura and continuing to the bottom of the image without loss of intensity (Figure 12.3)

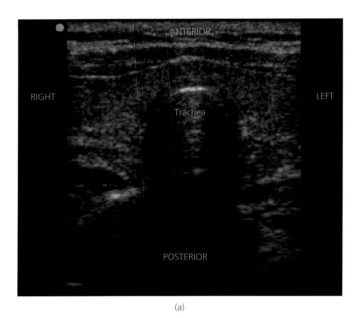

(a)

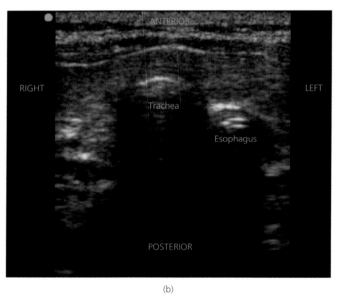

(b)

Figure 12.2 (a) Ultrasound scan (USS) of an endotracheal intubation. (b) USS of an oesophageal intubation. (Courtesy of Prof Sandra Werner, Case Western Reserve University School of Medicine, Cleveland, OH, USA).

The absence of these signs suggests there is a pneumothorax. The sensitivity of these signs for ruling out pneumothorax exceeds that for CXR and is close to that of the CT scan. A false-positive diagnosis is possible in the absence of respiration/mechanical ventilation as these signs rely on the presence of lung movement.

Method
A high-frequency linear transducer is used and is placed in longitudinal plane and moved down the chest wall, starting immediately inferior to the clavicle and moving down to the sixth or seventh intercostal space in the mid-axillary line, sampling in each one. The ribs are identified as echogenic structures with an acoustic shadow. The pleura lie 0.5 cm posterior to the rib margins.

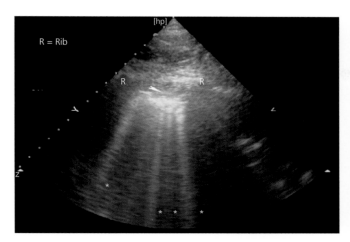

Figure 12.3 Chest ultrasound: comet tail artefacts (*) suggesting no pneumothorax is present.

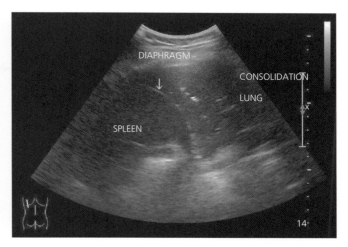

Figure 12.5 Chest ultrasound: consolidated lung (hepatinization). (Courtesy of Dr Joe Antony, MD, at www.ultrasound-images.com).

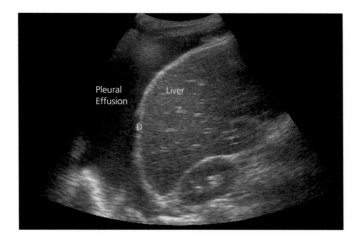

Figure 12.4 Chest ultrasound: a pleural effusion above the diaphragm (D).

attenuation so changing the USS image from chaotic scatter patter to a hypoechoic tissue structure akin to the appearance of the liver (Figure 12.5). Echogenic circular or tubular structures may be seen within the consolidated tissue, representing air-filled bronchi (ultrasound air bronchograms).

Alveolar interstitial syndrome

The sensitivity of the USS detection of pulmonary oedema in the setting of a dyspnoeic patient is up to 100% and specificity as high as 92%. An increased amount of fluid appears first in the interlobular septae (interstitial), and subsequently the alveolar spaces. The appearance is of vertical 'ultrasound lung comets' or B-lines. These move with respiration and transverse the full field of the ultrasound screen. These increase in number with increasing lung water and when multiple (>2 per intercostal space) are pathological (Figure 12.6). Multiple. B-lines 7 mm apart are caused

Pleural effusion

Pleural effusions (e.g. blood, exudate or transudate) appear anechoic on ultrasound (Figure 12.4). USS has sensitivity approaching CT (93%) and is better than plain chest film or clinical assessment for identifying pleural fluid.

Method

In the supine patient the chest may be assessed for pleural effusion using the curvilinear transducer as part of the focused assessment with sonography in trauma (FAST) examination (see later). The transducer should be moved superiorly one or two intercostal spaces from the position used for views of Morrison's pouch and the splenorenal angle in the mid-axillary line. The diaphragm appears as an echogenic line moving with respiration – pleural effusion appears as an anechoic area *above* this.

Lung consolidation

Consolidation may be due to lung oedema, bronchopneumonia, pulmonary contusion or lobar atelectasis. The non-aerated consolidated lung tissue allows transmission of ultrasound with minimal

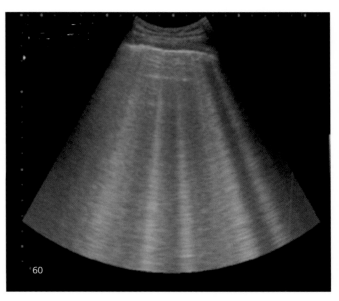

Figure 12.6 Chest ultrasound: multiple comet artefacts suggestive of pulmonary oedema.

by thickened interlobular septa characteristic of interstitial oedema. B-lines 3 mm apart, or closer, suggest alveolar oedema. The number of B lines that constitutes pathology is subject to ongoing trials.

C – The role of ultrasound in the assessment of circulation

USS can be used to assess the three components of the circulatory system: the heart, blood volume and blood vessels. A focused echo will give valuable information about the heart and volume status in cases of cardiac arrest and shock. A FAST scan may be useful in localizing intraperitoneal free fluid (e.g. blood) in the hypovolaemic patient. Blood vessels may also be imaged directly to facilitate intravenous line placement.

Focused echo

Knowledge of cardiac performance and chamber size can be critically important in the assessment of cardiac arrest and shock. The key questions answerable by focused echo are:

- Is there any cardiac activity?
- Is there a pericardial effusion/tamponade?
- Is there evidence of pressure loading of the right ventricle suggestive of massive pulmonary embolism?
- Is there evidence of hypovolaemia?

The absence of activity of the left ventricle denotes a dismal prognosis in cardiac arrest and may assist in deciding at which point to cease resuscitation.

The identification of a pericardial effusion is relatively easy, but identifying tamponade takes skill and experience. In the hypotensive trauma patient an effusion is likely to be causal. In medical patients in extremis any collapse of the right ventricle as it fills in diastole or paradoxical movement of the septum (into the left ventricular cavity) is evidence of tamponade.

If the right ventricle is pressure loaded and bigger than the left ventricle, especially if accompanied by paradoxical septal motion, this is suggestive of massive pulmonary embolus and may alert the clinician to the need for thrombolysis.

A hyperdynamic well-filled ventricle suggests sepsis. An empty left ventricle, suggested when the ventricular walls meet end systole, suggests profound hypovolaemia. This is further reinforced if the diameter of the inferior vena cava (IVC) is under 12 mm or collapsing completely with inspiration in the spontaneously ventilating patient. An IVC of greater than 25 mm suggests volume overload from PE, chronic lung disease or cardiac failure.

Method

The subcostal view is easily obtained with the patient lying flat on their back and so lends itself to the PHC environment (Figure 12.7). Curvilinear or phased-array probes both produce good subcostal images of the heart. The transducer is sited immediately inferior to the xiphisternum, flat with the abdominal wall and directed to the left clavicle. The views may be improved by deeper inspiration or angling/rotating the transducer. The pericardium is identified as a thick echogenic line within which the cardiac chambers are seen moving. A pericardial effusion separates them and appears anechoic. (Figure 12.8). The right ventricle lies against the liver separated from it by the pericardium and the diaphragm. Rotating the probe through 90 degrees over the right atrium will demonstrate the IVC in long axis (Figure 12.9). Assessment of IVC size and collapse is best measured in this view using B mode to enable measurements to be made at the same point along the IVC.

Alternative views such as the long axis parasternal and apical views require the use of a phased-array probe and greater degree of experience to obtain adequate views.

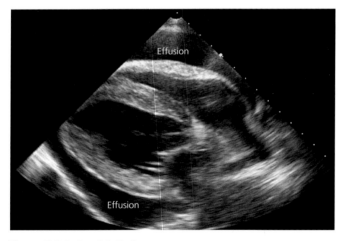

Figure 12.8 Pericardial effusion.

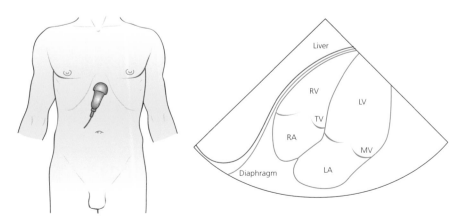

Figure 12.7 Subcostal view and probe position.

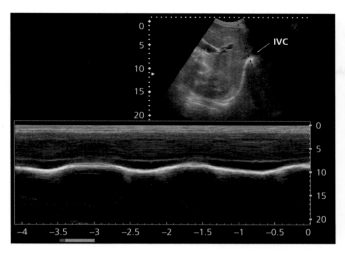

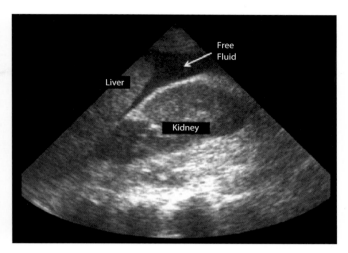

Figure 12.9 The inferior vena cava in B and M modes showing variation with respiration.

Figure 12.11 Free fluid in Morrison's pouch.

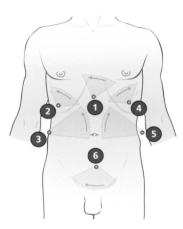

Figure 12.10 The eFAST examination probe positions.
(Source: Neil Robinson, *J Accid Emerg Med.* 2000;**17**:330–334).

Focused Assessment with sonography in trauma

The FAST examination has been studied in the PHC environment and images are similarly accurate to studies performed in hospital. It consists of three peritoneal windows together with the subcostal pericardial view described previously When used in combination with an assessment of the chest for pneumothorax and pleural effusion it is termed an extended-FAST or eFAST (Figure 12.10). The purpose of the eFAST is to identify sources of blood loss (and pneumothorax) in trauma patients – blood within the pericardium, the peritoneal cavity and/or the chest. It is most sensitive and specific in patients with haemorrhagic shock.

The FAST only identifies intraperitoneal blood in the most dependent areas of the abdomen and so does not exclude organ damage or have any utility in identifying hollow viscus injury or retroperitoneal injury. In PHC the pelvic view is thus more often positive whereas in the resuscitation room it is most commonly Morrison's pouch. In PHC it can alert the practitioner to important diagnoses such as pericardial or peritoneal fluid which may guide prehospital interventions such as thoracotomy and/or be reported to the receiving unit so that they can prepare (e.g. theatre on standby, specialist surgeon, massive transfusion).

Method

A curvilinear 3–5 MHz probe is used abdominally to provide a wide field of view. The subcostal pericardial view (position 1) has been described previously. The Morrison's pouch view (position 3) is obtained by moving the transducer to the mid-axillary line at the level of the xiphisternum. By adjusting the angle and rotation the right kidney and liver (hence Morrison's pouch) are bought into view. Fluid appears as an anechoic – black – stripe separating liver from kidney (Figure 12.11). The probe may then be moved cranially as described previously to allow the diaphragm and pleura (position 2) to be seen to assess for pleural effusion. The identical procedure is then performed on the left side to gain views of the spleen, left kidney (position 5) and chest (position 4). A more posterior approach is often required to gain sufficient views. Fluid appears anechoic surrounding the spleen or between it and the left kidney. Finally the transducer is placed just cranial to the pelvic rim (position 6) and the transducer angled towards the rectum. This requires a semi-full bladder to displace bowel, which would otherwise prevent the pelvis from being imaged. Fluid appears as a black stripe posterior and superior to the inferior bladder wall (Figure 12.12).

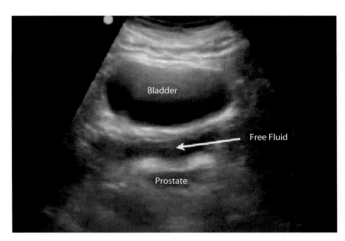

Figure 12.12 Free fluid in the pelvis.

Vascular access

Central venous access is rarely required in the prehospital environment and the sites are best preserved for sterile catheter placement in hospital. Prehospital and emergency placement is associated with high rates of misplacement of up to 38%. Central access may be indicated in cases of profound hypovolaemia. USS may be used to facilitate cannulation of the femoral vein and has been shown to reduce the number of attempts required for successful cannulation, failure rates, time to successful cannulation and complication rate. It may also be used to identify the position and patency of peripheral veins.

Method

To visualize the femoral vein a high-frequency linear transducer is placed just below and parallel to the inguinal sheath with the probe midline over the femoral pulse (Figure 12.13). The femoral vein is usually medial to the artery and is most reliably identified as it compresses under the probe at minimal pressure. The vein is cannulated, using either a Seldinger or direct method. The metal trocher of the cannula is echogenic and if 'jiggled' as advanced can be seen to move through the superficial tissues. The cannula is introduced steeply (45–60 degrees to the skin) compared with blind insertion.

D – The role of ultrasound in the assessment of disability?

Patients with traumatic brain injury are common in PHC. The early identification of patients with severe traumatic brain injury and raised intracranial pressure (ICP) is important. These patients require early institution of neurocritical care measures along with rapid transfer to a neurosurgical centre for urgent head CT and possible operative management. Clinical assessment for raised ICP is neither sensitive nor specific.

USS may be used to assess ICP. As ICP increases so the optic nerve and sheath become oedematous and swell. This may be measured by USS. There is emerging evidence that USS of the optic nerve can exclude a raised ICP if the diameter of the optic nerve is under 5 mm when measured 3.00 mm from the optic disc (Figure 12.14).

Method

The study is performed using a linear transducer held over the closed upper lid. An optic nerve sheath diameter >5 mm is sensitive but

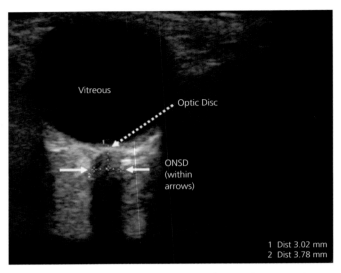

Figure 12.14 The measurement of optic nerve diameter 3 mm posterior to the optic disc (Source: Dr Vivek Tayal, *Annals of Emergency Medicine* 2007:**49**(4):509–514, with permission of the author).

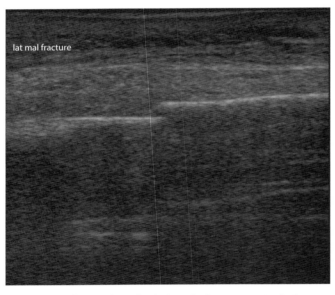

Figure 12.15 Ultrasound can clearly show the fracture as a step in the cortex – in this case a fractured fibula (Courtesy of Marieta Canagesabey and Prof Simon Carley, Manchester Royal Infirmary, Manchester, UK).

not specific for raised ICP. In one study these figures suggested 100% sensitivity for 5-mm-diameter optic sheath to detect patients with elevated ICP as judged by CT criteria. However, we need studies with greater numbers to confirm these findings.

E – The role of ultrasound in the evaluation of other injuries

Diagnosis of bone injury

USS has been shown to be useful in diagnosing fractures with a high sensitivity and specificity. This may be useful in the resource constrained environment (e.g. military, mass casualty)

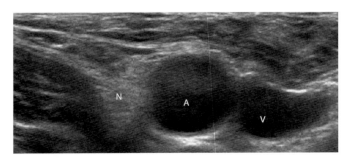

Figure 12.13 Ultrasound of the right femoral nerve (N), artery (A) and vein (V).

when radiographs are unavailable. It has also been used in the identification of dislocations and guide reduction with similar accuracy to plain films.

Method

Bone is an excellent reflector of USS energy and thus the cortex appears echogenic. Fractures are readily identifiable and appear as a step or irregularity in the cortical line (Figure 12.15). A linear high-frequency probe is used. Like plain films, images are obtained in two perpendicular plains but can also be moved around the bone to obtain the optimum view.

Tips from the field

- USS is highly user dependent but safe to learn for patients and practitioners alike – start as soon as you can!
- Before picking up the probe, think about how the results of the scan will change your management. If it won't – do not delay transfer!
- USS identifies pneumothoraces more accurately than chest films
- Don't always assume free fluid on FAST is blood (e.g. ascites, CAPD)
- USS is useful in the peri-arrest patient in defining the aetiology of hypotension/cardiac arrest not due to rhythm disturbance
- If you can't see anything use more gel, find a better acoustic window, and check your transducer, depth, and gain.

Further reading

Abboud PA, Kendall JL. Ultrasound guidance for vascular access. *Emerg Med Clin North Am* 2004;**22**:749–773.

Kimberly HH, Shah S, Marill K, Noble V. Correlation of optic Nerve Sheath Diameter with Direct Measurement of Intracranial Pressure. *Acad Emerg Med* 2008;**15**:201–204.

Lichtenstein DA, Meziere GA. Relevance of lung ultrasound in the diagnosis of acute respiratory failure: the BLUE protocol. *Chest* 2008;**134**:117–125

McNeil CR, McManus J, Mehta S. The Accuracy of Portable Ultrasonography to Diagnose Fractures in an Austere Environment. *Prehospital Emergency Care* 2009;**13**:50–52.

Perera P, Mailhot T, Riley D, Mandavia D. The RUSH exam: Rapid Ultrasound in Shock in the evaluation of the Critically ill. *Emerg Med Clin North Am* 2010;**28**:29–56.

Rose JS. Ultrasound in abdominal trauma. *Emerg Med Clin North Am* 2004;**22**:581–599.

Werner SL, Smith CE, Goldstein JR, *et al*. Pilot study to evaluate the accuracy of Ultrasonography in Confirming Endotracheal Tube Placement. *Ann Emerg Med* 2006;**49**:75–80.

Glossary

- **Anechoic:** No reflected ultrasound; appears black; suggests fluid.
- **Hypoehoic:** Little ultrasound reflected; appears dark grey.
- **Echogenic/hyperechoic:** Highly reflective of ultrasound; appears white.
- **Acoustic shadow:** The dark shadow under an echogenic structure due to little ultrasound energy reaching it.
- **Marker or active end of transducer:** Transducers have a mark to one end that corresponds to a mark on the screen. This is to assist the sonographer in orientation of the probe: convention is for the marked end to be orientated to the patient's right or cranially; unless performing a cardiac study when it is orientated to the patients left.

CHAPTER 13

Trauma: Head Injury

Jeremy Henning[1] and Clare Hammell[2]

[1]The James Cook University Hospital, Middlesbrough, UK
[2]Leighton Hospital, Crewe, UK

OVERVIEW

By the end of this chapter you should:

• Understand the pathophysiology of secondary brain injury

• Know which patients with minor head injury require secondary care and radiological investigation

• Understand the resuscitation end points and principles of management of severely head injured patients

• Appreciate the unique challenges in head injury management in the prehospital environment.

Introduction

Head injury is common with an incidence of 0.3% of the population and a mortality rate of 25 per 100 000 in North America and 9 per 100 000 in the UK. Severe head injury is associated with a high mortality rate (30–50%) and many survivors will have persistent severe neurological disability. Prompt identification and appropriate early management of such patients is necessary to ensure optimal long-term outcome. Managing such injuries in the field can pose many challenges. Patients may require extrication from vehicles, may be agitated and combative, or may require advanced airway management in a difficult environment. Coexisting injuries are common in patients with a severe head injury. Coordination between the various emergency services is essential to ensure that the patient is managed in a timely fashion.

Pathophysiology

Head injury can result from both relatively minor and high-velocity trauma. Primary brain injury occurs at the time of impact and includes injuries such as subdural and extradural haematomata, cerebral contusions, and axonal injury. These cerebral insults continue to evolve resulting in a secondary brain injury which is characterized by impaired regulation of cerebral blood flow and metabolism. This injury is exacerbated by exogenous factors which reduce cerebral oxygen supply and raise intracranial pressure (ICP) (Box 13.1). ICP will rise with an increase in volume of any of the cranial contents (blood, brain, cerebrospinal fluid) as the cranium is a rigid box (Monro–Kelly doctrine). It can be seen in the graph of intracranial volume versus pressure (Figure 13.1) that there is an inflection point (critical volume); this is important as it shows that very small changes of volume (from changing blood flow for example) can lead to big changes in pressure. When compensatory mechanisms are exhausted, sustained rises in ICP result in herniation of brain tissue (Figure 13.2). Modern head injury management focuses on preventing and managing the secondary insults.

Box 13.1 **Factors contributing to secondary brain injury**

Hypotension
Hypoxaemia
Hypocapnia
Hypoglycaemia
Hyperglycaemia

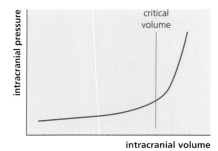

Figure 13.1 Intracranial volume pressure graph.
(Source: http://www.trauma.org/archive/neuro/icp.html).

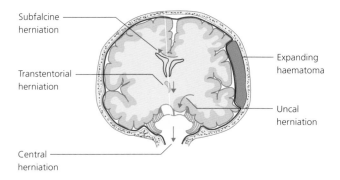

Figure 13.2 Herniation of brain tissue secondary to an expanding haematoma.

ABC of Prehospital Emergency Medicine, First Edition.
Edited by Tim Nutbeam and Matthew Boylan.
© 2013 John Wiley & Sons, Ltd. Published 2013 by John Wiley & Sons, Ltd.

Assessment

All patients should have their Glasgow Coma Score (GCS) calculated as part of their disability assessment (Box 13.2). The motor score is the most powerful predictor of outcome (except in cases of paralysis – therapeutic or traumatic). Abnormal posturing can be indicative of severe brain injury (Figure 13.3). Decorticate posturing, where the upper limbs flex and the lower limbs extend involuntarily, reflects injury at the level of midbrain or above (cerebral hemispheres, internal capsule, thalamus). Decerebrate posturing, where both the upper and lower limbs extend involuntarily reflects injury at the midbrain or below. The pupils should be

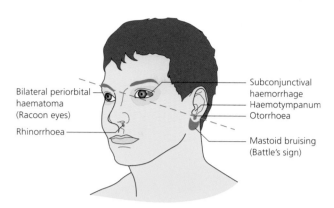

Figure 13.4 Signs of a basal skull fracture.

examined for signs of equality and reactivity. Any difference between the left and right side should raise a suspicion for significant head injury. Signs of basal skull fracture should be actively sought (Figure 13.4).

Minor head injury

Minor head injury ('concussion') occurs following trauma to the head in a patient who has a GCS of 14–15. It encompasses a wide spectrum of injury from those with minimal symptoms to those with significant amnesia or a period of unconsciousness. There is an increasing awareness that even these mild head injuries can lead to longer term morbidity (such as headache).

Assessment should include a witnessed account of the injury and a history from the patient if possible. The following points should be specifically enquired about or examined for as the presence of any of them increases the likelihood of a structural brain injury:

- GCS <15 on initial assessment
- loss of consciousness at any time
- focal neurological deficit
- retrograde or anterograde amnesia
- persistent headache
- vomiting or seizures post injury.

Relevant past medical history includes any previous neurosurgical interventions, use of anticoagulants (especially warfarin), clotting disorders or alcohol excess (acute or chronic). These increase the likelihood of structural brain injury after even minor trauma. Examination should focus on the presence of coexisting injuries; neurological state should be assessed by a GCS, the presence of focal neurology and pupillary size and reactions. Always check blood glucose. Patients exhibiting any of the above signs or symptoms should be referred on to the emergency department. Some patients may just require a period of observation but others will fulfil criteria for computed tomography scanning of the brain (Box 13.3).

It is also important to note that many sporting authorities have strict rules about returning to sport after mild head injury and the casualty should be advised to get an expert opinion.

Box 13.2 **Glasgow Coma Scale (score out of 15)**

Best verbal response

Orientated, converses normally	5
Confused	4
Utters inappropriate words	3
Incomprehensible sounds	2
Makes no sounds	1

Best motor response

Obeys commands	6
Localizes painful stimuli	5
Flexion/withdrawal to painful stimuli	4
Abnormal flexion to pain (decorticate)	3
Extension to pain (decerebrate)	2
Makes no movement	1

Best eye response

Open spontaneously	4
Eyes open to voice	3
Eyes open to pain	2
No eye opening	1

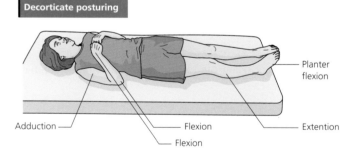

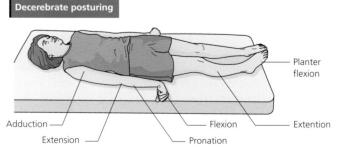

Figure 13.3 Abnormal posturing.

Box 13.3 **Who requires a CT brain scan following head injury?**

GCS <13 on initial assessment in the emergency department
GCS <15 at 2 hours after injury
Suspected open or depressed skull fracture
Any sign of basal skull fracture
Post-traumatic seizure
Focal neurological deficit
More than one episode of vomiting
Amnesia for events more than 30 minutes before impact.

Severe head injury

Assessment and management

Severe head injury implies a GCS <8. Many of these patients will have structural lesions on CT scanning and such patients have better outcomes if they receive early neurosurgical care. On-scene time should be kept to the absolute minimum required to address coexisting life-threatening injuries and to ensure an adequate airway and optimal ventilation and circulatory status.

Airway and ventilatory management

Airway obstruction and hypoventilation are common in severely head-injured patients. They quickly lead to hypoxaemia and hypercapnia, both of which contribute to the development of secondary brain injury. Initially basic airway adjuncts (jaw thrust and oropharyngeal airways) should be used along with administration of high-flow oxygen in patients that are unstable or have an SpO_2 ≤94%. Laryngeal mask airways can be inserted in unconscious patients and often provide reliable airway maintenance. They are especially useful in situations where patient access is limited. A subgroup of patients may require endotracheal intubation and ventilation at the scene (Box 13.4). Advantages of this include definitive airway control, improved oxygenation and improved control of arterial carbon dioxide levels. Endotracheal intubation usually requires the administration of anaesthetic agents and neuromuscular blocking drugs, even in patients who have a very low

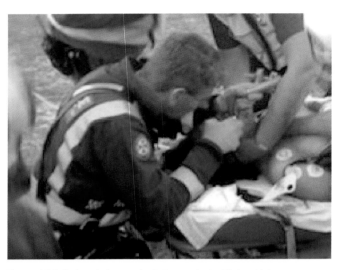

Figure 13.5 Prehospital anaesthesia in a patient with head injury.

GCS; therefore, this should only be undertaken by appropriately trained individuals with adequate patient monitoring in place (Figure 13.5). Always document GCS and pupil size prior to administration of sedative drugs. It is important to avoid post-intubation hyperventilation, as it leads to cerebral vasoconstriction and ischaemia. Head-injured patients who are hyperventilated have a worse outcome than patients ventilated to an arterial $PaCO_2$ of 4.5 kPa. Monitoring end tidal carbon dioxide reduces the incidence of hyperventilation by more than 50% and is now considered a routine standard of monitoring for all mechanically ventilated patients. The $ETCO_2$ target in the head injured patient should be 4.0 kPa (equivalent to a $PaCO_2$ of 4.5 kPA). Adequate post-intubation sedation and paralysis is essential to prevent ICP spikes from gagging or undersedation.

Circulatory management

Maintaining an adequate cerebral perfusion pressure (CPP) is a cornerstone of head injury management. Cerebral perfusion pressure is calculated by subtracting intracranial pressure from the mean arterial pressure.

Cerebral Perfusion Pressure (CPP)
= Mean Arterial Pressure–Intracranial Pressure (ICP)

Maintaining a CPP of 60–70 mmHg is the usual in-hospital target in severely head injured patients. Their ICP is often >20 mmHg, requiring a MAP of 80 mmHg or more. Patients with severe head injuries who become hypotensive have a doubled risk of mortality compared with normotensive patients (even after one single episode of hypotension). Hypotension results in reduced cerebral perfusion and neuronal ischaemia and is often multifactorial in origin in trauma patients. Always assume that hypotension is due to hypovolaemia until proven otherwise and search for the site of blood loss. Apply direct pressure to control external haemorrhage and splint the pelvis and any long bone fractures prior to induction

Box 13.4 **Indications for prehospital rapid sequence induction of anaesthesia in head injured patients**

Airway problems that cannot reliably be managed by simple manoeuvres
Respiratory insufficiency (SpO_2 <92%) despite 15 L/min oxygen or impending respiratory collapse due to exhaustion or pathology
Glasgow coma scale <9 or rapidly falling
Patients at risk of respiratory deterioration when access is difficult during transfer to definitive care (for example those with facial burns)
Patients needing sedation before transfer to hospital because they present a danger to themselves or attending staff, or for humanitarian reasons (for example to provide complete analgesia).

of anaesthesia if possible. MAP is not easily calculated in the prehospital environment so most guidelines use the systolic blood pressure (Box 13.5). A systolic blood pressure (SBP) of at least 90 mmHg is recommended in adults. Higher values (>100 mmHg) may be desirable in patients with isolated severe traumatic brain injury. In patients with multiple injuries and hypovolaemia a conflict exists between "permissive hypotension" resuscitative strategies to minimize blood loss and the need to maintain an adequate cerebral perfusion pressure to prevent secondary brain injury. A target SBP of 90 mmHg should be used. The ideal resuscitation fluid is unknown for patients with severe traumatic brain injury. Currently small boluses (250–500 mL) of crystalloid fluid, e.g. 0.9% sodium chloride, are utilized to maintain adequate blood pressure in the field, as use of vasopressors is often impractical during transport. Hypertonic crystalloid solutions may have a future role as the primary resuscitation fluid in this patient group due to their effects in reducing intracranial pressure.

Box 13.5 Resuscitation end goals for severely head injured patients

- SpO$_2$ >97%
- End tidal carbon dioxide (if ventilated) 4.0–4.5 kPa
- Systolic blood pressure
  - Adults: >90 mmHg (100 mmHg if isolated severe head injury)
  - Paediatrics: > (Age × 2) + 90 mmHg (Median normal value).

Management of raised intracranial pressure

Intracranial pressure is often raised in patients with severe traumatic brain injury and specific treatment should be given to lower it if clinical signs are present (for example, pupillary dilatation, systemic hypertension along with bradycardia) and if transfer time allows. Hypoxaemia, hypotension, hypercapnia and inadequate sedation (in an intubated patient) should all be addressed before specific treatment. Specific ICP-lowering agents include osmotic diuretics such as mannitol and hypertonic crystalloid fluids. Mannitol causes a reduction in ICP by reducing blood viscosity (immediate effect) and increasing serum osmolality (delayed effect). However, its diuretic effect will exacerbate hypovolaemia. Hypertonic saline solutions are increasingly first-line therapy for management of raised ICP. By increasing serum osmolality they promote movement of water from the intracellular to extracellular compartments. Hence they are beneficial in trauma patients with hypovolaemia as intravascular circulating volume and cardiac output are increased. Neither treatments have much evidence for their use in the field so far, but if osmotherapy is required to manage ICP then a single bolus of 3 mL/kg of 3% sodium chloride is most appropriate in this environment. A large randomized prehospital trial of hypertonic saline in traumatic brain injury is ongoing.

Hyperventilation to achieve arterial partial pressures of carbon dioxide of 3.5–4 kPa has previously been advocated as a treatment for raised ICP. Recent studies have demonstrated that although ICP may be reduced cerebral ischaemia is worsened and so this approach can no longer be recommended.

Immobilization

The presence of a head injury is the strongest independent risk factor for injury of the cervical spine. Suspect injury and immobilize the cervical spine in all patients with a GCS of <15, neck pain or tenderness, paraesthesia or focal neurology or in those with a high-risk mechanism of injury. Rigid cervical collars can be used but should not be so tight as to impede cerebral venous blood flow as this can increase intracranial pressure. Traditionally this has been followed with head blocks, tape and a long board to immobilize the thoracolumbar spine. Vacuum mattresses are being increasingly used for immobilization and have been shown to reduce body movements and improve patient comfort compared with long boards (Figure 13.6). Combative and agitated patients provide a challenge; in some it may be safer to leave just the cervical spine immobilized in a collar alone. Early in-hospital assessment of the cervical spine should be performed so that cervical collars can be removed. During transfer, severely head-injured patients should have at least a 15-degree head-up tilt to improve cerebral venous drainage.

Transfer

All head-injured patients need to be transferred to a hospital with facilities for computed tomography (CT) scanning. Ideally, severely head-injured patients should be transferred directly to a hospital with neurosurgical capabilities, as this avoids the need for subsequent secondary transfers. Current evidence also suggests that patients with such injuries have better outcomes if managed in specialist neurosurgical centres. The presence of other injuries and proximity to institutions should be considered when deciding which secondary care facility is appropriate. Transport will usually be by road but rotary wing air transport is appropriate in certain circumstances such as in remote locations or where a primary transfer to a neurosurgical centre is indicated, bypassing the local receiving hospital.

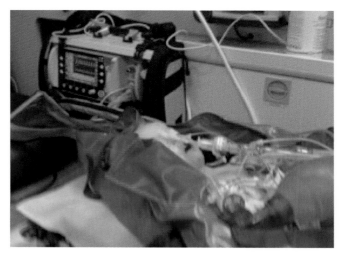

Figure 13.6 Packaging within a vacuum mattress (collar removed).

Tips from the field

- Management of severe traumatic brain injury is focused on rapid transfer to secondary care while preventing secondary brain injury
- Airway compromise and inadequate ventilation are common and should be addressed immediately
- Prehospital endotracheal intubation should be undertaken with the assistance of anaesthetic drugs by appropriately trained physicians
- Hypotension is a an independent risk factor for mortality; small boluses of isotonic crystalloid fluids should be given if it occurs
- Patients may be best managed in a neurosurgical centre where they should receive definitive neurosurgical treatment within 4 hours of injury.

Further reading

Association of Anaesthetists Great Britain and Ireland. Prehospital Anaesthesia. Association of Anaesthetists Great Britain and Ireland Safety Guideline www.aagbi.org/publications.

Brain Trauma Foundation. *Guidelines for the Prehospital Management of Severe Traumatic Brain Injury*, 2nd edn. The Brain Trauma Foundation www.braintrauma.org.

Guidelines for prehospital management of traumatic brain injury. *J Neurotrauma* 2002;**19**:111–174.

NICE. Head injury; triage, assessment, investigation and early management of head injury in adults, children and infants. National Institute for Health and Clinical Excellence Clinical guideline 2007 www.nice.org.uk/G056

CHAPTER 14

Trauma: Spinal Injuries

Lucas A. Myers[1], Christopher S. Russi[1], Matthew Boylan[2], and Tim Nutbeam[3]

[1]Mayo Clinic Medical Transport, Mayo Clinic, Rochester, MN, USA
[2]Royal Centre for Defence Medicine, University Hospitals Birmingham, Birmingham, UK
[3]Derriford Hospital, Plymouth Hospitals NHS Trust, Plymouth, UK

OVERVIEW

By the end of this chapter you should understand:

- The relevant spinal anatomy
- Different mechanisms of injury affecting the spine and cord
- Common injury patterns
- The management of injuries in the prehospital setting
- Patient selection for spinal immobilization.

Introduction

Spinal cord injury (SCI) can be a devastating and life-altering event. It is relatively rare with an incidence of approximately 800 cases per million population (in some countries this is significantly lower, e.g. the UK rate is approximately 10–15 per million). The most commonly affected group are young males with over 50% of injuries occurring in the 16–30 year age group and a male to female ratio of 4:1.

Over 90% of SCI are caused by trauma, with approximately 50% of these due to motor vehicle collisions The remaining trauma-related injuries are equally split between falls, interpersonal violence and sporting injuries. Up to 50% of adults who sustain SCI will be intoxicated at the time of injury.

Spinal anatomy

The vertebral column supports the upper body, including the head and neck, and keeps the body upright. It consists of 33 vertebrae: 7 cervical, 12 thoracic, 5 lumbar, 5 sacral and 4 coccygeal vertebrae. The stability of the spinal column is dependent upon the interspinal ligaments and discs. The vertebrae protect the vulnerable spinal cord within the spinal canal which extends from the foramen magnum to around L1 (T12–L3). Below this level the spinal canal is occupied by the cauda equina. The spinal cord is divided into 31 segments, each of which gives motor and sensory innervation to a specific myotome and dermatome (see Figure 14.1 and Box 14.1).

Autonomic nerve fibres originate from specific regions of the spinal cord. Sympathetic fibres originate from the T1–L3 segments,

ABC of Prehospital Emergency Medicine, First Edition.
Edited by Tim Nutbeam and Matthew Boylan.
© 2013 John Wiley & Sons, Ltd. Published 2013 by John Wiley & Sons, Ltd.

Figure 14.1 Dermatomes.

whereas parasympathetic fibres exit between S2–4. An in-depth knowledge of cord anatomy (e.g. descending motor and ascending sensory spinal tracts) is not required in the prehospital phase.

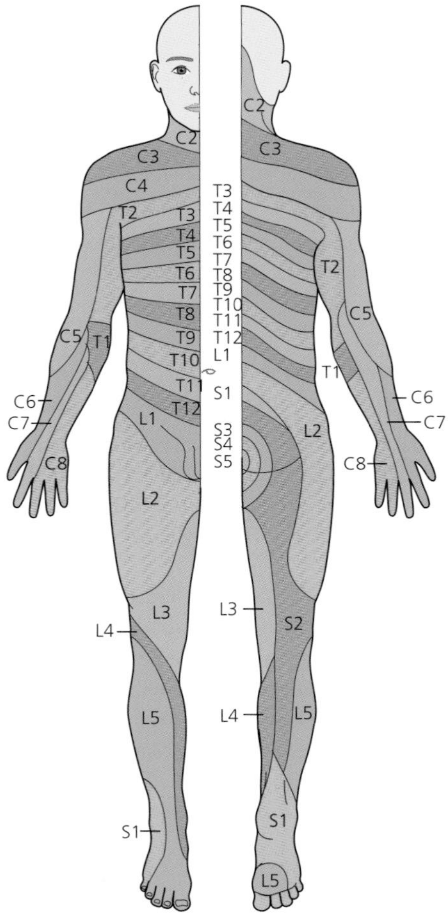

Pathophysiology

Primary cord Injury

Primary injury of the spinal cord occurs at the time of the impact by mechanical disruption, transection or distraction of the cord.

Box 14.1 **Myotomes**

C-5	Deltoid (biceps jerk C5, 6)
C-6	Wrist extensors (extensor carpi radialis longus/brevis)
C-7	Elbow/extensors/triceps jerk (triceps)
C-8	Finger flexors to middle finger (flexor digitorum profundus)
T-1	Little finger abductors (abductor digiti minimi)
L-2	Hip flexors (iliopsoas)
L-4	Knee extensors (quadriceps; knee jerk L3,4)
L-5	Ankle dorsi flectors (tibialis anterior)
S-1	Ankle planter flexors (gastrocnemius, soleus; ankle jerk S1,2)
S-5	Anal reflex

Table 14.1 Distribution of Spinal Injuries

Region	% injuries
Cervical	55
Thoracic	15
Thoracolumbar	15
Lumbosacral	15

The extent of the primary neurological damage depends on the spinal segments involved. The regional distribution of spinal injuries is shown in Table 14.1.

Secondary cord injury

Secondary injury occurs after the primary insult has occurred. The main contributory factors are hypoxia, hypoperfusion and further mechanical disturbance of the spine. All lead to worsening cord oedema, impaired cord perfusion and extension of the primary injury. The prehospital care of the spinal injured patient is directed towards preventing secondary injury from these three entities.

Spinal shock

Spinal shock is the complete loss of all neurological function below the level of the injury. The initial injury may be complete or partial. Clinically it presents as a flaccid paralysis with areflexia that can last up to 24–72 hours after injury. The full extent of neurological injury cannot be assessed until spinal shock has abated.

Neurogenic shock

Following cord injuries at or above the level of T6 there is significant loss of sympathetic autonomic outflow. The resultant loss of adrenergic stimulation leads to generalized vasodilatation and hypotension. Unopposed vagal parasympathetic tone causes a relative bradycardia. The resultant distributive shock state is termed neurogenic shock.

Mechanism of injury

Blunt Injury

The commonest mechanism for spinal trauma is the motor vehicle collision. Motor vehicle collisions are associated with a high risk of injury to all areas of the spinal cord.

Low-speed impacts may result in strain of the muscles of the posterior neck (whiplash) with resultant pain and stiffness. They can also result in significant cord injury in patients with pre-existing spondylosis, rheumatoid arthritis or instability (e.g. Down's syndrome).

High-speed crashes carry the highest risk for significant spinal cord injury. The transition zones tend to be injured with greater frequency (i.e. lumbosacral, thoracolumbar and cervicothoracic junctions).

Penetrating Injury

Traumatic, penetrating injuries are a less common cause of spinal cord injury. High-energy wounds (e.g. gunshot) involving the spinal cord are usually complete in nature and as such immobilization offers little benefit. Unstable vertebral column injuries with an intact cord are extremely rare. In fact, immobilization may mask important signs of penetrating vascular injury such as expanding haematoma. Low-energy transfer wounds (e.g. knife) may cause incomplete or complete spinal cord injuries. Again unstable vertebral injuries are rare without a complete cord transection and immobilization again offers little theoretical benefit.

Clinical assessment

Spinal injury should be suspected in all trauma patients. The symptoms of spinal cord injury vary, depending on the degree and the anatomic location of the injury.

Midline spinal pain may be reported by the patient and tenderness may be elicited during examination of the spine. A rapid assessment for movement and sensation in all four limbs should be performed during the primary survey and documented. This is particularly important if anaesthesia is to be induced. Any abnormality should be followed up with a more in depth examination to determine the presence of a motor or sensory level. The level of motor deficit is taken as the lowest muscle with power of 3/5 (American Spinal Injury Association scale). The level of sensory deficit is taken as the lowest dermatome bilaterally to have normal sensation. The ability to interpret incomplete cord injury patterns (i.e. anterior, lateral or central cord syndromes) prehospitally is not important and often not possible due to spinal shock or concomitant injuries.

The incidence of spinal cord injury is greatest in the unconscious trauma patient. The unconscious casualty will be unable to verbalize any motor-sensory deficit or midline pain. Other markers of spinal cord injury should be actively sought (Box 14.2).

Box 14.2 **Signs of spinal cord injury in the unconscious**

Neurogenic shock (Bradycardia and Hypotension)
Diaphragmatic breathing
Pain response above clavicles only
Priapism (often partial)
'Hands-up' flexed posture of the upper limbs.

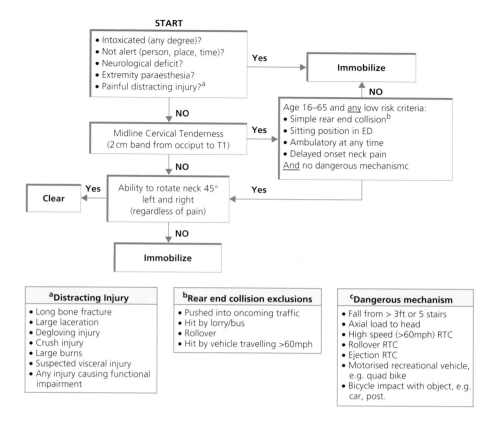

START

- Intoxicated (any degree)?
- Not alert (person, place, time)?
- Neurological deficit?
- Extremity paraesthesia?
- Painful distracting injury?[a]

Yes → **Immobilize**

NO

NO ↑

Age 16–65 and <u>any</u> low risk criteria:
- Simple rear end collision[b]
- Sitting position in ED
- Ambulatory at any time
- Delayed onset neck pain
<u>And</u> no dangerous mechanismc

Midline Cervical Tenderness (2 cm band from occiput to T1) — **Yes** →

NO

Clear ← **Yes** — Ability to rotate neck 45° left and right (regardless of pain) ← **Yes**

NO

Immobilize

[a]**Distracting Injury**	[b]**Rear end collision exclusions**	[c]**Dangerous mechanism**
• Long bone fracture • Large laceration • Degloving injury • Crush injury • Large burns • Suspected visceral injury • Any injury causing functional impairment	• Pushed into oncoming traffic • Hit by lorry/bus • Rollover • Hit by vehicle travelling >60mph	• Fall from > 3ft or 5 stairs • Axial load to head • High speed (>60mph) RTC • Rollover RTC • Ejection RTC • Motorised recreational vehicle, e.g. quad bike • Bicycle impact with object, e.g. car, post.

Figure 14.2 Selective immobilization pathway.

Identification of those patients at risk of spinal injury

Unnecessary immobilization places in a significant burden on limited prehospital and emergency department (ED) resources. Guidelines such as the Canadian C-Spine and NEXUS rules identify patients with significant cervical spine injury with a high sensitivity but low specificity. They can therefore be used to safely rule out significant cervical spine injury and allow selective spinal immobilization in the prehospital environment.

A suggested algorithm combining both NEXUS and Canadian C-spine rules is shown in Figure 14.2.

Management of spinal injuries

Prevention of hypoxia

Aggressive management of the airway and breathing is required to minimize hypoxic secondary injury to the cord. Where possible the spine should be immobilized concurrently. In the unconscious patient with suspected spinal injury, jaw thrust is the preferred airway-positioning technique as it limits movement of the cervical spine. Caution should be taken when suctioning or instrumenting the airway as unopposed vagal stimulation may precipitate severe bradycardia or cardiac arrest in patients with a high spinal cord injury. Atropine should be available and prophylactic use considered in those patients exhibiting signs of neurogenic shock. Intubation should be undertaken with manual in-line stabilization (MILS) in place to minimize the movement of the cervical spine during laryngoscopy. MILS is known to worsen the grade of view at laryngoscopy (Figure 14.3) and a bougie should be used in all cases.

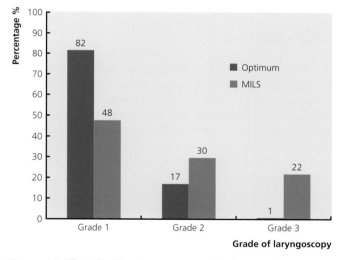

Figure 14.3 Effect of MILS on laryngoscopy grade. (Source: Nolan JP. *Anaesthesia* 1993;**48**:630–634).

High-flow oxygen should be applied, and concomitant chest injuries should be managed early. Ventilation should be monitored and supported where necessary. Loss of intercostal muscle function in high cord (C4–C8) injuries may reduce vital capacity to up to 10–20% of normal. Diaphragmatic breathing may be the only sign of this in the unconscious patient. Application of non-invasive capnography and the identification of progressive type II respiratory failure (rising $ETCO_2$) can aid the diagnosis and pre-empt the need for ventilatory support. Injuries above C4 often lead to rapid respiratory failure due to both diaphragmatic and intercostal paralysis, and early ventilatory support is essential.

Prevention of hypoperfusion

The triad of hypotension, bradycardia and peripheral vasodilatation should alert the prehospital practitioner to the presence of neurogenic shock. In the trauma patient other causes of shock (e.g. hypovolaemic or obstructive) must be excluded before attributing hypotension to neurogenic shock alone.

Initial resuscitation should begin with infusion of crystalloid to achieve a target systolic blood pressure of 90–100 mmHg. Mild neurogenic hypotension (systolic blood pressure <90 mmHg) often responds to crystalloid infusion alone. In contrast, severe neurogenic hypotension (systolic blood pressure <70 mmHg) often requires vasopressors (primarily α-agonists) and/or cardiac pacing to maintain target blood pressure and a heart rate of 60–10 beats/min.

Limit further spinal movement

In the absence of immediate dangers and life threats, patients must be carefully stabilized manually, and immobilization undertaken where appropriate. Basic management of the spine may consist of moving the patient into a neutral, in-line position, unless resistance is met, a deformity of the spine exists or movement causes a noticeable increase in pain. Hips and knees can be flexed slightly to minimize stress on the muscles, joints and spine.

Initial stabilization

MILS should be applied in the first instance. The neck should then be assessed for physical injury and cervical tenderness before then applying a cervical collar. Time should be taken to ensure an appropriate sized collar is fitted in line with the manufacturer's guidelines. A cervical collar will reduce movement of the neck, but even when correctly fitted will allow over 30 degrees of flexion/extension and rotation. MILS should therefore be maintained until the patient is fully secured to an immobilization device with head blocks and tape. In some cases deformity (e.g. ankylosing spondylitis) or anatomy (e.g. bull neck) may preclude the use of a cervical collar. Such patients must not be forced into a collar as this may worsen injury. Instead they should be splinted in the position found using padding to support them in their position of comfort (Figure 14.4).

Cervical collars should not be applied to those patient suspected of having a severe head injury as they have been shown to increase intracranial pressure by obstructing venous return from the head. Instead these patients should be immobilized in head blocks and tape alone as these have been shown to provide equivalent immobilization to the combination of head blocks, tape and a collar. Where a cervical collar is mandated by local policy it should be loosened.

Helmet removal

In some cases of sports-related injuries or bicycle/motorcycle accidents, patients may be wearing a helmet. Helmets should be

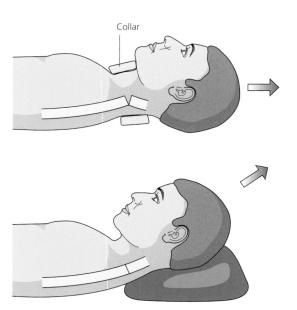

Figure 14.4 Collars may be detrimental in patients with kyphosis.

removed preferably by two trained persons to permit access to the airway and immobilization (Figure 14.5). The appropriate action to take will be based on the type of helmet and the ease of removing it. Sports helmets are equipped with face masks that are removable, whereas motorcycle helmets contain the airway and must be removed.

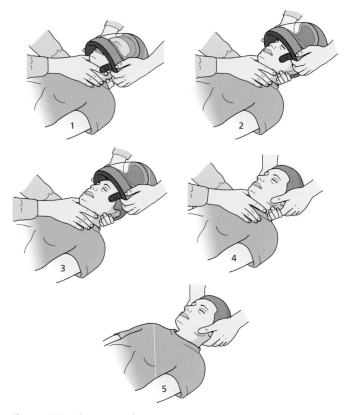

Figure 14.5 Helmet removal.

Movement of spinal patients

Movement during packaging should be minimized to reduce further mechanical disturbance of the spine. The same principles of minimal handling used for the bleeding patient apply to the spinal patient: early cutting of clothes, minimal log-rolling and skin-to-immobilization device packaging should be employed. The orthopaedic scoop device is ideal for this purpose as the blades can be applied individually using minimal rolls of 15 degrees each side in the supine patient. Where this is not available a single log-roll onto an extrication board is acceptable. It should be noted that if the latter method is employed one will often need to centralize the patient on the board after the initial roll. Any such movement must be performed in line with the long axis of the board and not by pulling/pushing laterally. As such it helps to position the patient on the board lower than is required on the initial roll to allow a single slide up and across to the centralized position when supine (Figure 14.6).

Immobilization of the spine

Movement during transfer should be minimized to reduce further mechanical disturbance of the spine. A combination of a rigid cervical collar and supportive head blocks on an immobilization device with straps is effective in reducing motion of the spine. A number of devices are available. With all devices the torso should be strapped before the head to prevent unwanted movement around the cervical spine. The advantages and disadvantages of common immobilization devices are shown in Table 14.2.

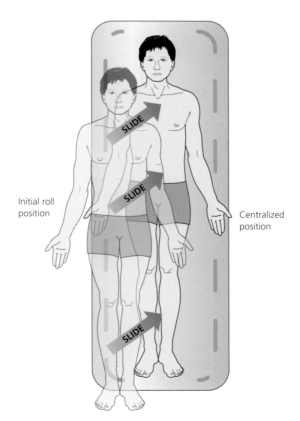

Figure 14.6 Repositioning on a long board.

Table 14.2 Clearer delineation between four devices and their relevant text bodies

Device	Advantages	Disadvantages
Scoop Stretcher	• Adjustable in length • No midline spinal pressure • Minimal rolling required for application & removal • Provides more lateral support than extrication board • Many fold in half saving space	• Allows lateral movement • Not all are radiolucent • Tendency to bend in the middle with heavy patients • Not suitable for carrying long distances • Pressure areas if on for prolonged periods • Cannot be dragged
Extrication Board (Long Spine Board)	• Commonly available • Robust • Smooth surface so excellent for sliding patients along during extrication • Handles for rope/strap attachment • May be dragged easily • Can fit a head immobilizer	• Midline spinal pressure • Allows lateral movement • Spinal padding required • Full roll or slide required for application/removal • Pressure areas if on for prolonged periods • More uncomfortable than scoop
Vacuum Mattress	• Increased comfort • Provides good lateral support • May help contain lines, etc. • Reduced pressure areas • Useful for long transfers • May be used with scoop stretcher or extrication board	• Vulnerable to puncture or being cut • Used alone is not sufficiently rigid to immobilize the spine • Take up a lot of space • Rely on presence of pumps or suction apparatus.
Extrication Device (KED*,TED*,RED*,KD2000*)	• Provides better cervical spine immobilization than a collar alone • Handles may be used for rotation and sliding • Useful for confined spaces • Useful for cockpits of aircraft or formula racing cars	• Impairs ventilation (reduced FEV^1, FVC) • Only immobilizes the c-spine • Often needs roof removal to apply to seated patient in car • Tendency to rise up if handles used to lift if not snug under armpits • Stable patients only

More specialized rescue stretchers (e.g. Chrysalis®, Reeves Sleeve®, MIBS®) are available for rescue at height, confined spaces and winching.

Certain patient groups may not tolerate full supine spinal immobilization and will require adaptation of normal procedures (Table 14.3). Application of a collar alone may be tolerated and will act as a marker for suspected cervical spine injury. In reality natural muscle spasm will provide protection that is far superior to any artificially imposed immobilization, and the position that the patient themselves finds most comfortable is likely to be the best for their particular injury. Patients prone to travel sickness may require prophylactic antiemetics prior to long transfers laid supine on an immobilization device.

Immobilization of children and infants

Children requiring spinal immobilization typically require a different device from an adult patient. Children aged between 2 and

Table 14.3 Patients unsuitable for conventional immobilization

Patient Group	Solution
Severe Cardiac or Pulmonary disease who are unable to lie flat	Apply collar and secure to stretcher bed with blocks, tape and straps in seated position if tolerated
Combative and agitated patients resisting immobilization	Apply collar alone
Paediatric patients resisting immobilization	Apply collar alone
Pregnant patients (>20 weeks) due to aortocaval compression	Immobilize supine then tilt board to the left lateral position during transfer, or Left lateral trauma position
Patients with active airway bleeding or atrisk airway	Left lateral trauma position

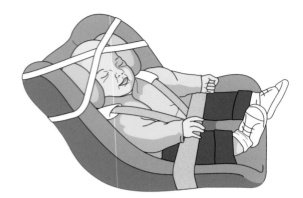

Figure 14.8 Immobilization of an infant in their car seat.

Hospital selection

Patients with pain from soft-tissue injury or isolated uncomplicated potential spinal fracture (no neurology) may be managed and investigated at a local/ district general hospital. Those with multisystem trauma, neurological findings and those with suspected unstable fractures will require management at a major trauma unit.

Tips from the field

- Routine use of a bougie for endotracheal intubation will mitigate C-spine manipulation
- Exclude other causes of shock before attributing hypotension to neurogenic shock
- Pregnant women secured to a long back board should be elevated on their right side by tilting the board 15–20 degrees and placing pillows or blankets beneath
- Small children in car seats can remain in the seat for transport to the hospital as long as there is no structural damage to the seat
- Long back boards using five straps will always secure a person to it better than using three straps.

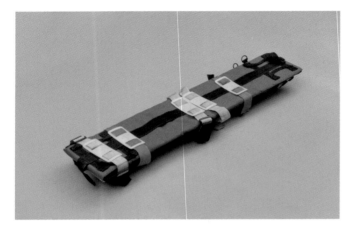

Figure 14.7 Ferno Pedi-Pac immobilizer® (Courtesy of Ferno).

10 years may be immobilized using a paediatric immobilization device, e.g. Pedi-Pac immobilizer® (Figure 14.7). Because it is narrower it reduces the lateral movement that may occur if a child is immobilized to an adult immobilization device. Additional shoulder padding is provided to compensate for the relatively large occiput of the younger child.

A degree of improvisation may be required to adequately immobilize a child for transport in the absence of a paediatric immobilization device. A useful alternative for the young child is the long leg box splint or vacuum splint. After a motor vehicle crash, infants in a car seat may be immobilized in the seat as long as it has no structural damage and the child does not have any apparent injuries that would require removal from the car seat. The head should be immobilized using padding and tape (Figure 14.8).

Further reading

Campbell J. *International Trauma Life Support for Prehospital Care Providers*, 6th edn. Chapter 11. Spinal Trauma. Brady Publishing.

Domeier RM, Evans RW, Swor RA, *et al*. The reliability of prehospital clinical evaulation for potential spinal injury is not affected by the mechanism of injury. *Prehosp Emerg Care* 1999;**3**:332–337.

Domeier RM, Swor RA, Evans RW, *et al*. Multicenter prospective validation of prehospital clinical spinal clearance guideline. *J Trauma* 2002;**53**:744–750.

Hoffman JR, Schriger DL, Mower W, *et al*. Low risk criteria for cervical-spine radiography in blunt trauma: a prospective study. *Ann Emerg Med* 1992;**21**:1454–1460.

CHAPTER 15

Trauma: Abdominal Injury

Keith Roberts

University Hospitals Birmingham, Birmingham, UK

OVERVIEW

By the end of this chapter you should:

- Appreciate the importance of mechanism of injury in blunt and penetrating abdominal trauma
- Understand how the abdomen should be assessed in the prehospital environment
- Understand how to manage abdominal injury in the prehospital environment.

Introduction

In Western countries abdominal injury is present in around one-fifth of major trauma cases. The majority are the result of road traffic collisions and frequently occur in the presence of other injuries. Unrecognized abdominal injury remains a significant cause of death. A high index of suspicion is required in order to recognize occult injury and manage it appropriately.

Mechanisms of injury

Up to 25% of serious abdominal injuries will be undetectable by clinical examination in the early stages (50% if the patient is unconscious). Only the mechanism of injury will give a clue as to the presence of such injuries.

Blunt trauma

Blunt abdominal trauma often results from compressive forces and/or deceleration. Low-energy localized compressive forces (e.g. a punch or kick) may cause significant damage to underlying solid organs. The kidneys, liver and spleen are particularly vulnerable to direct blows to the flank, right or left upper quadrants respectively (Figure 15.1). Sporting accidents, falls or assaults are responsible for the majority of these type of injuries and typically affect young adult males.

In blunt trauma involving forceful abdominal compression and/or deceleration (e.g. high-speed RTC or pedestrians hit by

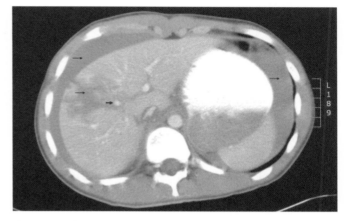

Figure 15.1 The patient's right hypochondrium struck a curb following a trip when running causing a Grade 4 liver laceration with haemoperitoneum (small arrows).

vehicles), although solid organ injury remains a common feature indirect injury due to deceleration must also be considered. Mesenteric tears are the commonest of these injuries, typically injuring the ileocolic vessels. Haemorrhage may occur acutely with the devascularization of associated bowel leading to delayed necrosis and bowel perforation. Similarly solid organs (e.g. spleen, kidneys, etc.) can be sheared off their vascular pedicle leading to bleeding and organ ischaemia. Significant abdominal compression, particularly with the use of lap belts, may also result in pancreatic, duodenal or diaphragmatic ruptures.

Penetrating trauma

The prevalence of penetrating trauma varies widely due to influences of society, welfare and firearms legislation. In the UK it accounts for between 5% and 20% of cases, whereas in the USA it can account for up to 50%. The injuries sustained are caused by the direct trauma as the penetrating item passes through the organs and tissues. Unfortunately, it is often impossible to tell from the appearance of a surface wound or the size of the penetrating implement, the extent of underlying damage. Gunshot wounds are three times more likely to damage major abdominal viscera than stab wounds and the commonest organs injured are the small bowel, colon and liver.

ABC of Prehospital Emergency Medicine, First Edition.
Edited by Tim Nutbeam and Matthew Boylan.
© 2013 John Wiley & Sons, Ltd. Published 2013 by John Wiley & Sons, Ltd.

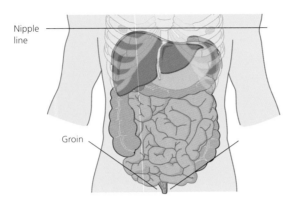

Figure 15.2 Extent of the abdominal cavity (anterior).

Assessment of the abdomen

The abdomen extends from the nipples to the groin crease anteriorly (Figure 15.2), and the tips of the scapulae to the gluteal skin crease posteriorly. Any blunt or penetrating injury within or through this region should raise the suspicion of abdominal injury.

It is essential to perform a thorough primary survey and not be distracted by any obvious injury. Upper abdominal injuries can cause a simple or tension pneumothorax or haemothorax, and cardiac tamponade may complicate penetrating cardiac injury in epigastric stab wounds. A rapid examination of the abdomen should form part of the primary survey circulatory assessment in the hypovolaemic patient as it is one of the four sites of hidden haemorrhage.

Clinical examination should include a full examination of the abdomen, flanks and back, particularly in cases of penetrating trauma. Abdominal distension or changes in girth **are rarely** seen with abdominal bleeding, even with massive haemorrhage. A rigid abdomen may reflect free intraperitoneal blood, contamination with bowel content or injury to the abdominal wall muscles, particular in young patients with large abdominal muscles. However, most patients with intraperitoneal haemorrhage will have minimal pain.

The presence of an abdominal abrasion from a seat or lap belt (Figure 15.3) carries a low sensitivity for intrabdominal injury.

Prehospital ultrasound may be used to identify intrabdominal free fluid in the trauma patient which usually represents free blood.

Prehospital management of abdominal injuries

Resuscitation

Suspected non-compressible abdominal haemorrhage resulting in hypotension should be managed by rapid evacuation to a surgical centre and permissive hypotension. Intravenous or intraosseus access should be obtained en route, and warmed intravenous fluid should be titrated using the patients level of consciousness (e.g. ability to talk to you) as an end point. This will permit a lower blood pressure than selecting an arbitrary systolic target or presence/absence of a peripheral pulse. The caveat to this is the

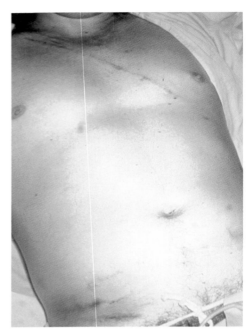

Figure 15.3 Seat belt bruising (Courtesy of Lifeinthefastlane.com).

intoxicated patient where a systolic of 60–70 mmHg should be the goal. Head injuries and injuries greater than 1 hour old are the only exceptions to this rule and in these patients normotension is the goal.

Analgesia

Opiate analgesia should be used to control visceral pain following abdominal trauma. It should not be withheld due to concerns of masking occult injury.

Evisceration

No attempt should be made to replace eviscerated bowel. Exposed bowel should be covered with saline soaked sterile pads or cling film to prevent it from drying out (Figure 15.4).

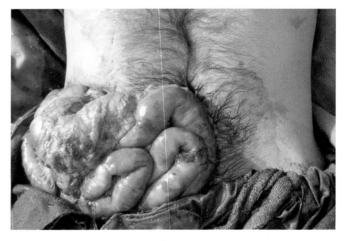

Figure 15.4 Evisceration following fragmentation injury.

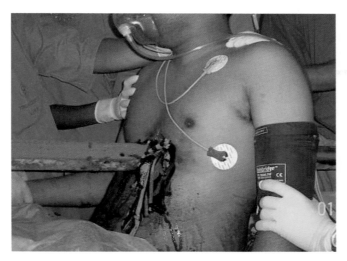

Figure 15.5 Impalement on a fence post (Courtesy of Dr Biplab Mishra).

Impalement

Removal of impaled objects may result in further trauma and uncontrollable bleeding. Such objects are therefore best left in place until they can be removed in the operating theatre under control. Long or fixed objects (e.g. fence posts or railings) may require cutting to permit evacuation and may preclude standard patient positioning during transfer (Figure 15.5).

Triage

Solid organ injury is best treated by conservative management wherever possible. This requires experienced and enthusiastic surgeons, access to 24 hour cross-sectional imaging and interventional radiology. These facilities will also enable occult injury to abdominal organs including the mesentery, duodenum or pancreas to be identified. Surgery is rarely required. Some procedures are less technically challenging, such as splenectomy or liver packing, than

others requiring specialist surgical input, such as vascular control of major haemorrhage and treatment of complex visceral or solid organ injury. It is not possible to predict in the prehospital phase which abdominal injuries a patient has. For these reasons major centres with suitable facilities should be selected where possible. When faced with a hypotensive patient (particularly in penetrating trauma), call ahead as early as possible in the prehospital phase to request senior surgical presence and blood products in the emergency department.

> **Tips from the field:**
>
> - Clinical assessment of the abdomen has a low sensitivity and specificity. Intoxication, head injury or distracting injuries may make clinical assessment of the abdomen even more unreliable
> - The presence of a physiologically normal patient does not exclude significant intra-abdominal injury
> - Abdominal distension rarely occurs with intrabdominal haemorrhage
> - Do not underestimate low-energy trauma direct to the abdomen – major solid organ injury can occur
> - The majority of solid organ injuries can be managed non-operatively in hospital. Interventional radiological and surgical expertise will be required for this; familiarize yourself with local hospital services.

Further reading

Demetriades D, Hadjizacharia P, Constantinou C, *et al*. Selective nonoperative management of penetrating abdominal solid organ injuries. *Ann Surg* 2006;**244**:620–628.

Boffard KD. *Manual of Definitive Surgical Trauma Care*, 3rd edn. London: Hodder Arnold, 2011.

Roberts K, Revell M, Youssef H, Bradbury AW, Adam DJ. Hypotensive resuscitation in patients with ruptured abdominal aortic aneurysm. *Eur J Vasc Endovasc Surg* 2006;**31**:339–344.

CHAPTER 16

Trauma: Pelvic Injury

Matt O'Meara[1,2], Keith Porter[2], and Tim Nutbeam[3]

[1]Queens Medical Centre, Nottingham, UK
[2]University of Birmingham, Birmingham, UK
[3]Derriford Hospital, Plymouth Hospitals NHS Trust, Plymouth, UK

> **OVERVIEW**
>
> By the end of this chapter you will:
> - Understand the mechanisms of injury associated with pelvic trauma
> - Understand the importance of applying a pelvic binders as part of the 'C' assessment
> - Understand how to avoid additional iatrogenic injury in these patient groups.

Aetiology

Pelvic fractures are associated with significant morbidity and mortality. They represent an application of significant force to the patient involved and are often found in association with multisystem trauma. Reported mortality rates are as high as 60%. Falls from height, motor vehicle collisions and accidents related to horse riding are common mechanisms of injuries in major pelvic injury. Low velocity falls in elderly people may cause significant life-threatening injury.

Injury classification

Pelvic fractures can be classified according to the mechanism of injury and the effect this has on destabilizing the 'ring' of the pelvis. These injuries do occur in combination (combined mechanical injury, CMI) and the treatment for each follows similar principles.

Anteroposterior injuries

Also known as 'open book' injuries. Significant force causes the pelvis to open causing (potentially) massive damage to the venous plexus, bladder, urethra and occasionally the internal iliac artery complex (Figure 16.1). Commonly associated with massive torso injuries and the resultant sequelae of this multisystem trauma: shock, sepsis, ARDS, etc.

Mechanism of injury: motorcyclists hitting their tank/trees, rolled on by horse, etc.

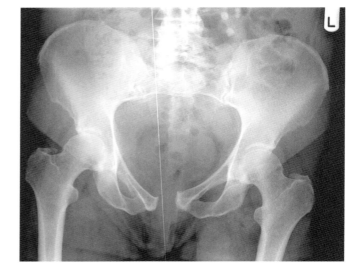

Figure 16.1 X-ray showing anteroposterior/open book injury.

Vertical shear injuries

Significant shearing forces applied to the pelvis often lead to unstable injuries. Damage to both anterior and posterior ligamentous complexes leads to vertical displacement of the hemipelvis (Figure 16.2). Often associated with lower long bone and spinal injury.

Mechanism of injury: falls from significant height landing on extended limb.

Lateral compression injuries

This most common form of pelvic fracture is most often associated with limb and head injuries. Fracture fragments may tear major vessels resulting in massive haemorrhage (Figure 16.3).

Mechanism of injury: falls and side impact motor vehicle collisions.

Haemorrhage

Massive haemorrhage is common in high force pelvic injury. Bleeding with arterial, venous plexus and bone injury often requires both massive transfusion and early definitive treatment: no clear consensus has been reached on angio-embolization versus surgical

ABC of Prehospital Emergency Medicine, First Edition.
Edited by Tim Nutbeam and Matthew Boylan.
© 2013 John Wiley & Sons, Ltd. Published 2013 by John Wiley & Sons, Ltd.

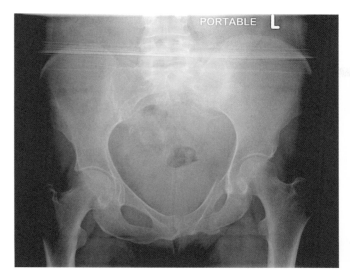

Figure 16.2 X-ray showing vertical shear fracture.

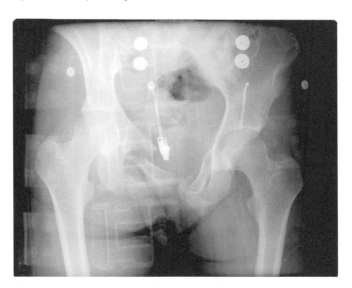

Figure 16.3 X-ray showing lateral compression fracture.

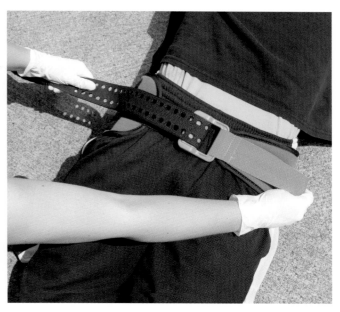

Figure 16.4 Pelvic binder: the SAM sling (Courtesy of SAM Medical Products).

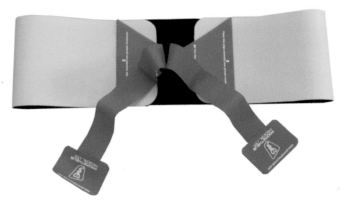

Figure 16.5 Pelvic binder: the Prometheus pelvic binder is suitable for all patient sizes (Courtesy of Prometheus Medical Ltd).

management of these patients; ideally the patient should be transported to a centre that offers both services.

Permissive hypotension is currently practised in the first stages of these patients' management – this is probably not appropriate for prolonged periods.

Pelvic binders

Pelvic binders should be applied at an early stage (as part of the 'C' assessment) and not removed until significant pelvic injury has been excluded (Figures 16.4 and 16.5). The binder performs two roles:

1 Anatomical reduction of the pelvis – reducing pelvic volume.
2 Stabilizing all forms of pelvic fracture limiting movement through mechanical splinting.

- Application: First correct shear by drawing feet level and binding feet/ankles and knees together. Then reduce A-P rotation through application of circumferential compression with binder at greater trochanter.
- Indications: All patients with a mechanism of injury which **may** have caused pelvic injury and are either (a) unevaluable (e.g. head injury, intoxication, intubated) or (b) complaining of back, pelvic or lower abdominal pain.
- Combined fractures: With suspected combined femoral and pelvic fractures, first apply manual traction to the legs drawing feet and ankles level. Next apply a pelvic binder before applying a Kendrick (or equivalent – see Chapter 17 on extremity injury) traction splint to each leg suspected of having a femoral fracture. Apply traction aiming for anatomical reduction. Bind feet together to prevent external rotation.

Avoiding iatrogenic injury

Pelvic fractures should be assumed to be unstable – additional iatrogenic injury may be caused by the movement of bone fragments and movement causing changes in pelvic volume and/or architecture.

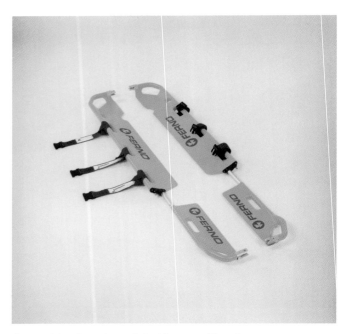

Figure 16.6 A Ferno Scoop Splint (Courtesy of Ferno).

Do not spring the pelvis – it adds little relevant clinical information but can cause significant damage.

Care must be taken when removing patient clothing, e.g. motorbike leathers. These clothes may be holding fractures in a reduced position – on removal significant damage may be caused by changes in pelvic volume/architecture.

Log-roll is not recommended and should be minimized (10–15 degrees maximum). A split scoop type stretcher is ideal for lifting and transporting patients (Figure 16.6).

Tips from the field

- Avoid iatrogenic injury by minimal handling techniques, avoidance of log-roll and not 'springing' the pelvis
- Have a high index of suspicion: if in doubt apply a pelvic binder
- PR or PV bleeding may represent an 'open' fracture into a hollow viscus; these have a mortality of >50%
- Pelvic binders need to be applied at the level of the greater trochanters (even though they may look better around the waist!)
- Do not allow anyone to mistake a pelvic binder for a board strap and accidentally unclip it!

Further reading

Joint Royal Colleges Ambulance Liaison Committee (JRCALC) *Prehospital Guidelines* 2006. Warwick: University of Warwick, 2006.

Lee C, Porter K. The prehospital management of pelvic fractures. *Emerg Med J* 2007;**24**:130–133.

CHAPTER 17

Trauma: Extremity Injury

Matt O'Meara[1,2], Keith Porter[2], and Tim Nutbeam[3]

[1]Queens Medical Centre, Nottingham, UK
[2]University of Birmingham, Birmingham, UK
[3]Derriford Hospital, Plymouth Hospitals NHS Trust, Plymouth, UK

OVERVIEW

By the end of this chapter you should:

- Understand the mechanisms of injury contributing to extremity trauma
- Understand the practical aspects of the management of extremity trauma in the prehospital environment
- Understand the indications for and principles of prehospital amputation.

Aetiology

Extremity trauma is common; alone and in combination with multisystem injury it represents a significant proportion of a prehospital practitioner's case load. Extremity trauma represents challenges in terms of assessment, management, packaging and transport: many of these challenges can be overcome through a systematic approach. Extremity trauma may be both life and limb threatening (Boxes 17.1 and 17.2).

Box 17.1 **Life-threatening extremity trauma**

- Pelvic fractures
- Traumatic amputation
- Open fractures (haemorrhage)
- Upper rib fractures (left-sided)
- Femoral fractures (especially bilateral)
- Crush injuries.

Box 17.2 **Limb-threatening extremity trauma**

- Joint dislocations
- Crush injuries
- Amputation
- Vascular injury
- Open fractures (infection).

ABC of Prehospital Emergency Medicine, First Edition.
Edited by Tim Nutbeam and Matthew Boylan.
© 2013 John Wiley & Sons, Ltd. Published 2013 by John Wiley & Sons, Ltd.

Mechanism of injury and injury pattern

Direct or indirect force through motor vehicle collisions, falls from height and sporting accidents account for the majority of extremity injuries. Crush, burn and blast injury though representing a small proportion of overall injuries present their own challenges (see individual chapters for detail). Attention should be paid to the likely mechanism of injury as this may identify otherwise occult significant injury (e.g. dashboard knee injury may cause proximal hip/femur/pelvic fracture).

Injury assessment

Ideally all extremity injuries would be identified and classified in the prehospital arena; however, this is often impractical. Time critical primary survey injuries, multisystem trauma and environmental conditions may lead (appropriately) to the delayed identification of injuries.

Injuries should be identified as open (compound) or closed – any abrasion or laceration may represent an occult open fracture. Injuries with associated neurovascular compromise may be time critical – early reduction may prevent further morbidity. A rapid assessment prior to rapid sequence induction may identify nerve injuries, which would otherwise be missed.

Analgesia

Give appropriate, rapid onset, intravenous analgesia early – titrate this to effect. Nerve blocks though purported to be useful are often impractical in the prehospital setting. Reducing periosteal stretch through early reduction of fractures further reduces patient pain.

Wound care

After haemostasis and if time allows, wounds should be rinsed clean and protected with an appropriate dressing. An antiseptic agent (e.g. povidone–iodine) should be applied. There may be a role for prehospital antibiotic use outside of battlefield wounds, but this has not yet been clearly defined.

In the case of traumatic amputation and if circumstances allow, the amputated part should be transported with the patient. If a 'complete' amputation wrap in a damp dressing and place in a watertight plastic bag (e.g. clinical waste bag). If ice is available this can be packed around the outside of the bag – this may prolong viability time for implantable tissue.

Reducing, splinting and packaging

Long bone fractures and some joints are suitable for reduction prehospitally. The aim should be to reduce pain, bleeding, vessel

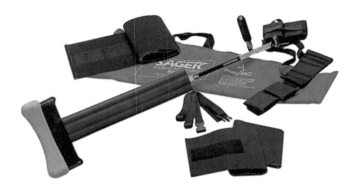

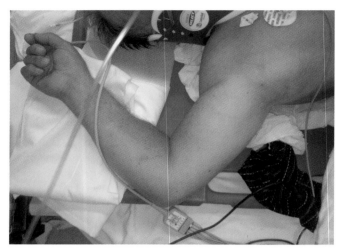

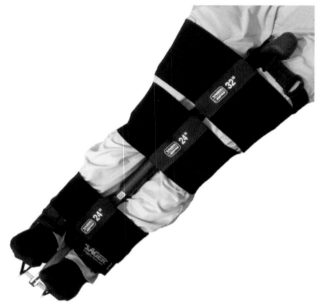

Figure 17.1 Luxatio erecta (inferior shoulder dislocation) may cause difficulties in patient packaging and transportation.

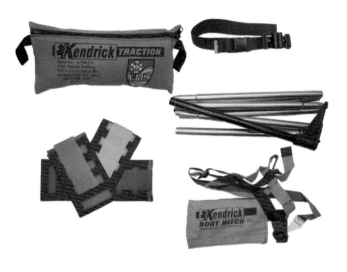

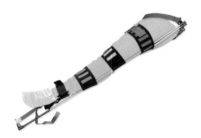

Figure 17.2 The Kendrick traction device (KTD), a portable device suitable for long bone traction and support. An advantage of the KTD is that it does not use counter traction on the pelvis to maintain limb traction.

Figure 17.3 The Sager traction device, suitable for bilateral femur fractures.

and nerve compromise. Larger joints (shoulder and hip) are often best left for in-hospital reduction – the exception to this rule may be where packaging and transport are compromised by limb position (Figure 17.1).

When an adequate level of analgesia with or without sedation has been achieved the limb should be brought into anatomical alignment: techniques for individual bones and joints vary and are beyond the scope of this chapter. The limb can initially be held in position manually – in selected patients this will occur with the primary survey, e.g. an unconscious patient with bilateral femoral fractures.

Various devices can be used to secure the limb in anatomical alignment (Figures 17.2 and 17.3).

Amputation

Prehospital amputation may be indicated in the following situations:

- An immediate and real risk to the patient's life due to a scene safety emergency.

- A deteriorating patient physically trapped by limb where they will almost certainly die during the time to secure extrication (Figure 17.4).
- A completely mutilated non-survivable limb retaining minimal attachment which is delaying extrication and evacuation from the scene in a non-immediate life-threatening situation.

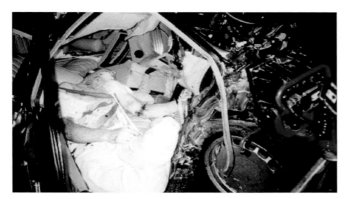

Figure 17.4 Severe limb entrapment. (Source: Keith M Porter, *Emerg Med J.* Dec 1, 2010, 27, 12).

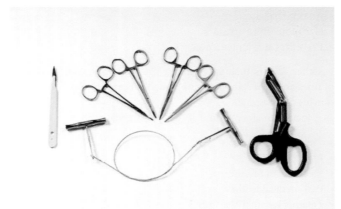

Figure 17.5 Surgical equipment required to perform prehospital amputation: scalpel, Gigli saw, Tuff cut scissors and several pairs of arterial forceps.

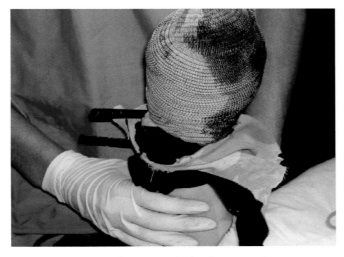

Figure 17.6 Dressing and tourniquets *in situ* after amputation.

- The patient is dead and their limbs are blocking access to potentially live casualties.

If time allows it is recommended that the decision to amputate is made with the agreement of two senior clinicians, one who will be performing the procedure. Figure 17.5 shows the basic equipment required. Deep sedation (with ketamine or similar) or general anaesthesia is mandatory. The principles of performing the procedure are outlined in Box 17.3. Following amputation the stump should be rinsed clean and dressed as described above (Figure 17.6).

Box 17.3 **Steps in performing prehospital amputation**

- Apply an effective proximal tourniquet (e.g. CAT tourniquet)
- Amputate as distally as possible
- Incise the skin circumferentially at the level of intended amputation with a scalpel
- Cut down through the subcutaneous tissues and open the fascia containing the underlying muscle groups
- Identify muscle groups using the gloved hand and divide with tuff cut scissors
- Apply arterial forceps to visible large blood vessels
- Divide the bone with a Gigli saw

Leave tourniquet *in situ* and dress the stump.

(Source: Keith M Porter, *Emerg Med J.* Dec 1, 2010, 27, 12).

Tips from the field

- Don't let impressive extremity injuries distract from a thorough, systematic primary survey
- Identification of all injuries may be difficult especially if the patient is obtunded: identify clinical priorities and move on
- Prehospital amputation involving more than cutting minimal soft-tissue bridges is rare: a decision made by two senior clinicians is advised
- Photographs of wounds/open fractures prior to reduction/dressing may be clinically useful
- Judicious pain management is crucial in reducing short- and long-term morbidity from extremity injury: it is often neglected, especially post RSI!
- If using a vacuum splint in a remote location remember to take the pump with you!

Further reading

Graces I, Porter K, Smith J. Consensus Statement on the management of crush injury and prevention of crush syndrome. *JRAMC* 2004;**150**:102–106.

Joint Royal Colleges Ambulance Liaison Committee (JRCALC) *Prehospital guidelines* 2006. Warwick: University of Warwick, 2006.

Porter K. *Prehospital amputation. Emerg Med J* 2010;**7**:940–942.

CHAPTER 18

Trauma: Burns

Alex Jones, Anna Barnard, and Keith Allison

The James Cook University Hospital, Middlesbrough, UK

OVERVIEW

By the end of this chapter you should know:

- The importance of burns in a prehospital setting
- A meaningful classification of prehospital burns
- How to assess burn size in the prehospital setting
- A prehospital approach to the management of the burn patient
- How to manage the prehospital burn patient with regard to airway and fluid management
- Referral pathways for burn patients
- The importance of triage in mass burn casualties.

Introduction

Burn injuries are incredibly common. Current World Health Organization (WHO) data suggest that fire deaths alone represent 5% of total global mortality due to trauma: this equates to more than 300 000 deaths per annum. Such figures exclude injuries from scalds, contact, chemical and electrical injuries, and therefore significantly underestimate the true incidence of and mortality from burn injuries.

Burn-related disability and disfigurement affects millions worldwide with great personal, social and economic impact. The frequency and pattern of such injuries varies with the socioeconomic status of individuals and the region or country.

Burn injuries can happen in isolation or in combination with other traumatic injuries; it is paramount that patients are assessed and treated methodically as advocated by courses like emergency management of severe burns (EMSB), advanced trauma life support (ATLS) and prehospital trauma life support (PHTLS). Numerous texts focus on the overall management of burns; however, this chapter will focus on those areas specific to prehospital care.

Types of burns

Burns often occur when there is a loss of control of the patient's environment through whatever cause. For example, a firefighter who deliberately tackles such situations, a toddler who has no understanding of the hot or cold tap, an epileptic or alcohol/drug-impaired patient who loses consciousness, or the elderly patient who becomes trapped through immobility.

Injury severity depends upon:

- Burn agent
- Duration of exposure
- Anatomical site
- Size of involved area
- Early first aid implemented

Other factors including patient age, general health or comorbidities are important in ongoing medical care and may be relevant outside the hospital.

A focused history should always be gained:

- Time of injury
- Place of injury
- Mechanism of injury
- Past medical history
- Tetanus vaccination status
- First aid already given

Burns should be classified by mechanism into three broad groups: thermal, chemical and electrical.

Thermal burns – These encompass a broad spectrum of injury mechanisms. They represent the most common cause of burns worldwide across all ages and comprise:

- Flame or flash burns associated with fires and explosions (Figure 18.1): it is important to note whether the patient or their clothing caught fire
- Scalds from hot liquids or steam: it is important to know the temperature
- Direct contact burns from hot objects
- Exposure to extremely low temperatures causing frostbite

Chemical burns – These can occur in the chemical and building industries as well as the domestic setting. They may follow direct contact with the chemical or through the air as a vapour. Chemical burns are subdivided into acid or alkali subtypes. Typical acids include sulphuric, hydrofluoric or hydrochloric and these are found in both the print and chemical industries. Typical alkalis

ABC of Prehospital Emergency Medicine, First Edition.
Edited by Tim Nutbeam and Matthew Boylan.
© 2013 John Wiley & Sons, Ltd. Published 2013 by John Wiley & Sons, Ltd.

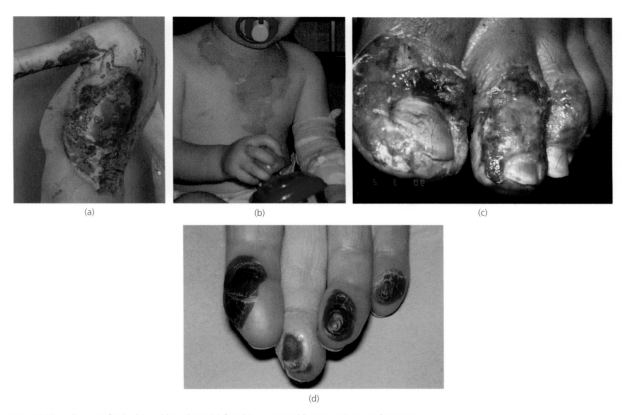

(a) (b) (c)

(d)

Figure 18.1 (a) Flame burn to flank; (b) scald to chest; (c) frostbite to toes; (d) contact burn to fingertips.

include household bleaches, oven cleaners, fertilizers and cement (Figure 18.2).

- Characteristic injury patterns are usually seen.
- Such burns can present many hours after the initial contact as often the patient is unaware of the contact at the time. This results in prolonged exposure and increased tissue damage.

Electrical burns – These are classified as either low or high voltage. The cut off for these descriptors is 1000 volts. Domestic injuries are typically low voltage and may occur where household wiring is inadequately insulated or earthed or stupidity intervenes for the DIY expert! Domestic voltage varies between countries. The pattern of injury usually involves a small area of deep burn (Figure 18.3).

High-voltage burns occur in industrial and recreational settings such as inadvertent earthed contact with overhead power lines or lightning strike. These often lead to extensive deep tissue damage necessitating aggressive surgery and amputation. Furthermore, there is a high risk of associated cardiac damage.

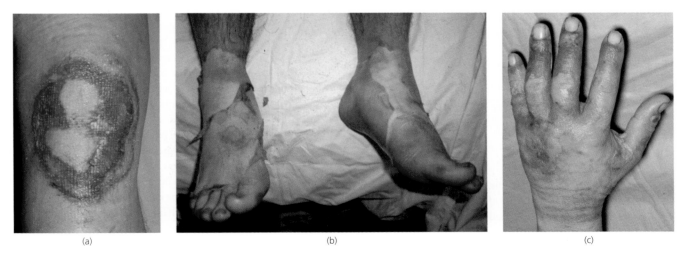

(a) (b) (c)

Figure 18.2 (a) Cement burn to knee showing patella sparing. (b) Chromic acid burn to feet. (c) Caustic soda burn to hand.

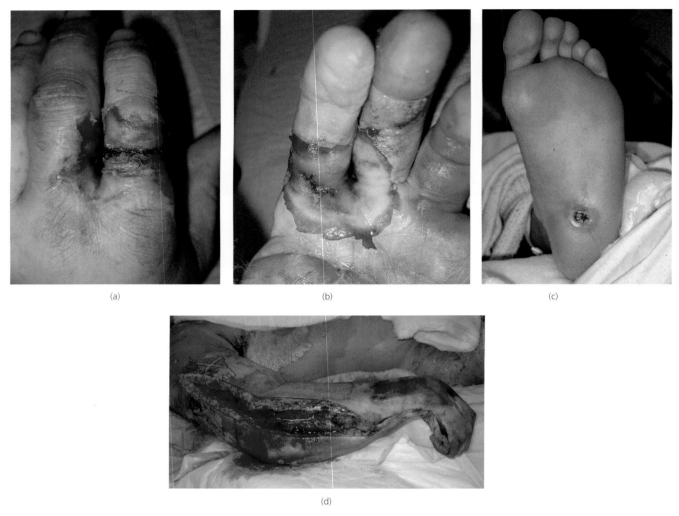

(a)   (b)   (c)

(d)

Figure 18.3 (a, b) Circumferential electrical burn with white finger. (c) Exit wound from high-voltage electrical injury. (d) Fasciotomy to right arm following high voltage electrical injury.

Assessing the burn: extent and depth

Within hospital, traditional teaching suggests the importance of two key factors in assessing and managing burns:

1 Extent
2 Depth.

In prehospital care, the relative importance of these differs as management decisions are driven by the burn extent. The ability to accurately assess extent is important as this influences initial fluid resuscitation and referral pathway.

How to assess burn extent

Extent relates to how much of the skin surface is involved. It is expressed as a proportion of the total body surface area (TBSA). The % TBSA can be estimated through:

• Serial halving
• Patient's palm and digits = 1%

• Rule of nines
• The use of a pictorial representation (e.g. Lund and Browder chart) is helpful for initial calculation and subsequent patient handover (Figure 18.4).

Serial halving is a recently described method where the patient is viewed from the front or the back and an estimate is made of whether the burn involves more or less than half the visible area. The assessment continues with an estimate of whether the burn involves more or less than half of that, i.e. a quarter TBSA and so on. Using this method can quickly enable a burn estimate to be reduced from <50% to <25% to <12.5% and provide an approximate range.

The rule of nines attempts to give a more exact burn size estimate rather than a range and is based on estimates of various body parts representing 9%. It relies on the assessor being able to recall the size of each area and also a reliance that the areas are the same proportion for all individuals, which they are not.

The 1% rule is flawed because there is no consensus on the precise representative proportion of the palm. For example, Lund

Area	Age 0	1	5	10	15	Adult
A = ½ head	9½	8½	6½	5½	4½	3½
B = ½ thigh	2¾	3¼	4	4¼	4½	4¾
C = ½ leg	2½	2½	2¾	3	3¼	3

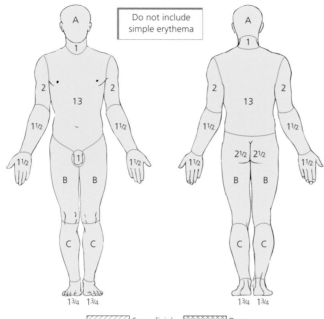

Region	% Burn
Neck	
Anterior trunk	
Posterior trunk	
Right arm	
Left arm	
Buttocks	
Genitalia	
Right leg	
Left leg	
Total burn	

Figure 18.4 Lund and Browder chart.

and Browder estimate this as 1.25% if the digits are included, whereas other authors claim it represents only 0.82% in children and 0.77% in adults. The ATLS guidelines (8th edition) state that the digits should be included in the 1% estimate. Body mass index (BMI) is another consideration as this will not be accurately assessed in the prehospital setting and yet this will also affect TBSA. As BMI increases, the proportional size of the hand reduces.

A UK study has suggested that in the prehospital setting there is little difference in accuracy of burn extent assessment between the rule of nines and the serial halving technique. Consider the use of the serial halving technique as this method provides a realistic ballpark figure from which to proceed.

Standard texts advise that erythema (redness) must not be included within the burn calculation. Erythema should be included when estimating extent in the prehospital setting because erythema may develop into deeper burn within the first 48 hours.

Burn extent can be difficult to accurately assess close to the time of injury and the patient will be reassessed multiple times

upon reaching hospital so treatment can be modified at this time if required. By taking such an approach, underestimation of burn extent and subsequent under resuscitation is avoided.

Burn depth

Standard burns texts describe different depths of burn, from superficial to deep. Sometimes the terms first degree, second degree and third degree are used. Accurate assessment of burn depth is notoriously difficult with considerable interperson variation even with experienced burn staff. Assessment of burn depth in the prehospital setting is largely irrelevant as management will be guided by extent in almost all cases. Exceptions include burns involving deep circumferential injury of the torso or limbs, which may affect ventilation or circulation respectively and when there is likely to be a protracted time (hours) to reach hospital for definitive care (see 'Fasciotomy and escharotomy').

Initial management of burns

The initial management of burns will depend on the severity of the burn injury and associated injuries (Box 18.1). It is best therefore to define burns as minor or significant.

Box 18.1 UK Consensus guidelines for prehospital management of burns

- SAFE approach
- Stop the burning process
- Cool the burn (but not the patient)
- Covering/dressing
- Assessment of AcBC (see Box 18.3)
- Assessment of burn severity
- Intravenous cannulation (and fluids)
- Analgesia
- Transport

Minor burns are those that involve small areas of the body in patients who are systemically well and are unlikely to require significant input from hospital staff. A significant burn therefore is any other! Significant burns will probably require specialist burn care skills such as resuscitation, surgery, ongoing management or prolonged rehabilitation.

Management of minor burns

These may be treated in the community without referral to hospital. These burns should be cooled if thermal or thoroughly irrigated if chemical, cleaned with soap and water then dressed with a simple composite dressing comprising a low-adherent base (such as Jelonet or Mepitel) and absorbent gauze. Evidence to support deroofing of blisters is weak but will assist burn assessment. A 48-hour review should be arranged for reassessment and simple low-adherent dressings used until re-epithelialization is complete. Minor burns to the face and scalp are best managed with application of petroleum-based jelly, as occlusive dressings are not practical in these areas.

Management of significant burns

The initial management of significant burns should be according to the advanced trauma life support guidelines, which have been adapted for burns (Box 18.2). Consensus guidelines have been drawn up in the UK for prehospital burn care and combine the ATLS principles with a common sense approach across all burn injuries.

Box 18.2 **Adapted ATLS approach to burns**

A Airway with cervical spine control
B Breathing and ventilation
C Circulation with haemorrhage control
D Disability–neurological status
E Exposure preventing hypothermia
F Fluid resuscitation

Cooling the burn, but not the patient

Cooling provides good initial analgesia and may decrease the inflammatory response to injury. There is no strong evidence to prove that early burn cooling will affect final outcome. In spite of this, cooling remains accepted good practice. Care must be taken to avoid cooling the patient overall, as evidence suggests mortality rates of burn victims increases with decreasing core body temperature. Once cooling has been performed, careful covering and warming of the patient is important.

Selection of burn dressings

In the prehospital setting use of dressings serves a number of key functions. They minimize fluid and temperature loss, keep the burnt area clean and reduce patient discomfort. The market is flooded with a huge variety of wound dressings and these vary greatly in their characteristics and cost. Burns dressings in the acute setting need to be simple, cheap and readily available. They need to start with of a low-adherent base layer that does not alter the clinical appearance of the burn (which could affect further burn depth assessments). Good examples include ClingFilm™, Seran wrap or petroleum impregnated gauze such as Jelonet. Alternatively for smaller burns, Mepitel a silicone-based dressing, may be useful. Because burns can be associated with significant fluid leak, an absorptive layer such as standard gauze over the burns is often useful.

Who needs fluid resuscitation?

This differs between adults and children. Traditional indications for fluid resuscitation are 10% TBSA for children and 15% TBSA for adults.

We suggest that in the prehospital setting, significant burn patients receive an initial volume of 1 l per hour for adults and 0.5 l per hour for children.

Mode of resuscitation: intravenous versus oral

Fluids are usually given intravenously and should be warmed to minimize patient cooling. Typical fluids are Hartmann's, Ringers Lactate or Normal Saline. Box 18.3 shows the recommended fluid resuscitation format.

Box 18.3 **In hospital recommended fluid resuscitation for major burns (adapted from the Australian and New Zealand Burns Association**

- Adults need resuscitation fluids for the first 24 hours
- Adults need resuscitation if their estimated burn exceeds 15% TBSA
- Suggested resuscitation fluids are 3–4 mL/kg/%TBSA/24 hours Divided in half with one half given in first 8 hours of injury and the second over the following 16 hours
- Children need resuscitation if their estimated burn exceeds 10% TBSA
- Children need additional maintenance fluids
- Maintenance fluids in children should be 100 mL/kg for the first 10 kg, then 50 mL/kg for the next 10 kg, and 20 mL/kg for further weight (over 24-hour period).

Oral rehydration

Oral rehydration following a burn is often overlooked as a concept. In the absence of other injuries, assuming the patient is able to drink and unlikely to require immediate surgery, then oral fluids should be commenced. Whether sufficient fluid intake can be achieved is of some debate. But taking a 15% TBSA burn for example we can see that the fluid requirement would be just over 3 L in 24 hours, so a significant proportion of this could feasibly be administered orally in a relatively short timeframe.

Example: 15% TBSA in a 70 kg adult.
Fluids $= 3$ mL $\times$ 70 kg $\times$ 15% TBSA $= 3.15$ L in 24 hours.

The airway and burn injury (suspected inhalational injury)

There is often confusion over the terms airway burn and inhalation injury. The two are distinct entities and should be managed accordingly.

Airway burns

Burns to the face, such as occurs during a flash burn (Figure 18.5) or explosion, will cause thermal injury to the head and neck region. This may also involve the upper airways (above the larynx) such as the mouth, nostrils and pharynx. During the first 48 hours after burn injury, these areas are subject to significant soft-tissue oedema, which may result in subsequent upper airway compromise.

Key signs of upper airway injury or potential for upper airway obstruction are facial burns, particularly involving the lips, mouth and nose, singed nasal hairs, sooty sputum, productive cough, difficulty breathing, hoarse voice and flaring of the nasal alae.

Standard teaching is that early intubation is indicated for those deemed at high risk of delayed airway compromise even when they may have a GCS of 15 and are systemically well. In reality, intubation can often be postponed until reaching hospital where full anaesthetic and surgical support services are available.

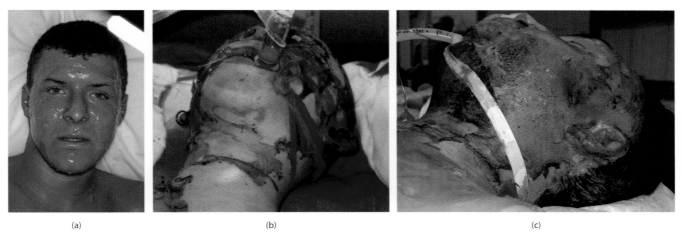

(a)　　　　　　　　　(b)　　　　　　　　　(c)

Figure 18.5 (a) Flash burn to face requiring observation but not intubation. (b, c) Severe facial burns requiring intubation.

If prehospital definitive airway management is required:

- This will often require either prehospital emergency anaesthesia or surgical airway under local anaesthetic and/or sedation.
- Use an uncut tube – cut tubes will not allow for subsequent facial swelling.
- Severe swelling may necessitate a smaller than calculated size endotracheal tube.
- Secure the tube with a suture through nose columella/septum (nasal intubation) or with interdental wire or suture (oral intubation). Adhesive tape often fails to stick to burnt skin. Ribbon tape or tube holders may be employed for short transfers, but may cut the face or lead to accidental extubation as the face swells.

Inhalational injury

Thermal injury to the lung and lower respiratory tract is rare due to the excellent heat filtering ability of the upper airway. However, where a patient is exposed to the by-products of combustion such as carbon monoxide, carbon dioxide, cyanide, ammonia, sulphur, nitrogen or phosphorus, a chemical injury to the lower respiratory tract and lung can occur and can be fatal.

Treatment involves giving the patient 100% oxygen in order to help flush out the carbon monoxide from their system. Assisted ventilation may be required if high flow oxygen alone is inadequate. Pulse oximetry is not reliable in patients with carbon monoxide poisoning and the reading may be artificially high.

Management of specific burns

Chemical burns

Chemical burns will continue to destroy tissues until removed by irrigation or neutralization. Consequently, all liquid chemical burns require very thorough irrigation early (ideally within 10 minutes of the burn) to limit tissue damage. Involved clothing must also be removed. Powder chemicals are better brushed off before irrigation and phosphorous must be kept damp otherwise it causes further injury. Prehospital carers must take care to protect

themselves from the contaminant by using gloves, eyewear and aprons.

Acids produce a coagulative necrosis, whereas alkalis produce a liquefactive necrosis.

Some chemicals can produce systemic toxicity. These include hypocalcaemia with hydrofluoric acid and inhalational injury with strong acids or ammonia. Table 18.1 shows some key agents that need special management.

Electrical burns (Box 18.4)

Tissue damage in electrical burns occurs secondary to heat generated by the resistance of the tissues. The resistance of skin is site dependent, i.e. glaborous skin as found on the foot soles and palms have higher resistance than thinner skin. Resistance differs according to tissue type with decreasing resistance seen going from bone to skin to fat to nerve or muscle. Hence bone involvement can result in a significant temperature rise with ongoing heat escape once the current has stopped. This results in significant local tissue damage.

Box 18.4 **Key concepts in prehospital management of electrical burns**

- High risk of C-spine damage (associated falls etc.)
- ECG is vital
- Assess involved limbs for compartment syndrome.

Fasciotomy and escharotomy

Escharotomy is an emergency procedure used in circumferential burns where there is vascular compromise to the affected limb secondary to a tourniquet effect of the burn in combination with tissue oedema. Circumferential chest burns may compromise ventilation in the same way. Escharotomy involves making a longitudinal incision through the burned area in the limb or chest wall. In contrast, fasciotomy defines the release of a subcutaneous fascial

Table 18.1 Specific agents to be aware of in prehospital management of burns

Agent	Problem/s	Treatment
Hydrofluoric acid	Highly corrosive and potentially fatal. Hydrogen ions damage skin then fluoride ions penetrate to cause deep damage. Arrhythmias may occur secondary to hypocalcaemia and hypomagnesaemia	Prompt water irrigation, trim fingernails, and inactivate free fluoride with topical calcium gluconate. ECG monitoring
Cement burns	Wet cement is caustic with pH up to 12.9. Pain and burning occur late	Prolonged irrigation with water (up to 1 hour)
Phosphorus burns	Oxidizes to phosphorus pentoxide. Particles of phosphorus can become embedded in the skin and cause deep burns	Copious water irrigation, remove particles, apply copper sulphate, which can facilitate particle removal
Petrol	Can be either ignition or immersion without ignition. This complex mixture of hydrocarbons can cause skin and airway damage	Irrigation/cooling as per standard treatment, but may require additional fluid resuscitation
Bitumen	Transported and used in liquid forms (Temperatures up to 150°C). Burns are due to the high temperature rather than the toxic effects	Cool with copious amounts of water
Tar	Burns by heat and phenol toxicity	Treat by cooling and remove with toluene
Eye involvement	Susceptible to damage due to thin	Copious irrigation and ophthalmology referral

compartment and compartment syndrome and this may also be part of the escharotomy procedure.

These procedures are ideally performed in a controlled environment under general anaesthetic with access to electrocautery for haemostasis and therefore the prehospital setting is rarely appropriate and may cause further injury. If situation, delay and geography dictate that this is necessary for preservation of life or limb then suitable analgesia and dressings will be required after the incisions are made until more advanced care is available.

Referral pathways: when to refer?

Patients with significant burns irrespective of mechanism should be referred to or taken to local accident and emergency departments for further assessment and treatment. All resuscitation burns should go to a burns unit/centre either directly or after initial treatment has begun in an emergency department

(Box 18.5). Any patient with a suspected non-accidental injury (Figure 18.6) should be taken to an appropriate burns center and a safeguarding referral initiated.

Box 18.5 **Other factors to guide referral to a burns centre**

- Extremes of age (children and elderly patients)
- Complex injuries, e.g. site of injury (face, hands, perineum and any flexure including neck or axillae, circumferential dermal or full thickness limb, torso, neck)
- Inhalational injury
- Mechanism: chemical >5% or hydrofluoric acid 1%
- Ionizing radiation
- High-pressure steam
- High-tension electrical
- Suspected non-accidental injury
- Large size >5% children 10% adults
- Coexisting conditions, i.e. medical/pregnancy/fractures, etc.

Mass casualties involving burn injury

Mass burn injury is more common and has repeatedly produced up to 300 hospital admissions in the civilian setting worldwide.

- Burns may coexist with other trauma injuries.
- High-risk environments for mass burns in particular include off-shore oil rigs, mines, nightclubs and enclosed spaces with public gatherings.

Recent examples include the Melbourne Bush Fires (2009 – 173 dead at scene), the Bali nightclub bombing (2002 – 411 casualties), the Piper Alpha oil-rig disaster (1988 – 228 casualties), the King's Cross Underground fire (1988 – 91 casualties), and the Bradford Football Stadium fire (1982 – 256 casualties).

The emergency response must be pre-planned and well communicated to be effective. There must be a reliable triage mechanism to prevent swamping of scarce specialist burns care facilities with injuries that can be adequately managed in a standard hospital setting.

Triage categories
- Minor injury: (small burns <10% TBSA, minimal other injury, delayed or no hospital attendance).
- Major injury requiring resuscitation and prompt general hospital care (burns 15–30% TBSA with or without other injuries).
- Severe injury requiring specialist burn facility care (burns >30% TBSA adults).
- Expectant – in mass casualty situations, this group will include patients who might survive given individual and prompt care, but this patient type is 'resource hungry' and distracts from caring for multiple other patients with better chances of survival.
- Dead at the scene.

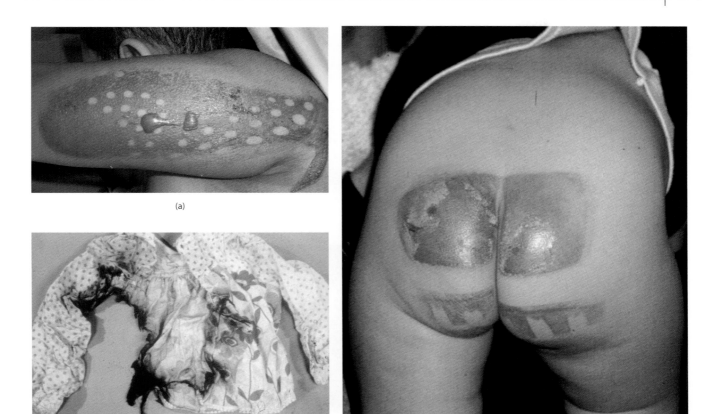

Figure 18.6 (a) Contact burn from iron in self-defence. (b) Potential non-accidental contact injury to child's bottom. (c) Corroborating evidence from the scene may clarify the history given.

Tips from the field

- Prehospital assessment of burn extent and depth is notoriously unreliable, if there is any doubt treat judiciously and transport to a specialist centre
- No international guidelines exist for advanced airway management in these patients: the decision will be multifactorial including: patient condition, transport times and the skill set of your prehospital team
- Cool the burn not the patient – hypothermia in large burns needs to be avoided
- Ketamine (intravenous, intramuscular, nasal) provides excellent pain relief
- Avoid circumferential application of cling film to burns.

Further reading

Allison K, Porter K. Consensus on the prehospital approach to burns patient management. *Emerg Med J* 2004;**21**:112–114.

American College of Surgeons. Chapter 9: Thermal Injuries. In: ACS Committee on Trauma, ed. Advanced Trauma Life Support for Doctors (ATLS), Eighth Edition, 211–224. 2008.

BLEVE video: http://www.youtube.com/watch?v=sl-JgyQA7u0

British Burn Association. *Emergency Management of severe burns course manual*. UK Version. Manchester: 2008.

Ching-Chuan L, Rossignol AM. Landmarks in burn prevention. *Burns* 2000; **26**, 5:422–434.

Enoch S, Roshan A, Shah M. Emergency and early management of burns and scalds. *BMJ* 2009:**338**;937–941.

Hettiaratchy S, Dziewulski P. ABC of Burns. *BMJ* 2004;**328**:1366–1429.

Muehlberger T, Ottomann C, Toman N, *et al*. Emergency prehospital care of burn patients. *Surgeon* 2010;**8**:101–104.

National Association of Emergency Medical technicians. *Prehospital Trauma Life support Manual*. 1994

National Burn Care review. National burn injury referral guidelines. In: *Standards and Strategy for Burn Care*. London: NBCR, 2001:6.

Smith J.J, Malyon AD, Scerri GV, Burge TS. A comparison of serial halving and the rule of nines as a prehospital assessment tool in burns. *BJPS* 2005;**58**:957–967.

Tobiasen J, Hiebert JM, Edlich RF. The abbreviated Burn Severity Index. *Ann Emerg Med* 1982;**11**:260–262.

WHO Facts about injuries http://www.who.int/violence_injury_prevention /publications/other_injury/en/burns_factsheet.pdf.

CHAPTER 19

Trauma: Suspension and Crush

Jason van der Velde

Cork University Hospital, Cork, Ireland

OVERVIEW

By the end of this chapter you should know:

- The haemodynamic effects of entrapment, suspension and subsequent rescue
- The pathophysiology of muscle and soft tissue trauma
- The management of a patient immobile for many hours
- How to release a crushed limb or someone suspended in a harness.

Introduction

Crush injury occurs when a prolonged static compressive force sufficient to interfere with normal tissue metabolic function is applied to a body part (Figure 19.1). The extremities are most commonly affected, with the lower limbs being more frequently involved than the upper limbs. Significant crush injuries to the head and torso often result in early death from other causes (e.g. traumatic brain injury, asphyxia, exsanguination).

When a crushed limb is released a predictable sequence of pathophysiological events occurs, known collectively as **crush syndrome**. These events include hypovolaemia, rescue cardioplegia, electrolyte and acid–base abnormalities, rhabdomyolysis and acute renal failure.

Suspension syncope occurs because of motionless vertical suspension and orthostatic pooling of blood in the lower extremities. The inability to regain a horizontal position and the resultant hypoperfusion of the brain leads to orthostatic syncope and, if uncorrected, death (Figure 19.2). The term **suspension trauma** defines a 'crush syndrome' resulting from compressive forces applied by a harness to the lower extremities during prolonged vertical suspension.

Rescue cardioplegia: the problem with uncontrolled limb release

Rescue cardioplegia describes the myocardial stunning that can occur on uncontrolled release of a compressing force, harness or tourniquet (Figure 19.3).

ABC of Prehospital Emergency Medicine, First Edition.
Edited by Tim Nutbeam and Matthew Boylan.
© 2013 John Wiley & Sons, Ltd. Published 2013 by John Wiley & Sons, Ltd.

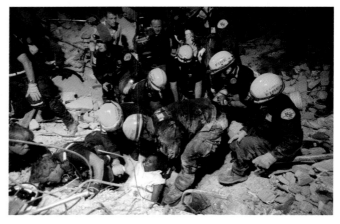

Figure 19.1 A Haitian woman is pulled from earthquake debris by members of LA County SAR. (U.S. Navy Photo by Mass Communication Specialist 2nd Class Justin Stumberg).

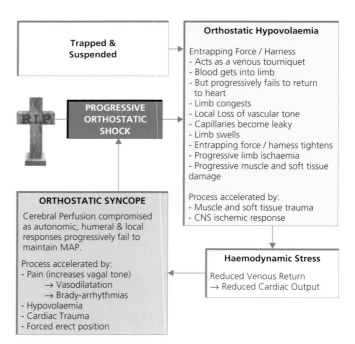

		Orthostatic Hypovolaemia
Trapped & Suspended		Entrapping Force / Harness - Acts as a venous tourniquet - Blood gets into limb - But progressively fails to return to heart - Limb congests - Local Loss of vascular tone - Capillaries become leaky - Limb swells - Entrapping force / harness tightens - Progressive limb ischaemia - Progressive muscle and soft tissue damage

PROGRESSIVE ORTHOSTATIC SHOCK

Process accelerated by:
- Muscle and soft tissue trauma
- CNS ischemic response

ORTHOSTATIC SYNCOPE

Cerebral Perfusion compromised as autonomic, humeral & local responses progressively fail to maintain MAP.

Process accelerated by:
- Pain (increases vagal tone)
  → Vasodilatation
  → Brady-arrhythmias
- Hypovolaemia
- Cardiac Trauma
- Forced erect position

Haemodynamic Stress

Reduced Venous Return
→ Reduced Cardiac Output

Figure 19.2 Mechanism of suspension syncope.

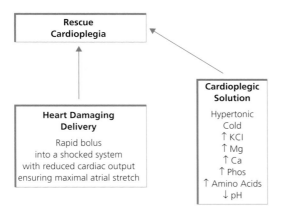

Figure 19.3 Mechanism of rescue cardioplegia.

As cold 'toxic' pooled blood under pressure in congested limbs is rapidly released back into the systemic circulation, a sudden, transient and considerable increase in preload to the right heart occurs. Increasing preload by so much and so rapidly results in sudden atrial stretch, which causes alterations in conduction properties, potentially stunning the myocardium into asystole or initiating atrial fibrillation. This occurs at the same time as afterload and systemic vascular resistance is rapidly reduced by allowing blood to flow again into the previously isolated limb. Even in the controlled conditions of the operating theatre, acute hypotension after tourniquet deflation is commonly observed.

Hypotension is further complicated by post-ischaemic reactive hyperaemia in the released limbs. This results in decreased venous return and a further rapid reduction in cardiac output. Taking the weight off a harness or releasing two limbs trapped by a dashboard may result in both limbs being suddenly released, and as such the reduction in cardiac output can in itself be fatal, particularly in the presence of a relatively fixed cardiac output from heart disease, drugs or pre-existing valvular heart defects.

Cardiac electrical activity functions in both a very narrow pH range and concentrations of intra- and extracellular ions, in particular calcium and potassium. There are a number of mechanisms that can illicit fatal cardioplegia. Damaged, congested, ischaemic limbs can quiet literally brew an 'ideal cardioplegic solution', which when released into circulation can precipitate a fatal arrhythmia, especially in combination with the haemodynamic effects described. It is well-recognized that these electrolyte abnormalities may develop over time as limb reperfusion is not an all or nothing effect, but rather a 'bolus' then tapering off 'infusion' or 'reperfusion' phenomena (Figure 19.4).

Muscle and soft-tissue trauma: whole system effects

Even if the initial trauma is insufficient to damage muscle and soft tissues, the combination of pressure, stasis and ischaemia underneath an entrapping force, harness or tourniquet will usually initiate some irreversible muscle death within an hour. A constant external mechanical pressure prevents muscle from adequately maintaining cell wall integrity by literally forcing extracellular cations and fluid against their normal electrochemical and osmotic gradients. Cell wall extrusion pumps eventually become overwhelmed, allowing water with dissociated sodium, chloride and calcium ions to enter the cell. Progressive tissue oedema ultimately leads to cell death.

Compartment syndrome occurs where intramuscular compartment forces act continually above the diastolic blood pressure resulting in compression and ultimately death of nerves, blood vessels and muscle inside their normal anatomical spaces within the body. An external entrapping force will nearly always compress more than one compartment.

With so many uncontrollable variables in the prehospital environment, it is impossible to accurately predict muscle viability against Ischaemia time. Lengthy entrapments will obviously have a detrimental effect, but it important to appreciate that there is absolutely no 'minimum' universally agreed time for 'safe' suspension or entrapment.

When the integrity of muscle cell walls are breeched by an external force, intracellular components leak extracellularly while water and extracellular ions will flow into the damaged tissue, so called **third space fluid loss**. Cell contents will literally be forced into the vascular compartment and, as such, an isolated insult has the potential to initiate a distal systemic effect, the principle effect being direct and indirect renal damage.

Acute kidney injury: an indirect effect of muscle damage

Direct renal damage result from the nephrotoxic properties of a variety of leaked intracellular substances such as proteases and purines. However, damage principally occurs indirectly as the kidneys attempt to filter acidotic plasma and the muscle protein, myoglobin (Figure 19.5).

It is very important, from a therapeutic perspective, to appreciate that myoglobin itself causes no renal damage. It is a small protein that is freely filtered and eliminated by the kidneys with no nephrotoxic properties. Myoglobin release unfortunately does not occur in isolation. Organic acids are released into the circulation during

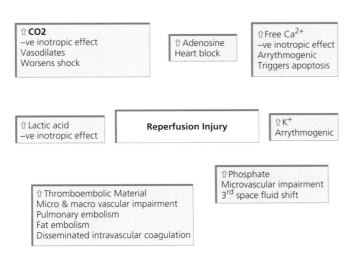

Figure 19.4 Mechanism of reperfusion injury.

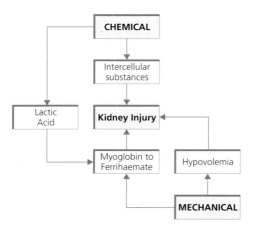

Figure 19.5 Mechanism of acute kidney injury.

cell death, while progressive muscle ischaemia results in lactic acid production. This by-product of anaerobic metabolism, together with other organic acids being released from cells, lowers the pH of urine. As the filtered myoglobin combines with urine below a pH of 5.6, it is converted to a larger protein, ferrihaemate. Ferrihaemate is both directly nephrotoxic to renal tubules and causes mechanical obstruction by precipitating within the lumen of nephrons. Inadequate circulating volume due to hypovolaemia and third space fluid shift will contribute significantly to the development of an acute kidney injury and subsequent renal failure as it reduces renal perfusion, just as the kidneys are seeking additional filtrate to dilute urine and wash away rapidly accumulating ferrihaemate and other mechanical obstructions.

Management

Isolate and move to a place of safety

By applying arterial tourniquets just proximal to a harness or entrapping force, one can prevent the massive haemorrhage or rescue cardioplegia frequently encountered with sudden release of an entrapment on scene; transferring the problem to a safer, controlled environment (Box 19.1). This ethos fits well within the established philosophy of 'scoop and run'. In the case of a suspended casualty, they should be rescued as soon as is safely possible and placed in the horizontal recovery position if consciousness is impaired. There is no evidence to support rescue in the semi-recumbent position.

Tourniquets must be purposefully designed for prehospital use, and ideally provide a broad, evenly distributed force, sufficient to isolate arterial supply to the limb. They will inevitably cause a degree of ischaemic reperfusion injury themselves, but the benefits greatly outweigh this risk, especially where ambulance transit times are short. If rescue has been completed without the application of a tourniquet and the patient remains stable then delayed application of a tourniquet is not required as 'washout' will have already occurred.

Where tourniquets have been applied, they should remain in place until the patient is fully resuscitated, potential haemorrhage points addressed and in a safe environment. Ideally this will be in the hospital resuscitation room or operating theatre, with full cardiovascular monitoring and support. There may be cases where there is a long delay to definitive care and in these cases 'staged release' should be employed.

Limb amputation may be indicated if the limb is deemed non-viable or if the patient's clinical condition deteriorates during rescue. Amputation prior to release will also prevent the sequelae of the reperfusion syndrome by removing the source of the problem.

Resuscitate the system

A haemodynamically stable system will handle a reperfusion injury better than a collapsed, shocked system. A great deal of thought needs to be applied to preparing the circulation prior to entrapment release. There is a wealth of data from disaster medicine literature to support early circulatory resuscitation prior to reperfusion. Spending time optimizing an entrapped person poses significant health and safety risks, the obvious being the stability of the entrapping structure and the potential for injury to personnel. Medical staff must work in close collaboration with rescue personnel, ideally as an integrated team, to understand differing roles and needs.

Systemic resuscitation prior to extrication in earthquake entrapment has been shown to significantly improve outcome. An initial 20 mL/kg bolus (10 mL/kg in elderly people) of 0.9% saline should be administered prior to release in patients trapped for over 1 hour. Ongoing fluid administration should continue at a rate of 5 ml/kg/hour with additional fluid boluses titrated against clinical response. Administration of potassium-containing solutions (e.g. Hartmann's) must be strictly avoided in the field to avoid hyperkalaemia. When the patient is collapsed in a confined space, intravenous access maybe challenging and intraosseous infusion should be considered.

For prolonged transfers the patient should have a urinary catheter placed to monitor urine output. Improving urine output is a good indication of end organ perfusion and that preventative management is starting to become effective. When this is not possible simple verification of urine output may be an acceptable compromise.

Analgesia

Pain is often minimal in the early post-crush phase because of circulating endorphins and pressure neuropraxia. As limbs become progressively more swollen and the intrinsic analgesic effects of endorphins wear off, pain will become more problematic. Judicious use of opiates and/or analgesic doses of ketamine (0.2 mg/kg) should be employed. Regional local anaesthetic blocks may also be useful in providing additional analgesia for the trapped limb, but avoid long acting agents which may mask the onset of compartment syndrome.

Staged tourniquet release strategy

Tourniquet application for longer than an hour causes further rhabdomyolysis, skin necrosis and neurovascular damage. A staged or staggered tourniquet release strategy (Figure 19.6) may therefore be considered when evacuation to hospital is likely to be prolonged (>1 hour). This allows for controlled washout and systemic redistribution of ischaemic metabolites during reperfusion. It should be employed on one limb at a time and the patient must be monitored closely. If at any point the patient becomes unstable, then the tourniquet should be immediately reapplied and the patient's cardiovascular state managed prior reinstituting the release strategy. Once optimal volume resuscitation has been achieved further hypotensive episodes may be treated with inotropic or vasopressive agent.

Management of hyperkalaemia

Post-release hyperkalaemic ECG changes (QRS widening) should be treated emergently with 10–30 mL of intravenous 10% calcium gluconate and an enema of sodium or calcium resonium if available. Calcium should only be given under these circumstances, as you run the risk of precipitating metastatic calcification and further muscle damage.

Standard medical management strategies for hyperkalaemia tend to be ineffective, as hyperkalaemia in a crush injury results from muscle wall damage, and not ionic or osmotic shifts. Patients must therefore be immediately transferred to an intensive care environment capable of haemofiltration.

In the event that prehospital anaesthesia is required as part of the resuscitative process, non-depolarizing muscle relaxants (e.g. rocuronium) should be used instead of suxamethonium to minimize avoidable elevations in serum potassium.

Alkaline diuresis

When evacuation times are prolonged (>4 hours) the use of alkaline diuresis may be considered. Alkaline diuresis will prevent the precipitation of toxic myoglobin metabolites in nephrons and help ameliorate acidosis and hyperkalaemia. A 50-mL bolus of 8.4% sodium bicarbonate can be added to each alternate litre of fluid administered, titrated to a urinary pH ≥6.5. If prolonged alkaline diuresis is planned, then 0.9% saline should be alternated with 5% dextrose to reduce the sodium load and risk of pulmonary oedema (particularly in the presence of pre-existing renal or heart failure). The risk of iatrogenic metabolic alkalosis and sodium overload is greater in the unmonitored prehospital environment and where possible alkaline diuresis should be left for the hospital environment where it can be titrated to urine output, urine pH and serum pH.

Triage

Where possible, all patients with significant crush injury or suspension trauma should be triaged to a facility capable of providing renal replacement therapy (haemofiltration).

Future considerations

Strong evidence is emerging that calcium antagonists, given either before the onset of ischaemia, or at the time of reperfusion, ameliorate myocardial 'stunning' by preventing excessive calcium uptake.

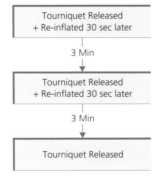

Figure 19.6 Staged tourniquet release strategy.

> **Tips from the field**
>
> - Resuscitate the system prior to release
> - Consider use of tourniquets to prevent rescue cardioplegia
> - Limb amputation may be considered in the non-viable limb
> - Prepare for clinical deterioration after release.

Further reading

Adisesh A, Lee C, Porter K. Harness suspension and first aid management: development of an evidence-based guideline. *Emerg Med J* 2011;**28**: 265–268.

Ashkenazi I, Isakovich B, Kluger Y, *et al*. Prehospital management of earthquake casualties buried under rubble. *Prehosp Disast Med* 2005;**20**:122–133.

Sever MS, Vanholder R, Lameire N. Management of crush-related injuries after disasters. *N Engl J Med* 2006;**354**:1052–1063.

Townsend HS, Goodman SB, Schurman DJ, *et al*. Tourniquet release: systemic and metabolic effects. *Acta Anaesthesiol Scand* 1996;**40**:1234–1237.

CHAPTER 20

Trauma: Ballistic and Blast

Matthew Boylan

Royal Centre for Defence Medicine, University Hospitals Birmingham, Birmingham, UK

OVERVIEW

By the end of this chapter you should:

- Understand the basic pathophysiology of firearms injuries and blast trauma
- Understand how to approach a ballistic scene
- Recognize that the level of treatment provided will be dictated by the threat level
- Understand how to manage the patient with blast or firearms injuries.

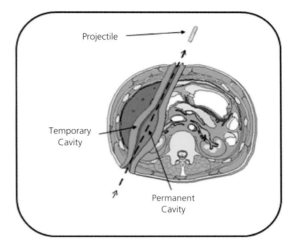

Figure 20.1 Cavitation.

Introduction

The term ballistic trauma encompasses any physical trauma sustained from the discharge of arms or munitions. The two main types of ballistic trauma likely to be experienced by prehospital practitioners are firearm and blast injury. The rise in terrorist activity over the last decade and the increased use of firearms during criminal acts means such injuries are becoming increasingly common.

Firearm injuries

Firearms are weapons designed to expel projectiles at high velocity through the confined burning of a propellant. The degree of injury produced by projectiles is determined by a number of factors including muzzle velocity, projectile mass, entrance profile, projectile construction (e.g. expanding tip), distance travelled within the body and the elasticity of the impacted tissues. As a projectile passes through the body it displaces tissue in its path resulting in laceration and crush injury. The clinical consequences of this will be determined by the structures traversed. If the projectile encounters a vital structure such as the brain, heart or great vessels the wound may prove lethal. Projectiles with higher energy, such as those fired by long-barrelled weapons (e.g. assault rifles), generate a shockwave which drives tissues radially from the wound track creating a temporary cavity (Figure 20.1). As this cavity expands it forms a vacuum which draws in contamination from outside. After

passage of the projectile the temporary cavity collapses down to leave a permanent cavity and in doing so trapping contamination deep within the wound. Different tissues tolerate cavitation in different ways. Cavitation within solid organs such as the liver, kidney and brain leads to massive tissue disruption. By comparison elastic tissues such as muscle and lung tissue have the ability to stretch and tolerate the effects of cavitation to a greater degree.

Projectiles may traverse body cavities and often take unpredictable courses. Attempting to predict the path and extent of internal injury from the size and location of the external wounds is therefore not recommended.

Blast injuries

Explosive detonation is the rapid chemical transformation of a solid or liquid into a gas. Under high pressure and temperatures this gas expands rapidly outwards as a wave of high pressure. Air is highly compressed at the leading edge creating a shock front called a **blast wave**. When unobstructed the blast wave rapidly loses its pressure and velocity with distance and time. If solid structures such as walls or buildings are encountered, the blast wave is reflected and amplified resulting in higher over-pressures and greater potential for injury. The blast wave interacts with body tissues by imparting stress and shear particularly at gas-tissue interfaces. This is termed

ABC of Prehospital Emergency Medicine, First Edition.
Edited by Tim Nutbeam and Matthew Boylan.
© 2013 John Wiley & Sons, Ltd. Published 2013 by John Wiley & Sons, Ltd.

primary blast injury. The tympanic membranes, lungs and bowel are particularly at risk (Box 20.1). Blast lung is the commonest cause of death in immediate survivors. In severe cases, primary blast injury can induce vagally mediated bradycardia, apnoea and hypotension. Survivors in this group are rare as a casualty close enough to an explosion to sustain this level of primary injury will commonly have other lethal injuries (secondary and/or tertiary).

Box 20.1 **Primary blast injury.**

Injury type	Pathophysiology	Clinical Features

Blast lung	*Blast wave damages causes:*
	• Interstitial haemorrhage/oedema
	• Intra-alveolar haemorrhage/oedema
	  ○ Pulmonary oedema
	• Parenchymal lacerations
	  ○ Pneumothorax
	• Alveolar-venous fistulas
	  ○ Air embolism
		• Dyspnoea
		• Chest pain
		• Haemoptysis
		• Wheeze
		• Crepitations
		• Severe { Apncea / Bradycardia / Hypotension

Blast bowel	*Blast wave damage causes:* • Bowel Contusion • Bowel perforation (may be delayed) • Intra-luminal bleeding Large bowel > Small bowel	• Abdominal pain • Malaena • Peritonitis • Shock Often delayed onset
Blast ear	*Blast wave damage causes:* • Rupture of the tympanic membrane • Ossicle dislocation • Inner ear damage	• Hearing loss • Ear pain • Vertigo
Blast brain	*Blast wave damage causes:* • Concussion syndrome • Intra/extra-axial haemorrhage	• Loss of consciousness • Amnesia • Disorientation

Blast waves and primary blast injury are seen following detonation of high-order explosives (e.g. Semtex, C-4, ammonium nitrate fuel oil). They are not a feature of low-order explosives (e.g. gunpowder, petroleum-based explosives) where gas expansion is subsonic.

Fragments of the explosive device itself (primary fragments) and other material energized by the blast (secondary fragments) are projected outwards and may cause penetrating injury. This is termed **secondary blast injury** and is seen with both high- and low-order explosives (Figure 20.2). Fragments tend to be irregular in shape, size and mass and therefore produce varying degrees of tissue injury and penetration depending upon their velocity and the site of impact. Biological material from victims such as bone may also form projectiles and cause penetrating injury further afield. Transmission of blood-borne viruses by this route has been reported and post-exposure prophylaxis is advised.

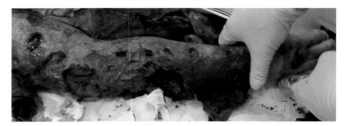

Figure 20.2 Secondary blast injury - fragmentation injury to arm.

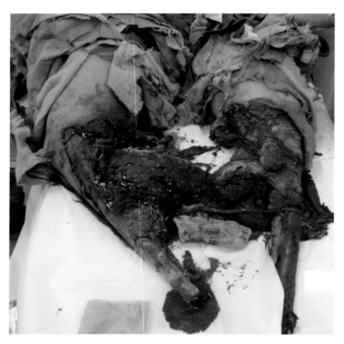

Figure 20.3 Tertiary blast injury - traumatic amputation lower limbs.

As the blast wave spreads out radially it accelerates the air through which it traverses causing turbulence and physical displacement of objects in its path. This is the **blast wind** and injuries resulting from it are termed **tertiary blast injury**. Bodies may be thrown against solid objects causing blunt injury, or limbs traumatically amputated (Figure 20.3). Structural collapse as a result of blast wind may result in crush and blunt trauma from falling debris. **Quaternary blast injury** is the term given to any other explosion-related injury including burns and psychological trauma.

Incident management

The potential threat to rescuers from active shooters, secondary explosive devices and damaged infrastructure (e.g. structural collapse, fire) should not be underestimated. Appropriate personal protective equipment (PPE), a safe scene approach and regular dynamic risk assessments on scene are essential in mitigating risk to the rescuer.

Personal protective equipment

Blast incidents commonly result in hazardous ground debris (e.g. broken glass, masonry, twisted metal), a risk of falling debris and

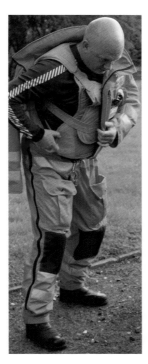

Figure 20.4 Application of lightweight ballistic jacket.

a respiratory hazard from hanging dust. Full PPE including eye and respiratory protection is therefore essential if deploying to such incidents. The possibility of an associated CBRN or HAZMAT release must be considered in all incidents involving blast. Personal radiation dosimeters should be worn and chemical escape hoods carried until the scene is declared safe.

Lightweight ballistic vests provide some protection against handgun, stab and low-velocity fragmentation. When available this should be applied prior to deployment to the scene of any ballistics incident (Figure 20.4).

Tactical medics deploying within the outer cordon of an active firearms incident (e.g. marauding terrorist firearms attack) should be provided with additional Kevlar ballistic helmets and ballistic vests with integral high-velocity plates for additional protection against high-velocity rounds. Such individuals should also have received additional training in tactical medicine.

Approach to scene

The police are responsible for the control of incidents involving firearms and/or blast. Their initial actions will follow the four Cs approach (Box 20.2).

Box 20.2 **Four Cs approach**

The four Cs:	
Confirm	Confirm the presence of the threat
Clear	Clear people away from the threat as quickly as practicable
Cordon	Create a cordon to keep people at a safe distance
Control	Create an Incident Control Point (ICP) to control the cordon

Where a local operating channel or talk group is in operation the prehospital practitioner should utilize this to optimize their situational awareness during the approach to an incident. An emergency service rendezvous point (RVP) should be designated by the coordinating police force at a location that is both remote and protected from the incident. It is critical that the prehospital provider obtains an accurate location for the RVP including the preferred route of access, prior to making their way to the incident. In the absence of an RVP, prehospital providers should not attempt to proceed towards the scene but instead hold off at a safe distance until one has been designated. Approach to the RVP should be made slowly and with emergency lights and sirens turned off where requested. Incidents do not always remain static and the RVP may have to be relocated if the threat moves. Ensure vehicles are parked in a manner to facilitate rapid evacuation. It is preferable for casualties to be brought to the RVP for triage, assessment and treatment. Where deployment forward of the RVP is required it should be in a level of PPE appropriate for the threat posed and with adequate police protection.

Dynamic risk assessment

Incidents involving firearms and blast are often dynamic in nature. They may involve multiple assailants and/or locations as well as the real risk of follow-up attacks or secondary explosive devices deliberately targeting emergency personnel. When attending a firearms or blast incident it is essential to remain observant at all times and not become complacent. When working as part of a prehospital team, one member should have designated responsibility for team safety. If at any point the practitioner feels at risk they should notify the nearest police officer and make immediate plans to retreat to the RVP, ideally with the patient. In the event of shots being discharged in the vicinity of the practitioner the immediate action should be to get low and move into hard cover (e.g. behind an earth mound, base of tree, wall or behind a ballistic shield) with the patient where possible. Vehicles provide cover from view but limited protection against high velocity rounds which can pass easily through bodywork into personnel sheltering behind. If this is the only available cover the engine block and wheels provides the greatest level of protection.

Be aware that assailants themselves may become casualties at blast and firearms incidents. Ensure the police have searched and disarmed all casualties prior to approaching. This includes injured officers who may through injury or fear of further attack lose their ability to make rational decisions regarding the discharge of their weapon.

Forensic considerations

All firearms and blast incidents are treated as scenes of crime by the police. Do not touch objects or disturb the environment except to treat patients to avoid contaminating the forensic evidence. Dead bodies should only be disturbed to give access to live casualties. When cutting clothing from casualties avoid cutting through points of penetration and do not dispose of any item of clothing. Finally, keep control of your equipment to prevent it being lost to the police forensic team particularly if death is declared on scene.

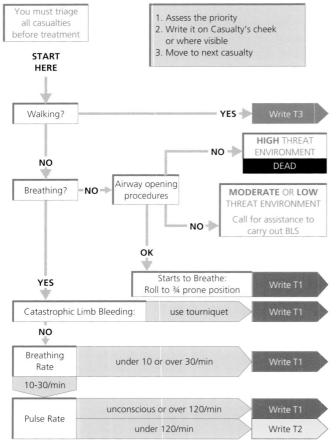

Figure 20.5 Triage sieve.

Triage

Mass shootings and bomb blasts often result in multiple casualties. Initial triage should be performed using a simple triage tool such as the triage sieve or START triage tool (Figure 20.5). Designed for patients with blunt trauma, these tools may under-triage a number of patients with significant ballistic or blast injury.

Reassessment and where necessary modification of the initial triage allocation should then be undertaken by experienced clinicians at the casualty clearing station. The characteristic physiological response to blood loss of increasing tachycardia can be less marked in penetrating trauma and often manifests with bradycardia or relative bradycardia. This patient group may be missed by triage tools using tachycardia as a marker for treatment prioritization. Similarly patients with airway burns and blast lung may be ambulatory in the early stages and inappropriately triaged to the delayed category. It is essential these patients are identified at this stage and receive appropriate upgrading.

Tympanic membrane rupture is indicative of blast wave exposure; however, its absence cannot be used to rule out primary blast injury. Patients presenting with both traumatic limb amputation and early signs of blast lung have a very high mortality and may be appropriate for expectant categorization in the mass casualty situation.

Management of ballistic trauma

The initial assessment and management of ballistic trauma should follow the standard <C>ABCDE approach. In most situations the level of threat to the rescuer will be low and the full spectrum of prehospital critical care intervention possible. In the event of an unexpected escalation in threat level (e.g. active shooter, secondary explosion) the degree of intervention should be restricted accordingly and primacy given to team safety (Figure 20.6).

Catastrophic haemorrhage control

Rapidly assess for exsanguinating limb haemorrhage and apply a tourniquet if indicated. The time of application should be noted. Where haemorrhage remains uncontrolled consider a second

HOT ZONE (HIGH Threat)	WARM ZONE (Moderate threat)	COLD ZONE (Low Threat)
There is a direct and immesiate threat to patients or responders	A potential hostile threat remains but is not direct or immediate	There is no significant danger or threat to responders or patients
Examples: • Active shooting–incoming fire • Imminent blast threat • Imminent structural collapse	**Examples:** • Active shooter–not in vicinity • Threat of secondary device • Structural damage evident	**Examples:** • Active shooter–police all clear • Explosion–bomb squad all clear • Emergency Services RVP

INTERVENTIONS
 	
Evacuate self from danger
 	
Evacuate casualty from danger
 	
<C> Tourniquet application
 	
A Position ¾ prone
 	
Provision of additional care would put rescuers at unnecessary risk
	INTERVENTIONS:
	
	Be prepared to evacuate
	<C> Tourniquet application
	   Novel Haemostatics
	
	A Airway positioning
	   Airway adjuncts
	
	B Chest seal
	   Needle decompression
	
	C Pressure dressings
	   Splinting fractures
	   Pelvic Binder
	
	D Immobilization if indicated
	
	E Hypothermia prevention
		INTERVENTIONS:
		
		Full **<C>ABCDE** Assessment
		
		Full Spectrum of Interventions
		
		Rapid transfer to definitive care

Figure 20.6 Staged care.

tourniquet above the first particularly on proximal limb injuries and/or amputations. Patients presenting in traumatic cardiac arrest or in a peri-arrest state with critical hypovolaemia following significant limb trauma should have tourniquets applied even in the absence of active bleeding as rebleeding is common with resuscitation and/or movement during packaging.

Catastrophic bleeding from junctional zones should be controlled immediately by a combination of novel haemostatics, pressure dressings and direct pressure.

Airway management

Penetrating injury or blast trauma to the face or neck may result in complete or partial airway obstruction as a result of bleeding, soft-tissue disruption, haematoma expansion or loss of bony support to the upper airway structures (Figure 20.7). Conscious patients will maintain themselves in the optimum position to maintain their own airway and drain secretions and blood. Where appropriate this position should be maintained during transfer to a facility capable of fibreoptic intubation and/or surgical tracheostomy. Patients should not be forced to lie supine. Obtunded or unconscious patients with significant facial bleeding and pooling of secretions should be maintained in a position to allow postural drainage (e.g. lateral trauma position) while an airway management plan is formed. Where transfer distances are short and the patient's injuries permit, patients should be maintained and transferred in the lateral position with high-flow oxygen and regular airway toilet. In cases where transfer time, persistent obstruction or other injuries dictate further airway intervention, the location and severity of injury will determine the type of intervention selected (Figure 20.8).

Cervical spine immobilization

Penetrating ballistic trauma to the neck involving the cervical spine is often fatal. Unstable cervical spine injuries are therefore extremely rare in survivors. For this reason routine cervical spine immobilization is not recommended for patients with penetrating head or neck trauma unless there is clear evidence of neurological deficit. In these cases head blocks only are recommended in order that the neck remains clear for vascular observation. In the presence of mixed blunt and penetrating injury (e.g. blast) immobilization should be undertaken.

Breathing management

The whole chest should be inspected for wounds. Roll the casualty so that posterior wounds are not missed and remember to check the axilla and neck. Do not be falsely reassured by lack of wounds to the chest, as projectiles may still traverse the thoracic cavity from remote wound sites. Sucking chest wounds should be sealed off as soon as they are found using occlusive or valved dressings. Assess for and rapidly treat tension pneumothorax with needle decompression and/or finger thoracostomy if ventilated. Insertion of an intercostal drain may be indicated if transfer distance and time is prolonged or if the patient is spontaneously breathing. Drains should not be inserted through existing wounds.

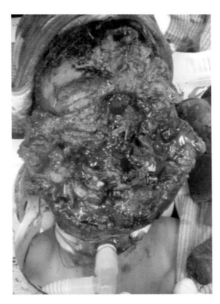

Figure 20.7 Facial blast injury requiring a primary surgical airway.

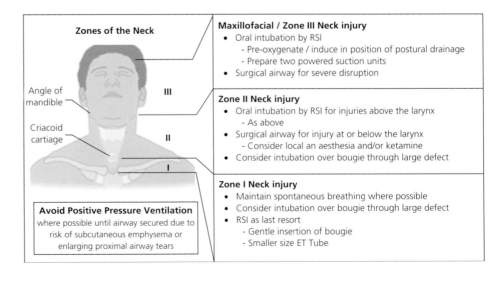

Figure 20.8 Ballistic airway management.

Zones of the Neck

Angle of mandible

Criacoid cartilage

III

II

I

Maxillofacial / Zone III Neck injury
- Oral intubation by RSI
  - Pre-oxygenate / induce in position of postural drainage
  - Prepare two powered suction units
- Surgical airway for severe disruption

Zone II Neck injury
- Oral intubation by RSI for injuries above the larynx
  - As above
- Surgical airway for injury at or below the larynx
  - Consider local an aesthesia and/or ketamine
- Consider intubation over bougie through large defect

Zone I Neck injury
- Maintain spontaneous breathing where possible
- Consider intubation over bougie through large defect
- RSI as last resort
  - Gentle insertion of bougie
  - Smaller size ET Tube

Avoid Positive Pressure Ventilation
where possible until airway secured due to risk of subcutaneous emphysema or enlarging proximal airway tears

Blast lung should be suspected in anyone presenting with dyspnoea, cough, haemoptysis or chest pain within 48 hours of a blast exposure. Management is supportive with supplementary oxygen, observation, judicious fluid resuscitation and ventilatory support if there are signs of respiratory failure. If ventilation is required, lung protective ventilation strategies should be employed including low tidal volumes (6–8 mL kg lbw^{-1}), conservative application of PEEP$_e$ and limitation of plateau pressures to less than 30 cmH$_2$O. Prophylactic bilateral thoracostomy should be considered due to the increased risk of barotrauma.

Circulation management

Circulatory volume should be preserved at all costs through the aggressive application of haemorrhage control techniques, splinting of fractures and minimal handling. Even simple wounds to the legs, particularly the upper thigh, can prove fatal as uncontrolled bleeding occurs into the large volume of the thigh. Patients presenting with shock and penetrating injury to the chest or abdomen should be evacuated immediately to a major trauma facility for surgical haemostasis. Unnecessary delays on scene will have a negative effect on survival. Fluid resuscitation may be initiated during transfer and should be targeted to a central pulse or verbal response in penetrating torso trauma. Care should be taken to avoid volume overload as this may exacerbate blast lung and cause rebleeding.

Patients with proximal lower limb amputations due to blast have a high incidence of associated pelvic injury and the early application of a pelvic binder is recommended in these cases. Intravenous access in patients with multiple limb amputations may also prove challenging - subclavian central venous access and sternal intraosseous access are useful points of access in these situations. Tranexamic acid should be given to all patients at risk of ongoing significant haemorrhage who are within 3 hours of their injury.

Disability

Head injury is common following blast injury and may be the result of primary (concussion), secondary (penetrating fragmentation) or tertiary (blunt trauma) blast mechanisms. Gunshot wounds to the head carry a high mortality, especially through-and-through wounds and those passing close to the brainstem. Penetrating brain injury is easy to miss unless wounds are actively sought (Figure 20.9). Management is focused on the prevention of secondary injury through effective management of the airway, breathing and circulation. The level of consciousness after resuscitation is the most useful indicator of survival (Box 20.3).

Box 20.3 **Penetrating brain injury: relationship between level of consciousness after resuscitation and mortality.**

Level of Consciousness	Mortality (%)
Alert (A)	11.5
Drowsy (V)	33.3
Responds to Pain (P)	79.1
Unresponsive (U)	100

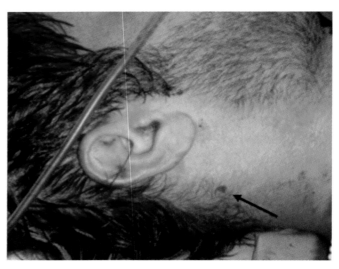

Figure 20.9 Gunshot entry wound to the posterior triangle – missed on initial assessment.

Exposure

It is vital that the patient is kept warm throughout the resuscitative process with appropriate use of blankets and vehicle heaters. All wounds and burns should be dressed and analgesia provided as necessary. Common sites for missed wounds include the back, buttocks, perineum, axilla and scalp. If broad spectrum prehospital antibiotics are carried, administration within 1 hour of wounding is recommended. Limbs amputated by blast or high calibre munitions are rarely suitable for reimplantation. They should however be bagged up and accompany the patient to preserve forensics. No specific intervention is required for suspected blast bowel or blast ear in the prehospital environment other than standard resuscitation and onward referral to hospital.

Tips from the field

- Never enter a ballistic scene before police arrival
- For the shocked patient with a ballistic airway injury, secure the airway early because airway bleeding may worsen with resuscitation
- Apply double tourniquets on proximal limb amputations
- Monitoring may be difficult in patients with multiple limb amputations:
  - defibrillator pads stick better to clammy skin than electrode leads
  - capnography trends can be used to guide fluid resuscitation
- Recheck dressings and tourniquets at regular intervals to ensure continued haemorrhage control during resuscitation.

Disclaimer

'The views and opinions expressed in this chapter are those of the authors and do not necessarily reflect the official policy or position of the MOD'

Further reading

Brooks AJ, Clasper J, Midwinter M, *et al. Ryan's Ballistic Trauma*, 3rd ed. London: Springer, 2011.

Irwin RJ, Lerner MR, Bealer JF, *et al.* Shock after blast wave injury is caused by a vagally mediated reflex. *J Trauma* 1999;**47**:105–110.

JRAMC. Special Issue: Wounds of Conflict, 2001.147(1).

Lichte P, Oberbeck R, Binnebösel M, *et al.* A civilian perspective on ballistic trauma and gunshot injuries. *Scand J Trauma Resusc Emerg Med* 2010; **18**:35.

CHAPTER 21

Trauma: Extrication of the Trapped Patient

Malcolm Q. Russell

Kent, Surrey & Sussex Air Ambulance Trust, UK

OVERVIEW

By the end of this chapter you should:

- Understand the concept of 'reading the wreckage'
- Know how to assess safety in casualty extrication scenarios
- Be able to formulate an 'A-plan' and a 'B-plan'
- Understand how to communicate the rescue plan
- Know the basic techniques available to the fire service to make space in order to free the casualty
- Know how to safely extricate a patient from a damaged vehicle.

Introduction

Motor vehicle collisions are common and produce a significant burden of death and morbidity in a largely young adult population. Managing patients effectively during the rescue phase can be complex and challenging but is possible with education and training. The whole rescue team should understand the processes involved and should be able to communicate with each other in a shared language. Regular joint training is essential if this care is to be optimal.

A structured approach to the management of motor vehicle collision casualties allows consistency and efficiency on scene. Although elements of collision scenes vary, many features are shared and allow for a generic approach to be made.

The rescue team's tasks are often divided into extrication and casualty care elements, with the senior fire officer taking overall lead informed by the senior medic present (Figure 21.1). The two functions are not necessarily provided exclusively by single services (e.g. a firefighter will often be part of the casualty care team). The teams must work to a shared plan, and each has its key priorities. Effective communication, coordination and command are essential in delivering a plan that works.

When approaching casualties, it is useful to observe the scene to assess how the incident happened and the rate of deceleration and other forces involved. This can help predict the severity and nature of injuries involved and is known as 'reading the wreckage', and is a skill that can be developed with experience (Figure 21.2).

ABC of Prehospital Emergency Medicine, First Edition.
Edited by Tim Nutbeam and Matthew Boylan.
© 2013 John Wiley & Sons, Ltd. Published 2013 by John Wiley & Sons, Ltd.

Activity is concurrent with the extrication team working physically on the vehicle and the medical team accessing and managing the casualty. The team leaders come together at regular intervals to ensure the overall plan is progressing and that each part of the team is aware of the other's constraints and progress.

Describing the anatomy of the car

Vehicles vary widely in their design and structure. It is useful to be able to describe standard parts of a vehicle and standard rescue techniques within your local rescue service using shared terminology.

The most common terms used in a rescue setting relate to the support structures that attach the roof. These are labelled, from the front, as the A-post, B-post and, in theory, alphabetically as far back as there are posts. It is commonly only the front two post (A and B) which are referred to (Figure 21.3).

Casualty care team (and shared) tasks

Safety

Safety is the shared first priority for the whole rescue team.

Think about safety from the perspective of yourself, the scene and the casualty. The medical team should be trained to work in this environment and be aware of the risks involved. They should wear appropriate personal protective equipment for the environment which can include:

- helmet
- eye protection ± face visor
- dust mask if working inside a vehicle where glass (particularly the windscreen) is being cut
- coveralls (ideally flame retardant material)
- boots with steel or composite toe protectors
- high-visibility waterproof over-jacket
- medical protective gloves
- 'debris' gloves (e.g. leather), which can be useful when gaining access to a patient, although the medical team should rarely be involved in handling the wreckage.

Safety of the scene is managed mainly by fire and police personnel and includes injury prevention while conducting the rescue, fire prevention (or control) and traffic management around the scene.

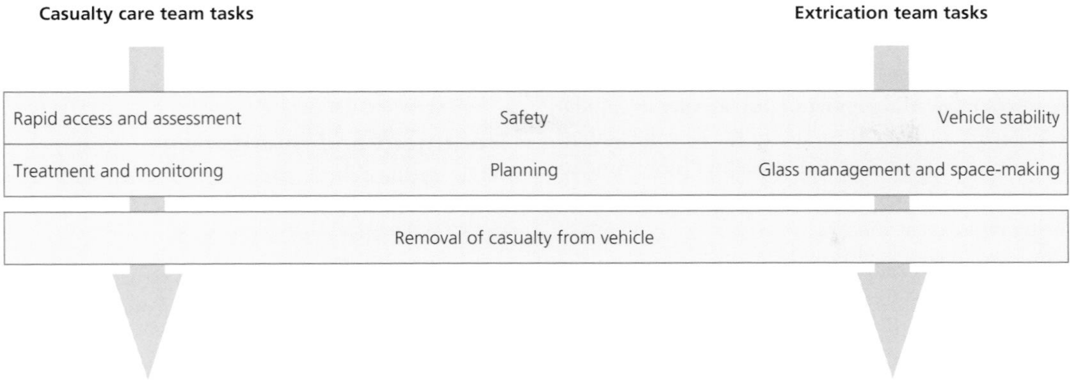

Casualty care team tasks		Extrication team tasks
Rapid access and assessment	Safety	Vehicle stability
Treatment and monitoring	Planning	Glass management and space-making
Removal of casualty from vehicle		

Figure 21.1 Division of tasks at an extrication.

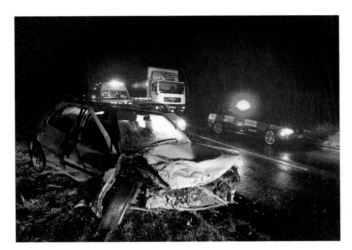

Figure 21.2 Severe frontal impact.

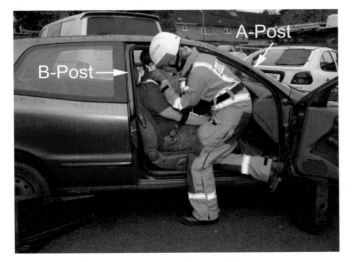

Figure 21.3 Car anatomy–key terms.

If the medical team is first on scene, simple measures should be carried out such as stopping traffic and removal of car keys to isolate the electrical system of a car. Be aware that un-deployed airbags may still be 'live' for several minutes after the ignition has been turned off. Consider too whether the vehicle is carrying any hazardous materials and react accordingly.

Safety of the patient may include using a plastic shield (commonly known as a 'tear-drop') when tools are being used in glass management or space creation. Think too about the risk of hypothermia using blankets, bubble-wrap, or chemical or electrical heating systems to keep the patient warm.

Vehicle-specific hazards

Modern vehicles often have multiple safety systems, some of which can present hazards to the rescue team during casualty rescue. These are managed by the fire service and are best demonstrated in practical exercises. Vehicle-specific hazards to consider include:

- airbags and their activation units (most modern cars have multiple air-bags in various parts of the car)
- gas struts which raise a hatchback door; these usually contain pressurized gas and fluid which may be released in an uncontrolled way if cut
- seat-belt pre-tensioning devices (may include pyrotechnic materials)
- hazardous chemicals and materials, especially if there has been a fire.

Rapid access and assessment

With safety in mind, access to the casualty should be gained as early as possible, and triage carried out for treatment and extrication. A primary survey should be completed noting whether the patient can move all four limbs, and the degree of physical entrapment (particularly the lower legs and feet). This information is then communicated to the medical team leader and treatment can begin as appropriate.

Tricks of the trade

Occupants of vehicles that have rolled are often ejected from their original positions. You may find them in the vehicle where you do not expect them (e.g. in the foot-wells, or the rear part of the passenger cell) or ejected from the vehicle itself. Ensure the surrounding area external to, and under, the vehicle is always searched to avoid missing any casualties.

Planning

When planning the extrication of a casualty, consideration should be given to the urgency of their release. Some scene or patient factors push the rescuer towards removing the casualty as rapidly as possible, possibly with some compromise in the way the patient is handled. Other considerations may favour taking more time to remove the patient to optimize control.

Factors favouring rapid extrication:

- occupant at immediate physical risk (e.g. significant risk of fire)
- unmanageable medical problem (e.g. obstructed airway that cannot be dealt with in situ).

Factors favouring a more thorough extrication (often slower):

- patient handling is more controlled (potential benefits for clot stability and spinal control)
- rescue team issues: taking a slower approach usually means more considered movement in and around a damaged vehicle which is generally safer for those in the team and may lead to a more stable platform for the patient.

These needs can conflict and the rescue team must make a dynamic risk assessment to determine the best course of action. Two main types of extrication are known as the A-plan and the B-plan (or plan-A and plan-B).

A-plan considerations

The A-plan is the controlled release of a casualty, taking great care by gentle handling and usually with full spinal immobilization, bringing the casualty out of the vehicle along their long axis. This typically means full roof removal and then bringing the patient out along a board.

The A-plan is often wrongly interpreted as a 'slow' or 'non-urgent' rescue. Both A-plans and B-plans should be conducted with an appropriate sense of urgency. Neither is slow.

B-plan considerations

The B-plan rescue is an immediate release of the casualty using a very simple plan and with minimal space-making. There is potential for more movement of the spine with the urgent nature of this rescue, so it is not without risks.

A sudden change from A-plan to B-plan must be communicated loudly and clearly, and usually occurs when the medical team identifies a critical deterioration in the patient. An effective B-plan should be carried out in less than 1–2 minutes. Do not be afraid of making this decision if you feel the circumstances merit it.

When planning the extrication of a casualty (usually following an A-plan), it is important *first* to identify or create a B-plan option and communicate this to the team. This may mean, for example, removal of an appropriate door initially so an escape route is clear. The B-plan may change as the extrication develops and more space is made, but the whole team should be ready to institute it at any moment if the scenario changes.

Tricks of the trade

In practice, B-plan rescues are often carried out too slowly, even when there is an immediate threat to life. Instituting a change from the A-plan to the B-plan necessitates clear (and usually loud) communication and demands a degree of physical leadership, i.e. the medical practitioner getting 'hands on' to demonstrate the required sense of urgency.

Treatment and monitoring

While in the vehicle, treatment and monitoring should be kept simple with only the most important interventions provided. Some examples of what may be reasonable are:

- Catastrophic compressible haemorrhage (rare in these incidents): direct pressure with or without tourniquet with or without topical haemostatic agent.
- Airway: simple adjuncts and suction required. Exceptionally, supraglottic device or surgical airway; there is no place for intubation within the confines of a damaged vehicle.
- Cervical spine control: manual in-line stabilization with or without semi-rigid collar.
- Breathing: needle decompression of tension pneumothorax usually possible. Chest drainage should be avoided unless absolutely necessary. Valved chest seal for the rare penetrating chest wound.
- Circulation: vascular access (intravenous or intraosseous) is useful to allow analgesics to be given and fluids where necessary. Bags of fluid and administration sets get in the way and should only be set up where there is an immediate need to give fluid.
- Neurological disability: pupils can be assessed and Glasgow Coma Score measured, with assessment of limb movement.
- Environment: assess risks to the casualty and protect where possible from hypothermia (e.g. shelter from rain, blankets or warming devices to slow the rate of heat loss).
- Monitoring: keep simple where possible, e.g. finger pulse oximeter.

Avoid using complex monitoring devices during the early phase of the rescue unless absolutely necessary. The process of applying monitoring often causes delay and complicates the rescue process with the 'spaghetti factor' of multiple cables running from patient, through wreckage, to the monitor. This is complicated by intravenous fluid lines and oxygen tubing. It is usually better to set up a casualty reception area a few metres from the vehicle where advanced monitoring can be laid out, ready to connect and minimize 'attachments' to the patient during the physical extrication.

Tricks of the trade

If the patient is vascularly 'shut down', usually due to a combination of shock and cold, intraosseous access can be very useful to give procedural sedation or analgesia where required. In these circumstances, the humeral head provides an ideal site being the most easy to access, easy to monitor and with good flow rates. Once in place, guard any intravenous or intraosseous device and ensure it is secured and protected: these are commonly dislodged when rescuers lift the casualty out of the vehicle.

Extrication team tasks

It is important to understand the basic approach and techniques used by the extrication team which are best learned by hands-on training with fire service colleagues in exercise scenarios.

Stability

The vehicle should be stabilized to prevent movement or vibration of the patient. This can help spinal immobilization, minimize movement of fractures (pain control) and assist haemorrhage control (clot stability).

To achieve this, the fire service may use tools including chocks and wedges, inflatable airbags and stabilization devices.

Glass management

The glass of a vehicle is 'managed' to allow space-making (such as roof removal) and to prevent any uncontrolled breakage which can risk the rescuers and the patient. Usually glass is broken in a controlled way, removed whole, or cut mechanically.

Space-making

The rescue team creates space to free the casualty using a range of tools to cut or spread the metalwork. Unnecessary work on the vehicle consumes time and resources so when the patient becomes free, space-making can usually stop.

Simple plans are usually the most effective. For a car on all four wheels, this usually means taking the whole roof off. Once access is made into the passenger cell, further space-making may be required such as a 'dash-roll' or 'dash-lift' to move the impacted dashboard off the patient's legs (Figure 21.4).

When a vehicle is on its side, access to occupants is often initially through the hatchback/rear door, through the windscreen or (with care and fire service control) through the 'upper' doors. The casualty can sometimes be extricated through the rear of the vehicle, and occasionally out through the windscreen once cut, particularly if a B-plan is required. The standard A-plan approach involves the 'roof fold-down' technique. In this technique, the upper supporting posts are cut (and sometimes some of the lower ones too) and the roof is laid down on the ground. This can give excellent access to the passenger cell (Figure 21.5).

When a vehicle is on its roof, there are a number of techniques that can be used to create space. Access can often be made through the rear door of a rolled hatchback (Figure 21.6), or by means of a 'B-post rip' (Figure 21.7). In this technique, the B-post is removed (with the rear door) by cutting it at the top and bottom. Sometimes, particularly where the roof has been crushed, further space-making is required using hydraulic rams to open up the side of the crushed vehicle: known as 'making an oyster'.

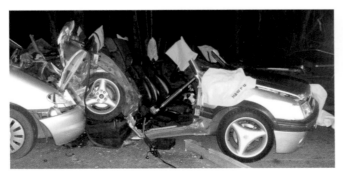

Figure 21.4 Dash-roll.

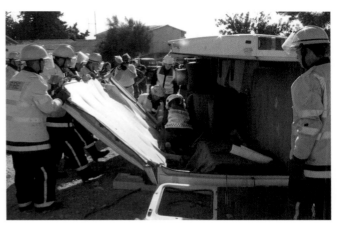

Figure 21.5 Roof fold-down.

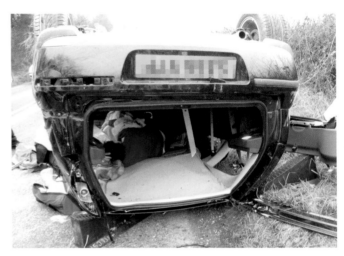

Figure 21.6 Access through rear hatch.

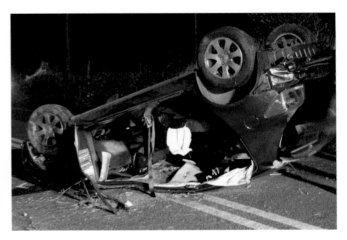

Figure 21.7 Access after B-post rip.

In extreme situations the fire service may consider rolling a vehicle back upright and then tackling the problem as if the car had been found on all four wheels. This technique is commonly used in some countries but rarely carried out in the UK.

Tricks of the trade

Before committing to 'space-making' to free a casualty's legs, ensure it is definitely needed. Sometimes limbs appear more trapped than they really are, or may be freed once adequate analgesia has been provided. It should be an experienced clinician who manipulates fractured limbs, and substantial time can often be saved at this stage. Consider even simpler measures such as removing the patient's shoes where feet appear to be trapped in the foot-well. That can sometimes be sufficient to free the patient.

It is difficult to set target times for casualty release, as scenarios are often complex with widely varying extrication challenges. With a single occupant trapped in a car on all four wheels, with good access and a well-trained team, 20 minutes is a reasonable target for releasing the casualty using a standard A-plan approach. It is useful for the rescue team, having assessed the situation, to agree a target time for A-plan and B-plan options.

Large vehicles

The principles for rescuing a casualty from a large vehicle such as a heavy goods vehicle are largely the same as for a car. The differences are most apparent in access (with the medic often on a ladder or access platform) and removal of a casualty from height. The extrication team will often require heavier cutting and lifting equipment to deal with the heavier vehicle and its structure. This may necessitate the dispatch of specialist rescue units which can impact on extrication time.

Removal of the patient from the vehicle

A-plan casualty removal

When following an A-plan, the roof of the vehicle is often removed to give better access to the patient.

If not possible earlier, an assessment of leg entrapment is usually made once the roof is off. If trapped by the dashboard of the vehicle, then space may be made with a 'dash-lift' or a 'dash-roll'.

Once the legs are free, a long-board is slid down between the patient's back and the back of the seat. The board is then held upright with the patient braced against it while the seat back is lowered back as far as possible. Additionally, if the mechanism is still intact, the whole seat may slide back horizontally creating more space. The casualty and board together are then lowered back as far as possible.

Tricks of the trade

Positioning the long board can be made easier by first sliding two 'tear-drops' down behind the patient's back. The long board is then guided between these, which act as introducers, making the process easier and often more comfortable for the patient (Figures 21.8, 21.9, 21.10, 21.11, 21.12, 21.13).

The casualty should then be moved along the length of the board in a series of small coordinated slides until fully on the board. The person providing manual in-line cervical stabilization is in control and should brief the team before giving give clear, loud instructions such as, 'Ready! Brace! Slide!' During this process, beware of un-deployed airbags.

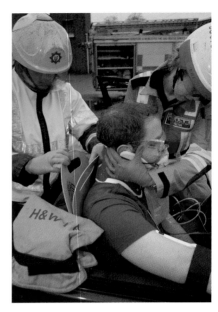

Figure 21.8 A-plan release: teardrops positioned.

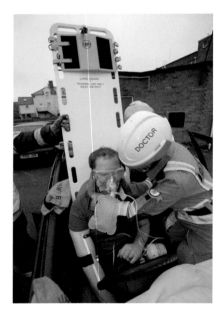

Figure 21.9 A-plan release: board introduced.

Typical roles during the movement of the casualty along the rescue board include:

- manual in-line cervical stabilization (this person in control)
- lifter: right shoulder
- lifter: left shoulder
- lifter: right hip
- lifter: left hip
- someone to disentangle legs and feet during early phase of move
- someone to take care of monitor and intravenous fluid lines (if attached).

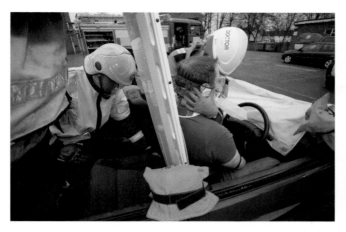

Figure 21.10 A-plan release: seat lowered.

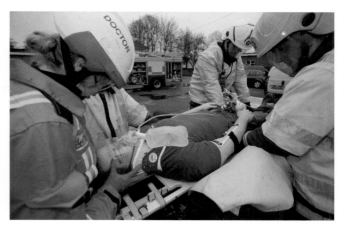

Figure 21.13 A-plan release: patient horizontal.

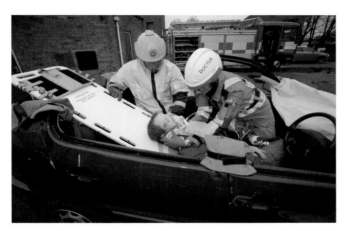

Figure 21.11 A-plan release: board fully lowered.

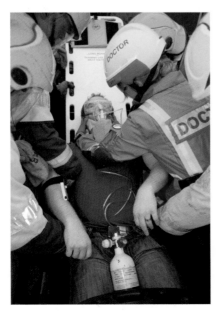

Figure 21.12 A-plan release: lifting positions.

With very little space and so many roles, think about temporarily disconnecting lines and cables. The oxygen cylinder is often placed on the board between the patient's legs. Vascular access points should be secured particularly well.

Once the patient is lying full-length against the board, it is lifted to the horizontal position and then slid out the back of the vehicle.

During the release of the casualty on a long-board, there is often a lull when the board becomes horizontal while the patient is strapped to it for 'control' or 'safety'. It is often neither of these. Strapping and blocking the patient on the board while half out of the vehicle is often precarious, takes time and can be poorly controlled. When the patient arrives at the reception area, they will need to have a full primary survey which necessitates strap removal anyway. It is usually much better to maintain manual control of spinal immobilization throughout this phase (with the exception of a semi-rigid collar which is usually in place already) with formal strap and block application later, in the casualty reception area.

B-plan casualty removal

The B-plan removal of the casualty is often done through the side door of a vehicle and follows similar principles of command and control. By its nature it tends to be much brisker and with less space so control is rarely as optimal as the A-plan approach. In the usual scenario, a rescue board is slid onto the patient's car seat and braced to provide a horizontal platform. The patient is then rotated and laid down on the board before being moved up along its length. In extremis, this procedure can be done without a board (Figures 21.14, 21.15, 21.16, 21.17).

Tricks of the trade

The scenario of a patient suspended upside down in a seatbelt can be particularly challenging. In practice the best solution is probably any that minimizes the time the patient is suspended while providing cervical spine protection as best as possible. Sometimes a firefighter can crawl below the patient's lap area, on their hands and knees, to support the patient as they are released from their seatbelt. Keep the plan simple and use as many hands as possible to

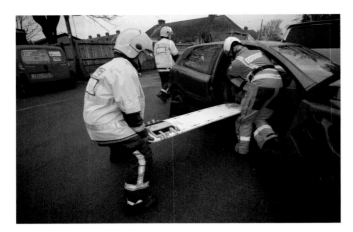

Figure 21.14 B-plan release.

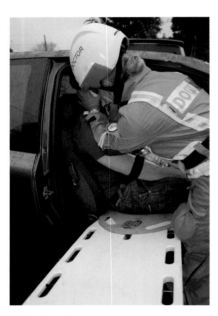

Figure 21.15 B-plan: board in place.

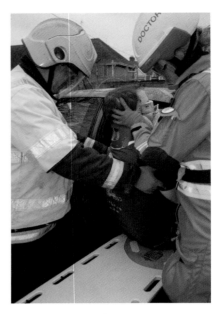

Figure 21.16 B-plan: patient rotated.

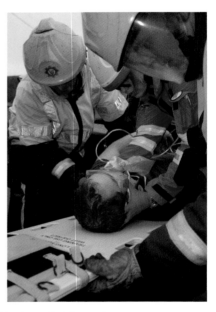

Figure 21.17 B-plan: patient lowered.

support the patient during the release. Once free, they are usually extricated as a B-plan option on a long board through the side of the vehicle.

Post-extrication care

Once free, the patient should be taken to a pre-designated casualty reception area. This is typically 5–10 metres away from the crashed vehicle and can be prepared in advance with ambulance trolley, monitor, suction and spare oxygen.

At the casualty reception area a rapid reassessment of the patient is made and immediately necessary interventions carried out. The patient is then packaged for transport. This involves securing them onto the trolley with formal spinal immobilization and monitoring, and protection from the cold. If interventions can be carried out in transit then this is preferable in order to minimize further on-scene delay.

The long board used for extrication of casualties is not designed as a transport device, but may be acceptable for very short journeys. Patients can often be packaged more comfortably and securely on a 'scoop-stretcher', which can also help minimize rolling required when transferred at hospital. For long journeys, consideration should be given to packaging on a vacuum mattress.

Summary

The management of entrapped patients is challenging and complex. The multi-agency rescue team can develop skills by training regularly together in order to develop skills leading to safe, efficient and reproducible rescue procedures which benefit patient care.

Tips from the field

- Safety is paramount
- Get early access to the patient(s) and make a plan
- Communicate with other emergency personnel and agree a target time for release
- Secure a B-plan option early
- Minimize unnecessary medical intervention in the vehicle
- Demonstrate effective leadership and communication skills throughout
- Be prepared to change the plan at any time
- Identify a casualty assessment area in which to carry out primary survey, essential treatment and packaging before transport.

Acknowledgements

Hereford and Worcester Fire and Rescue Service. Dr K White, Mercia Accident Rescue Service.

Further reading

Calland V. Extrication of the seriously injured road crash victim. *Emerg Med J* 2005;**22**:817–821.

Ersson A, Lundberg M, Wramby CO, Svensson H. Extrication of entrapped victims from motor vehicle accidents: the crew concept. *Eur J Emerg Med* 1999;**6**:41–47.

Mahoney PF, Carney CJ. Entrapment, extrication and immobilization. *Eur J Emerg Med* 1996;**3**:244–246.

Politis J, Dailey M. Extrication fundamentals. Proper care of the entrapped patient. *JEMS* 2010;**35**:41–47.

Wik L, Hansen TB, Kjensli K, Steen PA. Rapid extrication from a car wreck. *Injury* 2004;**35**:739–745.

Wilmink AB, Samra GS, Watson LM, Wilson AW. Vehicle entrapment rescue and pre-hospital trauma care. *Injury* 1996;**27**:21–25.

CHAPTER 22

Cardiac Arrest

Walter Kloeck[1], Efraim Kramer[2], Martin Botha[2], and David Kloeck[2,3]

[1]College of Emergency Medicine of South Africa, Rondebosch, South Africa
[2]University of the Witwatersrand, Johannesburg, South Africa
[3]Chris Hani Baragwanath Academic Hospital, Soweto, South Africa

OVERVIEW

By the end of this chapter, you should know

- How and why international cardiac arrest guidelines were developed
- The initial steps in performing cardiopulmonary resuscitation
- The major differences between in- and out-of-hospital resuscitation
- When to transport patients while performing CPR
- The specific considerations in the traumatic cardiac arrest victim
- How to perform an emergency thoracotomy
- When not to initiate CPR, and when to stop the resuscitation attempt
- What constitutes futile resuscitation.

International Cardiac Arrest Guidelines

Introduction

Since the original publication of successful closed-chest cardiac compressions by Kouwenhoven, Knickerbocker and Jude in 1960, numerous variations in cardiopulmonary resuscitation (CPR) have developed. In 1966 the American Heart Association published their first CPR guidelines, and this was followed by the development of resuscitation councils worldwide, each promoting their own unique set of recommendations. In view of the diverse variations that followed, in 1992 it was decided to form an International Liaison Committee on Resuscitation (ILCOR) comprising all major guideline-producing organizations (Table 22.1).

ILCOR's mission is to provide a mechanism by which the international science and knowledge relevant to CPR and emergency cardiovascular care is identified and reviewed. ILCOR has released more than 22 scientific Advisory Statements, and has published an International Consensus on Cardiopulmonary Resuscitation and Emergency Cardiovascular Care Science with Treatment Recommendations in 2000, 2005 and 2010, The 2010 International Consensus has been the most comprehensive ever, involving a review of several thousand articles by 313 resuscitation experts

Table 22.1 Member Organizations of the International Liaison Committee on Resuscitation (ILCOR)

American Heart Association (AHA)
Australia and New Zealand Committee on Resuscitation (ANZCOR)
European Resuscitation Council (ERC)
Heart and Stroke Foundation of Canada (HSFSA)
Inter-American Heart Foundation (IAHF)
Resuscitation Council of Asia (RCA)
Resuscitation Council of Southern Africa (RCSA)

from 30 countries. An ILCOR Universal Cardiac Arrest Algorithm was developed in 2010 (Figure 22.1) for use by member organisations, with the realisation that modifications and variations will be required based on economic, cultural, social and medico-legal differences in different regions and countries.

Initial actions

If the victim is unresponsive and not breathing or only having occasional gasps, immediately call for help and activate the Emergency Medical Services or appropriate Resuscitation Team. Gasping can persist for several minutes after cardiac arrest, and should not be a reason to delay starting CPR. Health-care professionals should take no more than 10 seconds to check for the presence of a pulse. If no definite pulse is detected, CPR is started, commencing with chest compressions.

CPR should be continued uninterrupted, using cycles of 30 compressions to two breaths until an automated external defibrillator (AED) or manual defibrillator is attached and ready to analyse the rhythm. If unwilling or unable to provide rescue breaths, rescuers should perform continuous chest compressions. Good-quality CPR entails pushing hard (at least 5 cm depth for an adult victim), pushing fast (at least 100/minute), ensuring complete chest recoil between compressions, minimizing interruptions and avoiding hyperventilation.

If a pulseless shockable rhythm is detected (**ventricular fibrillation or pulseless ventricular tachy**cardia), an immediate unsynchronized shock is delivered followed by 2 minutes of uninterrupted CPR. Chest compressions should be performed right until the shock is delivered, and resumed immediately after the shock in order to minimize pre- and post-shock pauses. If a biphasic defibrillator is being used, the shock should be delivered using

ABC of Prehospital Emergency Medicine, First Edition.
Edited by Tim Nutbeam and Matthew Boylan.
© 2013 John Wiley & Sons, Ltd. Published 2013 by John Wiley & Sons, Ltd.

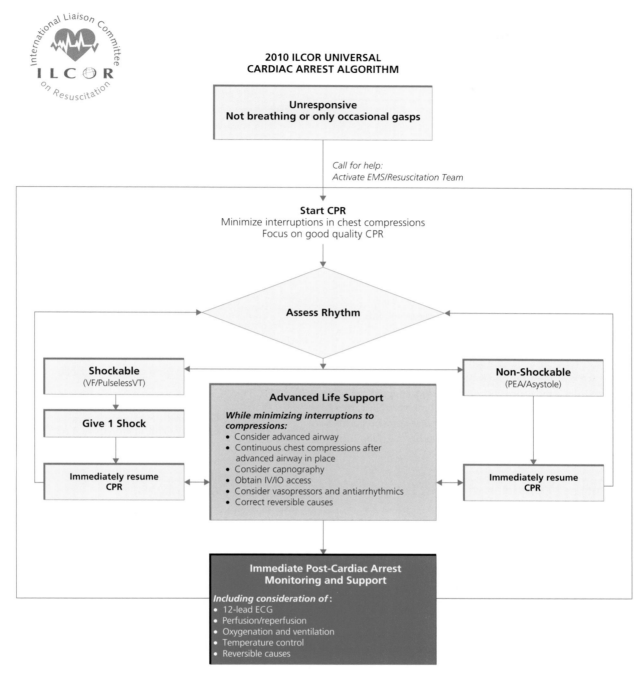

Figure 22.1 ILCOR Universal Cardiac Arrest Algorithm.

the manufacturer's recommended energy level. If unknown, use the maximum available energy setting, or use 360 joules if the defibrillator is monophasic.

If a non-shockable rhythm is detected (**pulseless electrical activity or a**systole), CPR is immediately resumed, starting with compressions, with reassessment of the rhythm occurring approximately every 2 minutes.

Insertion of an advanced airway (tracheal tube, combitube or laryngeal mask airway) can be considered provided that interruptions to compressions are minimized. Once an advanced airway is in place, continuous chest compressions can be performed, with an interposed breath being delivered every 6–8 seconds (8–10 breaths **per** minute).

Waveform capnography is highly recommended during CPR, not only to determine tracheal tube placement but also for the monitoring of CPR quality. A $P_{ET}CO_2$ level of <10 mmHg (1.3 kPa) indicates poor-quality CPR, and an abrupt sustained rise in $P_{ET}CO_2$ above 40 mmHg (5.3 kPa) suggests a return of spontaneous circulation.

Once intravenous or intraosseous access has been obtained, the administration of vasopressors and antiarrhythmics can be considered. Adrenaline (epinephrine) may be administered at a

Table 22.2 Reversible causes of cardiac arrest

Hypoxia	Tension pneumothorax
Hypovolaemia	Tamponade (cardiac)
Hypothermia	Toxins
Hypo-/hyperkalaemia	Thrombosis (cardiac)
Hydrogen ion imbalance	Thrombosis (pulmonary)

dose of 1 mg every 3–5 minutes once pulseless electrical activity (PEA) or asystole has been identified, or after the **second** or **third** shock if the rhythm is Ventricular fibrillation (VF) or pulseless vetricular tachycardia (VT). Tracheal administration is no longer routinely recommended, as absorption via this route is unreliable and unpredictable.

If the rhythm remains VF/VT despite defibrillation and adrenaline, amiodarone may be administered intravenously (IV)/intraosseously (IO) after the **third** shock at an initial dose of 300 mg, followed by 150 mg after 3–5 minutes if necessary. For torsades de pointes or suspected hypomagnesaemia, give 1–2 g of magnesium IV/IO (diluted in 10 mL of 5% dextrose water).

Crucial for cardiac arrest survival is the rapid identification and treatment of reversible causes of the cardiac arrest. This can conveniently be memorized as **the** 5 Hs and 5 Ts (Table 22.2).

Upon successful return of spontaneous circulation, intensive post-cardiac arrest monitoring and support is vital. A 12-lead ECG should be recorded, and perfusion, oxygenation and ventilation should be optimized. A meticulous search for reversible causes and correction thereof is paramount. Post-cardiac arrest reperfusion strategies and induced (therapeutic) hypothermia should be considered where indicated.

Cardiac arrest considerations in the prehospital environment

Introduction

The exhilaration and urgency of prehospital emergency care is nowhere more tangible than when confronted by a cardiac arrest victim. This demands from the rescuer several decisions, challenges and skills not routinely required by an in-hospital health-care provider:

1 **Scene safety** – The safety of the rescuer in the prehospital milieu is always one's first concern. Dead heroes save no lives. Crowd control without formal security is a routine challenge for EMS providers.
2 **Equipment** – The only equipment you have is the equipment you carry. Failing to plan is planning to fail. This means that one's kit must be well prepared, checked and cleaned prior to the call-out. Every item must have a particular place for ease of rapid access. Ideally the emergency bag should be packed exactly the same way every time.
3 **Limited resources and space** – Equipment must be robust, durable, light, easy to use and well maintained. Providers must be reflexively familiar with their equipment, and able to rapidly improvise if the need arises.
4 **Defibrillation** – It could be argued that basic life support (BLS) without defibrillation capacity has no place in EMS systems and

in optimal care of cardiac arrest victims. For optimal outcomes, CPR and defibrillation should be provided to the collapsed victim within 5 minutes.

5 **Back-up facilities** – Seldom in the prehospital environment is there a wide variety of extra equipment (or range of appropriate sizes) easily available, no extra personnel to back one up in a desperate situation, and no security personnel to protect one in a volatile situation. Responding alone and resuscitating a patient single-handedly, as occurs in many developing countries, is a challenging experience.
6 **Resuscitation ergonomics** – The positioning of equipment around the victim is important. If possible, for example, place the defibrillator at the left side of the patient. The victim is often found on the floor – an unusual position for those accustomed to resuscitating on a gurney or hospital bed. Space around the patient is often very limited.
7 **Urgency** – Responding to the scene, through traffic, often with poor address information, can be challenging. Gaining rapid access to the patient demands further urgency, which is dependant on proper, accurate emergency call-taking and dispatch instructions and systems.
8 **Undifferentiated patient and unknown circumstances** – One doesn't know the patient or their prior condition, and there is often no reliable history immediately available, or no time to elicit any.

The success of prehospital resuscitation is pivotal upon early access, early CPR, and early defibrillation by first responders. Early bystander CPR is vital, and unfortunately in many instances this has not been initiated, resulting in a low chance of survival.

CPR while transporting to hospital

For the most part, performing CPR while in transit to the emergency department is hazardous and merely serves to convert the place of death from prehospital to in-hospital. However, when the cause of the arrest can only be treated in-hospital, or when extenuating or particularly reversible conditions warrant prolonged resuscitation (such as persistent fibrillation or victims of drowning, lightning strike, accidental hypothermia, electrolyte abnormalities, anaphylaxis or drug-related arrests), CPR during transportation may be justified. The availability of a mechanical chest compression device might be an advantage in such situations.

Prehospital cardiac arrest in the trauma victim

Introduction

The provision of CPR in the prehospital environment in the trauma victim is generally associated with low survival rates. Penetrating trauma with single system injuries have higher survival rates compared to blunt polytrauma victims. With due regard to futility, it is often up to the treating healthcare professional to determine whether CPR will be initiated on scene in a trauma victim in cardiac arrest and if so, what resuscitative measures will be employed prior to transport of the victim to the nearest and most appropriate emergency department.

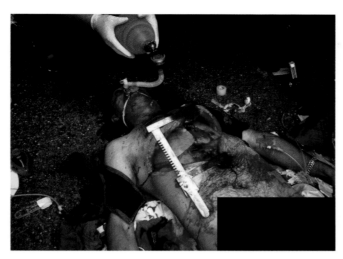

Figure 22.2 Prehospital emergency thoracotomy.

Owing to the possible presence of exanguinating haemorrhage (hypovolaemia), hypoxia, fractures to the anterior chest wall, open chest wounds, spinal column injuries and so forth, CPR in the trauma victim may require alterations in technique with regards to chest compressions, the requirement for rapid intravenous fluid administration, relief of pericardial tamponade, or even open cardiac massage via emergency thoracotomy. It is therefore necessary, when approaching the traumatic cardiac arrest victim, to consider the various alterations in technique and procedure that may be required in order to achieve a successful resuscitation (Figure 22.2).

1 Safety factors
  ○ Ensure that the **scene** is safe to enter (with due regard to traffic, gunfire, explosive devices, etc.).
  ○ Ensure that the **patient** is safe to touch and manage (electrical hazards, chemical contamination).
  ○ Ensure that the **rescuer** is adequately protected (full personal protective equipment).

2 Initiation of CPR
  ○ Absence of signs of life? Determine unresponsiveness and absence of normal breathing. Gasping is not a reason to withhold CPR.
  ○ How long have the signs of life been absent? Evidence of longstanding death such as rigor mortis, dependent livido or putrefaction are obvious indicators of futility.
  ○ What is the major mechanism of injury? Injuries incompatible with survival such as hemicorporectomy, severe head trauma and emaceration do not warrant resuscitation.
  ○ What is the initial rhythm on the ECG? Ventricular fibrillation or pulseless electrical activity would indicate potential viability as opposed to an asystolic rhythm.

3 Airway techniques
  Opening, maintaining and protecting the airway in a traumatic cardiac arrest victim may present challenges due to distortion of normal anatomy caused by the mechanism of injury. This may lead to the necessity of providing spinal protection and the early use of supraglottic, glottic or infraglottic devices to provide adequate oxygenation.

4 Breathing techniques
  The administration of supplemental oxygen to the traumatic cardiac arrest victim is mandatory as these patients are inevitably hypoxic from cardiac and/or respiratory causes.
  In addition to positive pressure ventilation and chest compressions, the following should be considered:
  ○ Closure of open chest wounds and control of active bleeding.
  ○ Performance of needle or tube or open thoracostomy when thoracic trauma or tension pneumothorax is evident or suspected.

5 Circulation techniques
  External chest compressions may not provide adequate cardiac output in the traumatic cardiac arrest victim with severe hypovolaemia, multiple rib fractures, exsanguinating haemorrhage or pericardial tamponade, and additional resuscitative measures may become necessary:
  ○ Rapid control of active bleeding.
  ○ Insertion of multiple large bore intravenous infusion lines for the rapid administration of fluids, either peripherally, centrally, intraosseously or via venous surgical cut-down.
  ○ Emergency thoracotomy in order to relieve pericardial tamponade, control major intrathoracic bleeding, compress or clamp the descending aorta to control sub-diaphragmatic haemorrhage, or to perform open cardiac massage. Should emergency thoracotomy be performed, fluid administration may be undertaken via the right atrium directly if necessary. Application of a pneumatic anti-shock device to control major abdominal haemorrhage.
  ○ Defibrillation of a victim with an open chest cavity will probably need to be performed transcutaneously by briefly closing the chest for the duration of the shock and using the maximum available energy setting, as the required internal paddles are unlikely to be available on scene (If internal paddles are available, start with 20 Joules).

6 Drug administration
  The administration of resuscitative drugs (e.g. adrenaline) in the post-traumatic cardiac arrest victim is similar to other causes of cardiac arrest when indicated. However, in the victim who undergoes emergency thoracotomy and develops a return of spontaneous circulation, hypnotic and analgesic agents may need to be administered in order to maintain the patient in a state of adequate anaesthesia prior to transport to the receiving emergency department.
  Care must be taken when calculating effective doses of medications and fluid administration in the post-traumatic cardiac arrest victim due to hypovolaemia and dilutional considerations. Once the pulse returns, it may be prudent to adopt a 'permissive hypotension' approach, maintaining the systolic blood pressure at approximately 90 mmHg (or until a radial pulse can just be felt), until uncontrolled haemorrhage has been managed.

7 Evacuation to hospital
  The post-traumatic cardiac arrest victim who has a return of spontaneous circulation, or who has a specific in-hospital medically or surgically correctible cause of cardiac arrest, will require transportation to the nearest and most appropriate emergency department or specialist surgical/trauma unit as expeditiously

and as safely possible. When undertaking such transfer, decisions regarding mode, duration and route of transport need to be considered:

- Adequate and safe packaging of the victim.
- Adequate immobilization of patient and equipment.
- Haemorrhage control en route, particularly following return of spontaneous circulation.
- Appropriate fluid administration en route, with due consideration to permissive hypotension.
- How defibrillation will be undertaken en route if required.
- How safe, yet effective, chest compressions will be undertaken en route if necessary.
- How effective positive pressure ventilation will be undertaken en route.

Prehospital emergency thoracotomy

Introduction

Prehospital emergency thoracotomy, although still a controversial subject, has a definitive role in the resuscitation of the critically injured patient when performed by an appropriately trained and resourced healthcare professional, working within approved protocols and policies, especially when each procedure is reviewed by the appropriate trauma system clinical governance programme. This systemized approach ensures that guidance is available in the decision-making process, safety is maintained during the operative procedure, adequate assistance is always on-hand, and hospital definitive care is activated timeously, all of which is geared towards patient resuscitation, stabilisation and hospital discharge neurologically intact. In this type of setting, the generally quoted success rates of 9–12% for penetrating trauma can be increased to as high as 38%.

Indications and relative contraindications

The indications and relative contraindications for prehospital emergency thoracotomy are listed in Table 22.3 and Table 22.4 respectively.

Equipment

The equipment required for on-scene resuscitative thoracotomy must be safe, simple and effective for use in an environment which is limited in resources, generally unsterile, and open to the elements. The minimum equipment required is listed in Table 22.5, but a pre-packed thoracotomy set would be ideal if available (Table 22.6).

Table 22.3 Indications for prehospital emergency thoracotomy

Penetrating trauma, particularly to the chest. Individual decisions will be required for blunt polytrauma patients where survival rates approximate only 1–2%.
The presence of signs of life on or within 10 minutes of arrival.
The travel duration from injury to specialist surgical hospital care is greater than 10 minutes.
Resuscitative procedures required include:
- Release of pericardial tamponade
- Control of massive intrathoracic haemorrhage
- Control of massive air embolism
- Occlusion of the descending aorta
- Provision of internal cardiac massage.

Table 22.4 Relative contraindications for prehospital thoracotomy

Blunt polytrauma, e.g. motor vehicle collision
Cardiopulmonary resuscitation >5 minutes with no return of spontaneous circulation
Associated severe head injury
Inadequate rescuer training, equipment, assistance or system resources
Inadequate emergency department or specialist surgical support within a reasonable distance or time.

Table 22.5 Minimum requirements for prehospital thoracotomy

Personal protective equipment (long-limb gloves, safety glasses, facial masks, etc.)
Scalpel with no. 10 blades
Large rescue-type scissors
Large sharp-pointed scissors
Artery forceps or equivalent
Foley catheter
3/0 non-absorbable suture on a curved needle or staples
Numerous large abdominal type swabs.

Table 22.6 An ideal pre-packed thoracotomy set

Gigli saw
Finochietto rib spreader
Curved Mayo scissors
Toothed forceps
Large vascular clamp (e.g. Satinsky)
Aortic clamp (e.g. De Bakey)
Needle holders (long and short)
Selection of sutures

Operative technique

A left anterolateral surgical approach is the classical method of entry, extending from the left parasternal costochondral junction in the fifth or sixth intercostal space to the mid-axillary line laterally, following the upper border of the rib. This limited technique is usually adequate for immediate relief of a cardiac tamponade, 'digital' clamping of the aorta or internal cardiac massage. However, it is far more practical to extend the incision across the sternum (clamshell incision) into a bilateral anterior thoracotomy because of the access that it provides to the pericardium, pleura and rest of the mediastinum, thus facilitating surgical release of a pericardial tamponade, compression of exsanguinating haemorrhage, cross-clamping of the aorta and cross-clamping of the hilum when indicated. Once spontaneous cardiac rhythm has been restored, haemorrhage from incised vessels, including the internal mammary artery, will require ligation or compression in order to avoid further exsanguination en route to the delegated emergency department nearby.

Paediatric resuscitation

The principles of high-quality CPR, i.e. push hard and fast, allow complete chest recoil and minimize interruptions, are similar to that of adults, but with a few specific differences:

- If there is no breathing or only gasping, a carotid pulse check is performed for a child, but a brachial pulse is felt for in an infant

(<1 year old). CPR should be started if no definitive pulse is felt within 10 seconds.

- There are local and international variations regarding the recommended sequencing with respect to the initiation of rescue breaths. The European Resuscitation Council recommends an initial five rescue breaths prior to performing chest compressions, as hypoxia is the main determinant of cardiac arrest in children. The American Heart Association recommends starting with 30 chest compressions prior to giving two initial rescue breaths, as with adult CPR, for ease of teaching and memory retention, and to avoid delays in starting CPR caused by having to retrieve, assemble and properly position a ventilatory device; 30 compressions will result in a delay of only 18 seconds or less prior to delivering initial rescue breaths.
- Chest compressions on a child should be performed using one or two hands placed in the centre of the chest on the lower half of the sternum. For infants, the tips of two or three fingers may be used if you are a lone rescuer, although if two rescuers are present, it is preferable to encircle the chest with both hands, allowing the thumbs to align next to each other on the lower half of the infant's sternum.
- The depth of compressions should be at least one-third of the anterior-posterior diameter of the chest wall. This would equate to approximately 5 cm in the child and approximately 4 cm in an infant.
- A ratio of 30 compressions followed by two breaths should be performed if you are a lone rescuer, but if a second rescuer is available, the ratio should be 15:2, to provide more oxygenation while minimizing delays in chest compressions.
- Once a defibrillator is attached and a shockable rhythm is detected, an initial shock at 2–4 joules/kg should be administered. Subsequent shocks at 4 joules/kg or higher (up to a maximum of 10 joules/kg: do not exceed adult dosage) may be administered after every 2 minutes of CPR if indicated.
- If a manual defibrillator is not available, an AED with a paediatric dose attenuator should be used. If paediatric pads or attenuator is not available, then the adult pads should be used.
- Adrenaline (0.01 mg/kg) may be administered every 3–5 minutes intravenously or intraosseous during cardiac arrest, and amiodarone (5 mg/kg) may be given after the third shock and repeated after the fifth and seventh shock if necessary (not to exceed 300 mg/dose or a maximum total dose of 2.2 g).
- If a pulse is detected but the child is not breathing, ventilations should be given at a rate of one every 3–5 seconds (12–20/minute). Post-resuscitation induced (therapeutic) hypothermia should be considered where appropriate.
- An aggressive search and correction of reversible causes of cardiac arrest (Hs and Ts) should be conducted before, during and after the arrest to optimize outcomes.

The ethics of resuscitation: difficult and demanding decisions

Introduction
The clinical ethics regarding the decision to start CPR or not, when to stop CPR and when it is futile demands a practical approach to morally defensible decision making. When confronted with these clinical conundrums in an emergency, decisions and actions must be swift and purposeful.

Criteria for not starting CPR
Futile resuscitation is not medically or ethically justifiable. Resuscitation should not be started if the patient has a valid Do Not Resuscitate (DNR) order, is obviously and irreversibly dead (rigor mortis, dependent lividity, putrefaction), has injuries incompatible with life or if no recovery can be expected because vital organs have irreversibly collapsed despite maximal therapy.

Do Not Resuscitate orders
DNR orders, more recently becoming known in some countries *as* AND (Allow Natural Death) and DNA-CPR (Do Not Attempt CPR), have thus been developed to pre-empt the initiation of reflexive resuscitation efforts in patients with no reasonable prospect of recovery, and are appropriate where the prevailing medical condition is a terminal illness and further treatment is unlikely to restore the patient to a meaningful quality of life. If this has been unequivocally established, then there is no reasonable duty to continue or start resuscitation. However, while any withdrawal of existing treatment which could hasten the patient's death would not be sanctioned, withholding of care may well be appropriate.

The right to withhold care is applicable in and outside the hospital. The imperative is to respect patient autonomy. However, if there is any doubt, start resuscitation immediately – one can always stop once one has obtained sufficient evidence and confirmed the veracity of the information at hand. Always err on the side of commission when it comes to resuscitation decisions.

Advance directives, living wills and patient self-determination
An 'advance directive' is an expression of a person's thoughts, wishes or preferences for their end-of-life care. Advance directives can be based on conversations, written directives, living wills or durable powers of attorney. The legal validity of the various forms of advance directives varies, but courts tend to consider written advance directives to be more trustworthy than recollections of conversations. Prehospital providers must be thoroughly familiar with their own local protocols and regulations.

A 'living will' is a patient's written directive to physicians about medical care the patient would approve when the patient can no longer take part in decisions for their own future. The living will is not a DNR order – it is devised to stand as a declaration of one's non-consent to prolonged artificial life support. It generally only comes into effect when there is no reasonable prospect of recovery, such as terminal illness or irreversible coma. It constitutes clear evidence of the patient's wishes, spelling out exactly the type of interventions allowed.

Surrogate decision makers may act on behalf of the patient when the patient is unable to decide for themselves. However, if there is any doubt, one generally does not require permission from the surrogates to start or to stop resuscitation.

Terminating resuscitative efforts

Following careful consideration of several factors, the decision to terminate resuscitative efforts rests with the emergency care provider. These factors include critical time intervals such as time to initiating CPR, time to defibrillation, co-morbid disease, pre-arrest state and the initial arrest rhythm. None of these factors alone or in combination is clearly predictive of outcome. However, witnessed collapse, bystander CPR and a short time interval from collapse to arrival of professional care significantly improve the chances of a successful resuscitation.

The decision to withhold or terminate resuscitation attempts in the field is always a difficult one, and perhaps even more daunting in the case if a child. EMS providers should be thoroughly familiar with their specific guidelines and protocols regarding withholding or terminating resuscitative efforts. Remember to take excellent notes and record your actions.

After resuscitating for approximately 20 minutes with no return of spontaneous circulation, termination of the resuscitation can be considered provided reversible causes for the cardiac arrest have been aggressively hunted for and managed (Box 22.1). Predictors of poor outcome and clinical decision aids can be found in Box 22.2.

Box 22.1 Reversible causes of cardiac arrest

Hypoxia	A systematic search for hypoxia extends from the oxygen source to the alveolus: Is the oxygen cylinder full? / Is the wall mount properly connected? Is the oxygen turned on? / Is there a leak? Is the oxygen tubing attached? / Is it kinked? Does the bag-valve resuscitator have a reservoir? / Is it inflated? Is the bag-valve resuscitator intact? / Is the pressure release closed? Is the face mask size appropriate? / Is the advanced airway correctly placed? Is the seal adequate? / Is the cuff adequately inflated? Is the mouth clear of secretions, blood or vomitus? / Is there a foreign body? Is the patient cyanosed? / Is a CO_2 detector available? Is the chest visibly rising? / Is it symmetrical? Is the air entry adequate? / Is it equal bilaterally?
Hypovolaemia	Evidence of relative or absolute fluid loss should be searched for and corrected: History of vomiting and / or diarrhoea? Visible bleeding? / Occult bleeding in chest, abdomen, pelvis, limbs? Evidence of distributive shock (anaphylactic / septic / neurogenic)?
Hypothermia	Obtain an accurate temperature reading and re-warm as necessary: Is a low reading thermometer being used? Was a core temperature reading taken?
Hypo-/Hyper-kalaemia	Abnormalities in serum potassium levels should be corrected: ECG – small T-waves or large U-waves (suggesting low potassium)? ECG – large peaked T-waves and absent P-waves (suggesting high potassium)?
H+ imbalance	Acidosis can be respiratory or metabolic in origin: High pCO_2 – Is intubation or chest tension decompression indicated? Low pCO_2 – With a pH <7,0, sodium bicarbonate might be indicated?
Tension Pneumothorax	Watch for asymmetrical chest rise and / or absent breath sounds: Has needle decompression been performed? Has an intercostal drain been inserted and is it draining adequately?
Tamponade (Cardiac)	Look for evidence of blunt or penetrating chest trauma: Are the ECG QRS complexes small or alternating in amplitude? Is sonography available to confirm and to facilitate decompression?
Toxins	Antidotes or prolonged resuscitation may be indicated: Is the patient taking any drugs (orally, rectally, IM or IV)? Has the patient been given any medications recently? Are any medications present in the patient's pockets? Is there evidence of needlestick or puncture wounds? Is there evidence of chemical contamination?
Thrombosis (Cardiac)	Look for evidence of cardiovascular pathology: Ischaemic changes on the ECG? Risk factors for coronary artery disease?
Thrombosis (Pulmonary)	Look for evidence of venous stasis: Are the patient's calves swollen? Is there a history of inactivity or peripheral vascular disease?

The pupils should be fixed and dilated with no response to light (remembering that adrenaline dilates the pupils) – the use of a magnifying glass here may improve the assessment accuracy. Asystole should be confirmed on all three limb leads, ensuring that the ECG amplitude (gain setting) is on maximum and that all leads are securely attached to both the patient and the machine to avoid artefactual error.

Although the family's permission to terminate the resuscitation is not ordinarily required, it is wise to involve them in the process, explaining actions and providing feedback about progress. Invariably onlookers will appreciate your labours more than you realize, and will be assured that everything possible was attempted. The rescuer's efforts are thereafter directed at comforting and supporting the family who have just witnessed a tragic event.

Box 22.2 **Predictors of poor outcome in patients in cardiac arrest**

Termination Guideline BLS

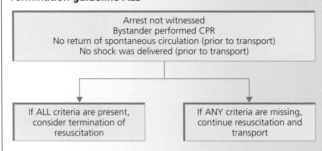

| Arrest not witnessed by emergency medical services personnel |
| No return of spontaneous circulation (prior to transport) |
| No AED shock was delivered (prior to transport) |

| If ALL criteria are present, consider termination of resuscitation | If ANY criteria are missing, continue resuscitation and transport |

Termination guideline ALS

| Arrest not witnessed |
| Bystander performed CPR |
| No return of spontaneous circulation (prior to transport) |
| No shock was delivered (prior to transport) |

| If ALL criteria are present, consider termination of resuscitation | If ANY criteria are missing, continue resuscitation and transport |

(Source: Laurie J. Morrison, Gerald Kierzek; Douglas S. Diekema et al. *Circulation* 2010; **122**: S665–S675).

Additional predictors of poor outcome

Asystole for >20 minutes

No cardiac activity on prehsopital ultrasound at any point during resuscitation

A maximum end-tidal carbon dioxide (ETCO2) of 10 mmHg during CPR

Tips from the field

- Scene safety, patient safety and rescuer safety are prime considerations in the prehospital environment
- Gasping is not a reason to delay starting CPR
- Commence CPR with chest compressions
- Focus on good quality CPR with minimal interruptions
- Early defibrillation, minimizing pre- and post-shock pauses, and rapid correction of reversible causes are vital for a successful outcome
- Waveform capnography is strongly recommended in order to monitor CPR quality
- Traumatic cardiac arrest victims require specific modifications with regard to airway, breathing, circulation, defibrillation, evacuation and fluid resuscitation
- Err on the side of commission: if you are uncertain about whether to start resuscitation … START!
- Stop resuscitation only when you are convinced the patient is clinically and irreversibly dead
- Futile resuscitation is ethically, medically and economically difficult to justify
- EMS systems are diametrically different in different parts of the world – know your local protocols and regulations
- Take excellent notes to record your actions.

Further reading

American Heart Association Guidelines for Cardiopulmonary Resuscitation and Emergency Cardiovascular Care, 2010. *Circulation* 2010;**122**:S639–946.

European Resuscitation Council Guidelines, 2010. *Resuscitation* **2010**: 1219–1451.

Hunt PA, Greaves I, Owens WA. Emergency Thoracotomy in Thoracic Trauma – a Review. *Injury.* 2006;**37**:1–19.

International Consensus on Cardiopulmonary Resuscitation and Emergency Cardiovascular Care Science with Treatment Recommendations, 2010. Resuscitation 2010;81(Supplement):e1–e330. (www.ILCOR.org).

Wise D, Davies G, Coats T, *et al.* Emergency thoracotomy: 'How to do it'. *Emerg Med J* 2005;**22**:22–24.

CHAPTER 23

Acute Medical Emergencies

Adam Low[1] and Tim Nutbeam[2]

[1]West Midlands Deanery, Birmingham, UK
[2]Derriford Hospital, Plymouth Hospitals NHS Trust, Plymouth, UK

OVERVIEW

By the end of this chapter you will:

- Have a general overview of some common and important medical conditions
- Understand the prehospital interventions, transport considerations and destination decision making for these conditions.

Introduction

This chapter focuses on medical emergencies in prehospital care. It covers the recognition and emergency treatment of these conditions within the prehospital environment and considerations such as patient destination and transport method. Many excellent textbooks cover the in-hospital emergency management of these conditions in further detail. Cardiac arrest and end-of-life decision making are covered in Chapter 13.

The ethos of doing simple things well, with timely, safe transfer to a definitive treatment facility is key. Think carefully about interventions such as intravenous cannulation in terms of subsequent risk, e.g. line-associated sepsis.

It is essential to elicit pertinent features of the medical history and perform a focused yet thorough examination in all patients. Collateral histories are important and must be documented and conveyed to the receiving hospital. An ABCDE approach is as applicable to medical patients as it is to trauma patients and scene safety should still be considered. Many trauma patients will have concurrent medical conditions that may require prehospital treatment in addition to their traumatic injuries. Furthermore trauma can mask an exacerbation of a medical condition and vice versa.

Respiratory emergencies

Asthma
Identification
Respiratory distress with expiratory wheeze. The severity of the attack can be assessed using the clinical symptoms (Table 23.1).

ABC of Prehospital Emergency Medicine, First Edition.
Edited by Tim Nutbeam and Matthew Boylan.
© 2013 John Wiley & Sons, Ltd. Published 2013 by John Wiley & Sons, Ltd.

Table 23.1 Levels of severity of acute asthma exacerbations

Near-fatal asthma	Raised $PaCO_2$ and/or requiring mechanical ventilation with raised inflation pressures
Life threatening asthma	Any one of the following in a patient with severe asthma:

Clinical signs	**Measurements**
Altered conscious level	PEF < 33% best or predicted
Exhaustion	SpO_2 < 92%
Arrhythmia	PaO_2 < 8 kPa
Hypotension	"normal" $PaCO_2$ (4.6–6.0 kPa)
Cyanosis	
Silent chest	
Poor respiratory effort	

Acute severe asthma	Any one of: • PEF 33–50% best or predicted • respiratory rate ≥ 25/min • heart rate ≥ 110/min • inability to complete sentences in one breath
Moderate asthma exacerbation	• Increasing symptoms • PEF > 50–75% best or predicted • no features of acute severe asthma
Brittle asthma	• Type 1: wide PEF variability (> 40% diurnal variation for > 50% of the time over a period > 150 days) despite intense therapy • Type 2: sudden severe attacks on a background of apparently well controlled asthma

An asthma-specific history includes frequency of severe exacerbations requiring hospital admission, any admissions to ITU/HDU, recent oral steroids, drugs required to control symptoms (stepwise approach to management usually taken) and non-steroidal anti-inflammatory drug (NSAID) sensitivity. Patients under respiratory physician outpatient care normally have poorer symptom control/more severe disease – beware the 'brittle' asthmatic. Most deaths from acute severe asthma occur prehospitally and the majority are considered potentially preventable.

Differential/concurrent diagnosis
Beware of concurrent pneumothorax and shock. A coexisting infective trigger such as pneumonia may need treatment as for sepsis. Differentiating between heart failure (cardiac asthma) and 'normal' asthma can be difficult.

Transport considerations

Beware of expansion of occult pneumothorax if travelling at altitude.

Destination considerations

Severe and brittle asthmatics may need transporting to centres with advanced ICU facilities.

Treatment

Oxygen, nebulised salbutamol (Adult dose 5 mg) with or without ipratropium bromide (Adult dose 500 mcg). Early use of oral prednisolone (adult dose 40–50 mg) or intravenous hydrocortisone (adult dose 100 mg). Intravenous or nebulised magnesium in severe attacks (with cardiac monitoring). Allow over 20 minutes as it may cause hypotension. Repeated doses of magnesium in spontaneously ventilating patients may cause muscle weakness making things worse. Aminophylline is not usually warranted in the prehospital setting unless other treatments are failing and there is a prolonged transfer time. Pay particular attention to dose calculation (narrow therapeutic range) and cardiac monitoring for arrhythmias if starting aminophylline.

Considerations for intubation and ventilation: Indications: coma, severe refractory hypoxaemia, respiratory or cardiac arrest, extreme fatigue and pneumothorax. This is a high-risk intervention in a high risk patient – the risks and benefits must be carefully weighed up. Fluid loading pre-intubation is essential due to risk of cardiovascular collapse. Ketamine is a good option for induction and maintenance of anaesthesia as it aids bronchodilatation. Use volume-controlled ventilation as pressure controlled may lead to dangerous increases in tidal volumes as bronchospasm eases. Use a low respiratory rate (e.g. 8), 4–8 mL/kg tidal volume with adequate expiratory time (1:2–4) in case of air trapping, with no PEEP. Beware of 'breath-stacking' leading to cardiovascular compromise. If in doubt disconnect the ventilator and hand ventilate.

Clinical tip: End tidal carbon dioxide monitoring even in unintubated asthmatics will provide useful information in transfer – changes in waveform from baseline may indicate worsening bronchospasm (though will not be as obvious as in ventilated capnographs), and it is a good overall marker of respiratory rate and sufficiency (Figure 23.1).

COPD/COAD (chronic obstructive pulmonary/airway disease)

Identification

Respiratory distress, cyanosis, wheeze with or without collaborative history.

Differential/concurrent diagnosis

Chronic condition; exacerbation normally related to trigger, e.g. concurrent infection, sputum retention, deterioration of cardiac function (e.g. arrhythmia). Can be difficult to distinguish from pulmonary oedema. Specific history: home nebuliser or long-term oxygen therapy, number of infectious exacerbations a year, exercise tolerance, ability to perform activities of daily living (ADLs).

Transport considerations

Transport sitting up.

Destination considerations

Hospital with appropriate services, e.g. respiratory consultant, chest physiotherapy and BiPAP services.

Treatment

Oxygen if hypoxic (aim for saturations of 88–92%). Nebulised salbutamol with or without ipatropium bromide. Early steroids (oral or intravenous as above). Facial BiPAP may assist – though many ventilators have significant oxygen requirements. Exclude

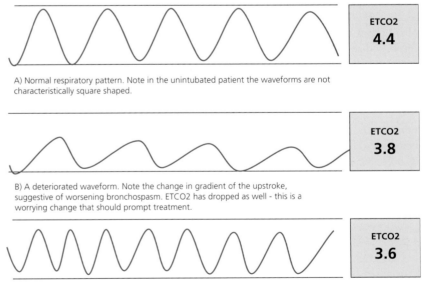

A) Normal respiratory pattern. Note in the unintubated patient the waveforms are not characteristically square shaped.

B) A deteriorated waveform. Note the change in gradient of the upstroke, suggestive of worsening bronchospasm. ETCO2 has dropped as well - this is a worrying change that should prompt treatment.

C) This example shows an acute change in respiratory rate - there is marked increase with decreased ETCO2 associated with hyperventilation

Figure 23.1 Capnogram traces in asthmatic patient.

pneumothorax. Ideally decision-making regarding invasive ventilation should be deferred until arrival in hospital.

Pneumothorax
Identification
Respiratory distress, pleuritic chest pain on affected side. Can be
'primary' (for example in tall, thin males) or 'secondary': associated
with pre-existing lung disease (which may also need treatment).
Examination may show decreased breath sounds on the affected
side and hyperesonance to percussion. Tracheal deviation is a late
sign. Absence of the 'sliding sign' on ultrasound has high sensitivity.

Differential/concurrent diagnosis
Any cause or consequence of chest trauma, pulmonary embolism.

Transport considerations
If travelling at significant altitude in an unpressurized cabin an
intercostal chest drain must be inserted.

Destination considerations
Hospital with appropriate services, e.g. if traumatic cardiothoracic
services, if secondary to diving, hyperbaric chamber.

Treatment
A small pneumothorax will probably not need treatment prehospitally. A large or tension pneumothorax should be decompressed as
described in Chapter 7.

Cardiac emergencies

Acute coronary syndromes and myocardial infarction
Identification
Classical central crushing chest pain radiating to the left arm
is neither sensitive nor specific for myocardial infarction. No
feature of the history or examination is pathognomonic – the index
of suspicion must be high (especially with strong family history,
smokers, diabetic, ethnicity, obese, known ischaemic heart disease).
A 12-lead electrocardiogram should be performed if it will alter
your immediate management/choice of destination or you work in
a region with a prehospital thrombolysis policy.

Differential/concurrent diagnosis
Potentially deadly differential diagnoses include pulmonary
embolism and dissecting aortic aneurysm (classically pain radiating
to the back between the scapulae).

Clinical tip: Check for significant blood pressure differences in
either arm that occurs with thoracic aortic dissection.

Monitor for arrhythmias. Concurrent treatment for heart failure
may be needed.

Transport considerations
Three-lead monitoring, or five-lead (CM5), as illustrated in
Figure 23.2, depending on personal expertise. Defibrillator

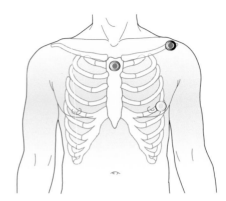

Figure 23.2 CM5 ECG monitoring.

pads *in situ* is recommended. Rapid transfer to an appropriate
destination is crucial: time is myocardium. The additional stress of
helicopter/aeromed transfer in phobic patients must be weighed
against time (and muscle) saved.

Destination considerations
Local resources and the availability of thrombolysis, percutaneous
coronary intervention (PCI) and a dedicated coronary care unit
will dictate destination.

Treatment
Oxygen if hypoxic or travelling by air, aspirin, nitrates and if
required parental analgesia (e.g. morphine) are the mainstay of
treatment. Use of beta-blockers, antiplatelet agents and heparin
must be guided by local policy and practice – you must be familiar
with these. Prehospital thrombolysis *may be* appropriate if transfer
to a centre providing PCI is likely to be prolonged/delayed or
unavailable – follow local policy. Thrombolysis + PCI remains
controversial. If the patient arrests, advanced life support algorithms
should be followed.

Clinical tip: Beware the patient with dental pain or epigas-
tric/indigestion pain: always consider myocardial ischaemia high in
your differential diagnoses.

Acute pulmonary oedema
Identification
Respiratory distress, wheeze with fine crackles at the lung bases with
or without collaborative history. Raised JVP and pedal oedema are
helpful associated signs to look for.

Differential/concurrent diagnosis
Can be difficult to distinguish from COAD. Beware of both tachy-
and bradyarrhythmias.

Transport considerations
Three-lead monitoring with defibrillator pads *in situ* is recommended. Patients should be transported sitting up.

Destination considerations
Hospital with appropriate services.

Treatment

Oxygen and sublingual nitrates if systolic BP >90 (remove if BP drops). Intravenous furosemide is probably not as effective as first thought. Consider giving sublingual ACE inhibitor and oral aspirin. Opiates though traditionally administered may be associated with a higher morbidity and mortality and should only be used if there is associated pain. Monitor for and treat arrhythmias. Intubation may be required depending on transfer time. Non-invasive ventilatory support can be considered with appropriate equipment (e.g. Oxylog 3000) but beware of high flows required – careful oxygen calculation is a must.

Arrhythmias

Identification

Arrhythmias are identified using a three-lead or 12-lead ECG.

Clinical tip: Get a print off of the rhythm strip to analyse, as well as for part of your contemporaneous records.

Differential/concurrent diagnosis

Beware of atrial fibrillation with a coexisting bundle branch block.

Transport considerations

Three-lead monitoring with defibrillator pads *in situ* is recommended – transcutaneous pacing may become necessary or defibrillation.

Destination considerations

Local resources and the availability of a dedicated coronary care unit will dictate destination.

Treatment

Treatment should be administered according to the local adaptation of the International Liaison Committee on Resuscitation (ILCOR) guidelines and presence of adverse clinical signs. Use of specific treatments such as adenosine or amiodarone will depend on the above and practitioner familiarity. Never give a drug you are unfamiliar with for the first time in the prehospital setting. DC cardioversion should only be attempted if you have the skill set for safe sedation, in the presence of severe adverse signs and prolonged transfer time – always weigh up the risks against the potential benefits.

Anaphylaxis

Identification

- CVS: Tachycardia/hypotension. Most common presentation.
- R/S: Wheeze and tachypnoea.
- GIT: Vomiting and diarrhoea.
- Skin: Oedema – typically facial and associated flushing.
- History of allergy and recent exposure to certain foodstuff (e.g. nuts, shell fish or drugs – e.g. antibiotics).

Differential/concurrent diagnosis

Urticaria/Hives. Note some medications can cause swelling without other features of anaphylaxis, for example ACE inhibitors can cause tongue or facial swelling (angioedema). Beware of patients with hereditary angioneurotic oedema (C1 esterase inhibitor deficiency) as they may not respond as well to adrenaline and steroids. History is vital in these cases and consideration given to which hospital to take them to – EDs with known local populations with C1 esterase deficiency will stock synthetic C1 esterase inhibitor making management easier – this information needs to be sought from collateral history and presence of medical alert bracelets/cards.

Transport considerations

True anaphylaxis carries a high risk for rapid deterioration. Airway is likely to be difficult to manage – allow the patient to position themselves if possible.

Destination considerations

Nearest hospital with emergency facilities and intensive care.

Treatment

Early recognition is key. Support the airway as necessary. If airway obstructs be prepared to perform prompt surgical cricothyroidotomy. Volume resuscitate with crystalloids. IM adrenaline – use patient's own EpiPen if they have one and it is in date. Repeat doses as needed (0.3–0.5 ml of 1:1000 adrenaline (epinephrine) intramuscularly). Intravenous hydrocortisone/chlorpheniramine if time permits. Do NOT delay on scene.

Neurological emergencies

The fitting patient

Identification

Many seizure types and presentations exist. Self-limiting seizures do not require emergency prehospital intervention. Continuous seizure types fall into two categories: generalized status epilepticus (including tonic–clonic, tonic, clonic, myoclonic and absence seizures) and focal status epilepticus (also known as partial seizures). Collateral history is vital. Pseudoseizure is NOT a prehospital diagnosis. Patients are at risk of traumatic injuries as a result of the seizure. Severe tonic–clonic seizures can result in posterior shoulder dislocation.

Differential/concurrent diagnosis

Attempt to identify and treat 'trigger', e.g. fever (especially in infants), infection, hypoglycaemia, poisoning, and head trauma. Assess and document initial GCS and pupil responses.

Transport considerations

Actively fitting patients are unsafe to transport. Have your drugs drawn up, a cannula in situ and a flush line running for those who are at risk of seizure/recurrent seizures. Elective RSI may be the safe choice for high-risk/prolonged transfers.

Destination considerations

A hospital with appropriate facilities to treat the cause of the fit.

Treatment

Prolonged seizures can be treated with intravenous benzodiazepines, e.g. lorazapam. Intravenous phenytoin may be administered during a prolonged transfer/on scene time (but not if seizures are associate with tricyclic overdose). Ensure the airway is patent. Does the cervical spine need protecting? Rapid sequence induction with thiopentone should be considered for those who do not respond to conventional treatment/are in status epilepticus.

Clinical tip: Midazolam can be given via the buccal or intranasal routes. Diazapam can be given rectally. Respiratory support may be needed following treatment with benzodiazepines.

Cerebrovascular accident
Identification

The FAST acronym/mnemonic is widely used amongst health professionals and lay-people to identify potential cerebrovascular accidents (CVAs): **F**acial weakness, **A**rm weakness, **S**peech difficulty, and **T**ime to act/**T**est.

Differential/concurrent diagnosis

Arrhythmias, hypoglycaemia and other causes of seizures are commonly mistaken for CVAs.

Transport considerations

As for the fitting patient.

Destination considerations

Rapid transfer to an appropriate centre offering thrombolysis or embolectomy within the locally defined time window is crucial.

Treatment

The development of point of care testing which accurately distinguishes between ischaemic and haemorrhagic stroke may lead to prehospital thrombolysis. Treatment currently consists of supportive management and rapid transfer.

Metabolic emergencies

High blood sugar including diabetic ketoacidosis and hyperosmolar states
Identification

A high blood sugar on point of care testing accompanied by autonomic symptoms: tachycardia, Kussmauls respiration, sweet smelling/pear drop breath (ketones).

Differential/concurrent diagnosis

Attempt to find and treat trigger, e.g. infection, myocardial infarction, CVA. All patients are intravascularly dehydrated. Be aware of arrhythmias caused by hyperkalaemia.

Transport considerations

Monitor for arrhythmias.

Destination considerations

A hospital with appropriate facilities.

Treatment

Intravenous isotonic fluid resuscitation. Insulin is probably only appropriate with prolonged prehospital times and when the potassium level can be measured. Treat concurrent infection.

Hypoglycaemia
Identification

Diagnosis confirmed by point of care testing. Patient may appear intoxicated or aggressive, exhibit signs of CVA, be suffering from seizures or even be unconscious.

Differential/concurrent diagnosis

Consider infection as a cause. Be aware of purposeful insulin overdose.

Transport considerations

In the case of agitated and confused patients correct this before transporting them. Recovery position is appropriate for those that can protect their own airway.

Destination considerations

A hospital with appropriate facilities.

Treatment

Oral glucose followed by complex carbohydrate if conscious and compliant. Consider IV 10% dextrose (2 ml/kg) and/or Glucagon (adult dose 1 mg) or hypostop gels. Block excision of the injection site may be life saving in massive insulin overdose.

Clinical tip: Though tempting to discharge on scene these patients have a high relapse rate so are best transferred to hospital for observation.

Poisoning
Identification

In the absence of a reliable and/or collaborative history, poisoning may be a difficult diagnosis. Consider in all patients with altered levels of consciousness, unexplained arrhythmia or unusual clinical manifestations. Combinations of toxidromes can further complicate identification (Table 23.2).

Differential/concurrent diagnosis

Need to consider both alternative causes of the clinical presentation (hypoxia, hypoglycemia etc.) and concurrent medical problems that may be masked by the poisoning, e.g. head injury.

Transport considerations

Will depend upon the specific toxidrome. Cardiac monitoring is sensible in case of tricyclic antidepressant overdose.

Destination considerations

Rare poisonings and those requiring specialist intervention may benefit from early transportation to a dedicated poisons centre.

Table 23.2 Toxidromes

Toxidrome	Site of action	Signs and symptoms
Opioid	Opioid receptor	Sedation, miosis, decreased bowel sounds, decreased respirations
Anticholinergic	muscurinic acetylcholine receptors	Altered mental status, sedation, hallucinations, mydriasis, dry skin, dry mucous membranes, decreased bowel sounds and urinary retention
Sedative-hypnotic	gamma-aminobutyric acid receptors	sedation, normal pupils, decreased respirations
Sympathomimetic	alpha and beta adrenergic receptors	agitation, mydriasis, tachycardia, hypertension, hyperthermia, diaphoresis
Cholinergic	nicotinic and muscurinic acetylcholine receptors	altered mental status, seizures, miosis, lacrimation, diaphoresis, bronchospasm, bronchorrhea, vomiting, diarrhoea, bradycardia
Serotonin syndrome	serotonin receptors	altered mental status, tachycardia, hypertension, hyperreflexia, clonus, hyperthermia

Source: Boyle J, Bechtel L, Holstege C. *Scandinavian Journal of Trauma, Resuscitation and Emergency Medicine* 2009, 17:29.

Awareness of the availability of rarely stocked antidotes may dictate destination.

Treatment

Rapidly remove the patient from any potential further contamination. Some poisons have specific antidotes – these are rarely administered in the prehospital environment. Activated charcoal can be administered in most cases of poisoning with a few exclusions (Box 23.1). The mainstay of prehospital treatment consists of symptomatic treatment and safe transfer.

Box 23.1 **Contraindications to activated charcoal**

Contraindications

- Decreased level of consciousness
- Acids
- Alkalis
- Alcohols
- Glycols
- Hydrocarbons
- Metals and Ionic Compounds
- iron, fluoride, potassium, mercury, lithium.

Remember to collect any 'evidence' of potential sources of poisoning at the scene – this may be the only opportunity to gather this valuable information. Past medical history or that of family members may also give clues as to potential medications taken as part of a mixed overdose.

Psychiatric emergencies/acute psychoses
Recognition

The patient may already have a psychiatric diagnosis. Careful communication and non-threatening body language are essential. Always have an escape route/plan. Your own safety is paramount. High risk patients include those with associated alcohol/drug abuse. Cases may include deliberate self harm or attempted suicide, with associated trauma or overdose.

Differential/concurrent diagnosis

Hypoglycaemia, transient ischaemic attack or stroke, epilepsy, thyrotoxic crisis.

Transport considerations

Team safety. Is the patient willing to go to hospital? If not do you require a police escort? Patients unwilling to travel to hospital are likely to require sectioning under the Mental Health act (or local equivalent). The police may intervene to protect the general public or the patient themselves. It is not safe to transport acutely disturbed patients by air.

Destination considerations

If the patient is known to a psychiatric facility it is best to take them to the associated hospital for continuity of care where feasible.

Treatment

You may have to assess the patient's capacity to consent to or refuse treatment. Minimize interventions to those necessary for safe transfer. If sedation is necessary, then this must be safe, and never so deep that the airway becomes compromised. The patient should be fully monitored: end tidal carbon dioxide monitoring is strongly advised. Choice of sedative agent will depend upon the presentation and practitioner familiarity.

Infection/sepsis
Identification

A prehospital sepsis screening tool (Figure 23.3) can be used to identify sepsis – those with systemic infection who require urgent treatment. Any immunosuppressed patient is at high risk of sepsis.

Differential/concurrent diagnosis

Consider likely source and type of infection.

Transport considerations

Depends on the source and symptoms of sepsis.

Destination considerations

A hospital with appropriate facilities.

Treatment

Early antibiotics and fluids are life saving. The 'sepsis six' has been modified for the prehospital environment (Figure 23.3).

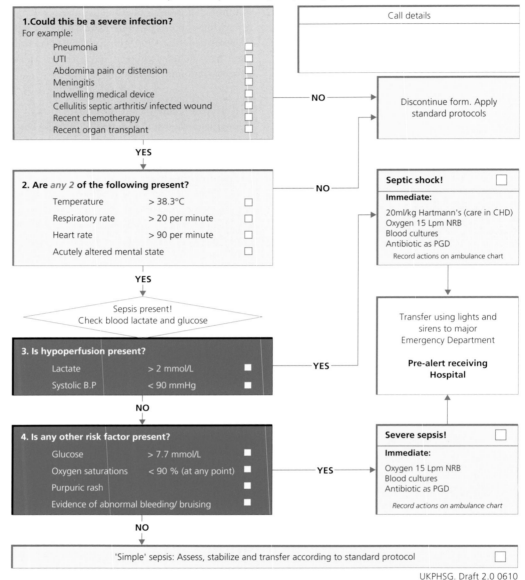

Figure 23.3 Prehospital sepsis screening and treatment tool. (Source: reproduced with permission of the United Kingdom Prehospital Sepsis Group.)

Tips from the field

- Oxygen is for hypoxaemia not breathlessness!
- Hypotensive resuscitation is for Trauma patients: many medical patients will benefit from IV fluids
- Early intravenous fluids and, if your system allows it, antibiotics can be life saving to a patient with sepsis
- Prealert the receiving emergency department for sick patients. Ensure quality care for arrival and handover
- Don't be pressured by systems or economics to discharge at scene without the necessary tests or investigations

- ACS, PE and dissecting aortic aneurysm cannot be safely excluded in the prehospital environment
- Less than 15% of patients with a life threatening condition will present 'classically', your index of suspicion must be high.

Further reading

Crocco T. Streamlining Stroke care: from symptom onset to emergency department. *J Emerg Med* 2007;**33**:255–260.

Ghosh R, Pepe P. The Critical care cascade: a systems approach. *Curr Opin Crit Care* 2009;**15**:279–283.

Goldstein P, Weil J. Management of prehospital thrombolytic therapy in ST-segment elevation acute coronary syndrome (<12 hours). *Minerva Anesthiolog* 2005;**71**:297–302.

Mattu A, Lawner B. PreHospital management of congestive heart failure. *Heart Failure Clin* 2009;**5**:19–24.

Mebazza A, Gheorghiade M, Piña I, *et al.* Practical recommendations for prehospital and early in-hospital management of patients presenting with acute heart failure syndromes. *Crit Care Med* 2008;**36**: S129–139.

Mental Health Act 2007. www.legislation.gov.uk/ukpga/2007/12/contents.

Michael G, O'Connor R. The diagnosis and management of seizures and status epilepticus in the prehospital setting. *Emerg Med Clin North Am* 2011;**29**:29–39.

O'Driscoll B, Howard L, Davison A. British Thoracic Society guideline for emergency oxygen use in adult patients. *Thorax* 2008;**63**;1–68.

Workgroup on EMS Management of Asthma Exacerbations. A model protocol for emergency medical services management of asthma exacerbations. *Prehosp Emerg Care* 2006;**10**:418–429.

CHAPTER 24

Environmental Injuries

Peter Aitken[1], Mark Little[1], Ian Norton[2], and Andrew Pearce[3]

[1] James Cook University, Townsville, QLD, Australia
[2] Royal Darwin Hospital, Darwin, NT, Australia
[3] Royal Adelaide Hospital, Adelaide, SA, Australia

OVERVIEW

By the end of this chapter you should know the:

- Types of environmental injury and generic approaches to prevention for the patient and prehospital team
- Types of cold related illness and injury and initial management in the prehospital environment
- Types of heat related injury and illness and initial management in the prehospital environment
- Basic envenomation syndromes and principles of early management.

Introduction

Prehospital care usually involves exposure to the elements. This introduces the environment as a potential cause of the initial injury or illness, a contributor to secondary effects on a patient with other illness or injury and the risk of environmental injury to personnel providing care. There are multiple types of environmental injury (Table 24.1). Many are discussed in other chapters (e.g. altitude, diving, drowning) while this chapter focuses on cold and heat injury and envenomation. It is worth remembering that people are also part of the environment and often the least predictable and most dangerous element.

Prehospital personnel should have a sound knowledge of environmental injury and its management. They also need to maintain an awareness of environmental risks to ensure the welfare of both the patient and team members and include preventive measures in their pre-planning.

Cold injury

Injuries due to cold exposure can be life threatening and debilitating. The human body has relatively tight thermoregulatory control of body temperature with diurnal variations of only 1°C. Hypothermia is a clinical condition defined as a core body temperature <35°C and may be classed as mild, moderate and severe (Table 24.2).

Table 24.1 Environmental injuries/illness in the prehospital environment

Grouping	Environmental injury/illness
Climate	Heat injury and illness Cold injury and illness
Flora and fauna	Envenomation Bite/sting Large animal encounters
Geography	Falls from heights Rockfalls/avalanches Drowning (Chapter 26) Altitude illness (Chapter 25)
Specific hazards	Environmental toxicology Burns (Chapter 18)
Human elements	Diving/dysbarism (Chapter 27) Crowd behaviour and bystanders (Chapter 35) Traffic and transport related (Chapter 23) CBRN (Chapter 34)

Table 24.2 Signs and symptoms of hypothermia

	Mild	Moderate	Severe
Core temperature	32–35°C	29–32°C	<29°C
Thermogenesis	Still possible	Progressive failure of thermogenesis	Adoption of the temperature of the surrounding environment
Signs	Shivering, apathy, ataxia, dysarthria, tachycardia	Loss of shivering, altered mental state, muscular rigidity, bradycardia, hypotension	Signs of life almost undetectable, coma, fixed and dilated pupils, areflexia, profound bradycardia and hypotension

Body heat is lost in four main ways – conduction, radiation, evaporation and convection. This is important in the development and management of both hypothermia and hyperthermia. Risk factors for development of hypothermia relate to environmental exposure, specific disease processes producing hypothermia and patients with predisposing conditions (Table 24.3). Many of these also need to

ABC of Prehospital Emergency Medicine, First Edition.
Edited by Tim Nutbeam and Matthew Boylan.
© 2013 John Wiley & Sons, Ltd. Published 2013 by John Wiley & Sons, Ltd.

Table 24.3 Risk factors for cold and heat injury/illness

Grouping	Cold injury/illness	Heat illness/injury
Weather Factors	Cold weather Rain, snow Wind chill effects	Hot weather Direct sun exposure Increased humidity High WBGT
Patient characteristics – behaviour	Period exposure Immersion Lack of acclimitization Clothing – lack or wet Sleep deprivation Dehydration Fatigue	Period exposure Exercise Lack of acclimitization Inappropriate clothing Combative behaviour Dehydration Increased physical activity Microclimate, e.g. inside CBRN suits, firefighting gear, etc.
Patient characteristics – health	Extremes of age CVA Paraplegia Parkinsons Hypoglycaemia Hypothyroidism Hypoadrenalism Sepsis Malnutrition	Extremes of age Obesity Seizures Cardiovascular disease Diabetic Ketoacidosis Thyrotoxicosis Febrile illness Neuroleptic malignant syndrome
Patient characteristics – drugs	Alcohol Benzodiazepines Phenothiazines (impair shivering)	Alcohol Amphetamines Cocaine Salicylates SSRIs Diuretics Anticholinergics Phenothiazines Malignant hyperpyrexia (suxamethonium + halothane) Allergic drug reactions
Trauma	Major trauma – entrapment, resuscitation, head injury, burns Minor trauma – immobility	
Transport factors	Open transport platform Lack of heating	Enclosed transport platform Lack of air conditioning or ventilation

Table 24.4 Frostbite classification

	Frostnip	Superficial frostbite	Deep frostbite
Depth	Short lived superficial freezing	Superficial skin layers only affected	Full thickness
Appearance		Clear blisters form 24–48 hours after injury Tissue beneath surface remains pliable and soft	Blood filled blisters form after 1–3 weeks Underlying tissues are woody and stony
Outcome	Responds rapidly to warming No residual swelling		Bad prognosis Loss of digits likely

be considered as part of the differential diagnosis. Elderly patients with pre-existing medical conditions are at particular risk from falls, lying on cold floors or the ground for long periods, until discovered hypothermic or deceased.

Cold tolerance depends on the individual, their fitness and preparation for the environment as well as the temperature, wind-chill factor and whether they are wet. While wind chill is measured differently in the southern and northern hemispheres, the point is that cold, windy and wet equates to increased propensity for cold injury and hypothermia.

Once energy is depleted, the individual is susceptible to hypothermia even at relatively mild temperatures. The hypothermic patient has impaired judgement that can lead to poor decision making and

inability to prevent further temperature loss. Paradoxical removal of clothing is seen in cases of severe hypothermia which correlates with the 'umbles' of hypothermia (stumbles, mumbles, grumbles, jumbles). The clinical signs and symptoms of hypothermia are described in Table 24.2. There is progressive 'slowing' of function as initial efforts to keep warm cease and the patient becomes 'one with the surrounding environment'. The ECG is characteristic with slow AF and 'J waves' seen. J waves are an extra positive deflection after the normal S wave and seen most commonly in leads II and V3–6, with the height of the J wave roughly proportional to the degree of hypothermia (Figure 24.1). The Glasgow Coma Scale (GCS) is not prognostic of outcome and patients with a low GCS may walk from hospital with timely and correct treatment.

Localized injury is a clinical spectrum from frostnip through the degrees of frostbite, from reversible to irreversible tissue damage (Table 24.4 and Figure 24.2). Non-freezing cold injuries such as chilblain, pernio and trench foot are also a spectrum from reversible to irreversible and result from having cold wet extremities for an extended period and can cause extreme pain and disability.

The prehospital management considerations can be broken down into consideration of immediate first aid and advanced medical care. Patients who are hypothermic and/or cold injured need to be treated in a medical facility while following the steps listed in Table 24.5 to avoid causing further injury. The adage that 'you are not dead until you are warm and dead' needs to be interpreted with caution. There needs to be an awareness of periods of exposure and ambient temperatures and should be realistic so as not to put rescuers at risk. In tropical environments, cold and dead is usually dead. Management of local tissue cold injury is described in Table 24.6.

The key to cold injuries is prevention (Table 24.7). Unfortunate scenarios in which lives have been lost due to cold exposure may have been prevented simply by correct clothing, adequate communications, weather checks, acclimatization and familiarization. Frostbite is not common in those adequately prepared, clothed and aware of the conditions. As health professionals, ensuring that we listen to the history and look for signs of cold injury in susceptible populations to ensure early goal directed therapy is the key to good patient outcomes.

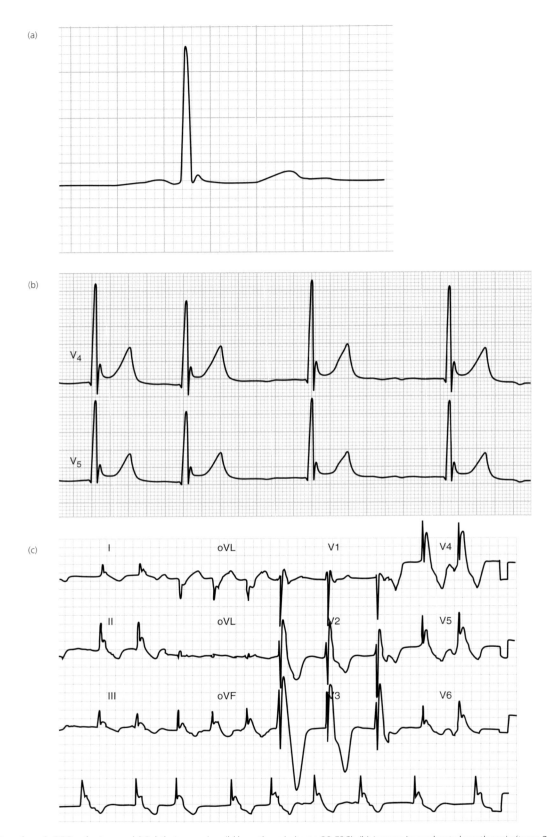

Figure 24.1 Hypothermia ECG – the J wave. (a) Subtle J waves in mild hypothermia (temp 32.5°C). (b) J waves in moderate hypothermia (temp 30°C). (c) Marked J waves in severe hypothermia (temp <27°C).

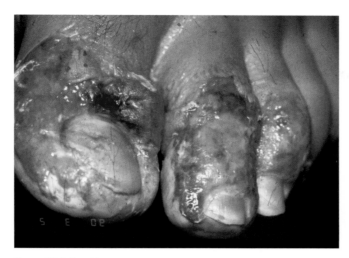

Figure 24.2 Frostbite.

Table 24.5 Management of hypothermia

Immediate first aid

Safety of self, scene then survivor

Call for help, emergency services

If possible remove from cold, take off wet clothes and dry

Check for a pulse up to several minutes, if no pulse start CPR and continue until care handed over

Cover and protect the head from further heat loss

Warm the patient, whether blankets, shelter, sleeping bag

If possible warm high calorie fluids drinks (avoid alcohol and caffeine)

Advanced life support

Check for airway and consider cervical spine precautions

Check for breathing and administer high-flow oxygen (humidified if possible)

Check for circulation

Any pulse however faint negates the need for CPR

Apply monitoring

Obtain intravenous access where possible and check blood glucose level

Fluid requirements are vastly underestimated working in cold climates and dehydration is common.

Other

Look at pupils and consider opioid antagonist if indicated

Measure core temperature (oesophageal/rectal low reading thermometer)

Heat packs to hands and feet

Gentle handling to reduce inducing ventricular fibrillation

Notify receiving facility of patient's condition and requirements on arrival

Table 24.6 Management of local cold injury

Do not rub the affected area

Splint the affected area and wrap in loose dry clothing

Do not start thawing unless able to continue as refreezing may cause more tissue damage

Once able rapid rewarming of affected area should begin at 40–42°C

This is extremely painful and in most cases will require analgesia such as ketamine or narcotics

Early surgical intervention has no role in the initial management of frostbite with the initial treatment focussed on preserving as much tissue as possible

Table 24.7 Prevention strategies for patients and personnel

Strategy	Intervention
Bulletins and warning	Public health bulletins regarding cold/hot weather and how to stay warm/cool
Community	Checking on neighbours
Social services	Social services (and cooling) for the elderly and vulnerable
Power supplies	Adequate power supplies to deal with surges in demand (air conditioning and heating)
Alarms	Monitored personal alarms for at risk patients
PPE	Including high heat loss areas and extremities in cold climates and sun protection/breathable in hot climates
Work rosters	Work rest ratios and active cooling/warming in high risk work groups (defence, emergency services workers)
Hydration	Adequate hydration (avoid greater than 2% dehydration for optimum work rates and decreased risk of illness)
Acclimitization	Care with staff from other regions not used to environment

Heat injury

Heat illness can be defined as an inability of normal regulatory mechanisms to cope with heat stress. It is a continuum of disease from mild 'heat cramps' through 'heat exhaustion' to life-threatening 'heat stroke'. All are characterized by hyperthermia, but with gradually worsening multi-organ impairment and eventually failure (Table 24.8). CNS dysfunction is the key differentiator between heat exhaustion and heat stroke and gradually worsens as the temperature rises and/or exposure time lengthens. Mortality rates range from 10% to 70%, depending on background health, age and length and severity of exposure.

Heatwave is defined as a prolonged period of excessive heat relative to the normal temperatures of that region. Local definitions recognize acclimitization, meaning heatwaves occur at lower temperatures in the UK than tropical Australia. Heat waves kill more people than floods and hurricanes/cyclones combined.

Table 24.8 Heat illness types/classification

System	Heat cramps	Heat exhaustion	Heat stroke
Temperature		>38°C	>40.5°C or 104.9°F
Skin temperature	Normal	Normal or cool and clammy	Hot and dry (50% cases)
Sweat rate	Increased	Increased or decreased	Decreased
Urine output	Normal	Oliguria	Anuria
GI	Thirst	Nausea ± vomiting	Nausea and vomiting
CVS	Tachycardia	Hypotension	± Circulatory collapse
CNS	Nil	Uncoordinated, Irritable or confused	Delirium/seizure/coma
Other	Thirst		Renal failure Liver failure DIC

Temperature alone is a poor indicator of risk. The level of heat discomfort is determined by a combination of factors including meteorological (air temperature, humidity, wind, direct sunshine); cultural (clothing, occupation, accommodation); and physiological (health, fitness, age, level of acclimatization). Patient risk factors for environmental heat illness are described in Table 24.3.

To account for meteorological effects other than temperature the WBGT (wet bulb globe temperature) was developed in the 1950s for US marines who were required to train in full sun and high humidity (Box 24.1). It is an easily measured heat stress index often used in guidelines for work in hot environments. The American College of Sports Medicine recommends cancellation of events if the WBGT is greater than 28°C. Prehospital practitioners at sporting events and mass gatherings can also expect heat illness presentations in at-risk groups at a lower WBGT.

Box 24.1 **Wet bulb globe temperature**

$WBGT = (0.7 \times Tnwb) + (0.2 \times Tg) + (0.1 \times Ta)$

Tnwb = natural wet bulb temperature (represents integrated effects of humidity, radiation + wind)

Tg = black globe temperature (represents integrated effects of radiation + wind)

Ta = ambient temperature.

A useful approach to diagnosis of hyperthermia is to recognize risk factors and alternative diagnoses (Table 24.3) and determine severity of heat illness (Table 24.8). Heat illness is primarily caused by hyperthermia, with hydration status a secondary factor, and sufferers may present in either an overhydrated (hyponatraemic) or dehydrated state.

Management of heat illness must start with cooling. ABCs are supported as this occurs, and hydration and replacement of electrolytes can occur concomitantly, but will not save the patient without cooling. The patient should be removed from the heat source and clothing removed, in particular any PPE. Cooling should begin by any practical means with cooling methods described in Table 24.9. Evaporative cooling using water applied to skin while fanning is the most powerful cooling method. Application of ice packs to neck, axilla and groin if available is partially useful. Both immersion and ice packs can cause adverse shivering and limit their efficacy while evaporative cooling dissipates seven times as much heat as the melting of ice. Expensive cooling devices and invasive techniques have little use in prehospital settings, although cold intravenous fluids have shown promise. The aim is to cool the patient to between 38.5 and 39°C to avoid overshoot hypothermia. Antipyretics have no role. The use of induced hypothermia after resuscitative efforts mandates prehospital clinicians have a thorough understanding of cooling techniques.

Prevention is a key element in management of heat illness with a number of strategies described in Table 24.9. Acclimatization allows a gradual increased tolerance to heat stress. It occurs over 7–60 days and is aided by routine exposure to ambient heat and a core temperature rise (over 38.5°C). Heat adaptations include increased sweat rates, lower temperature triggers for sweating, increased plasma volume and extracellular fluid and decreased heart rate at rest.

Table 24.9 Rewarming strategies and cooling methods

	Rewarming strategies	Cooling methods
Non-invasive	Remove all clothing* Warm, dry, wind free environment* Body to body contact Forced air blankets Heat packs (axilla, groin, neck)* Immersion (warm water)†§	Remove all clothing* Evaporative*‡ Ice packs (axilla, groin, neck)* Immersion (cool to cold water)†
Invasive	Warm intravenous fluids* Warm water gastric lavage Warm water bladder irrigation Warm water peritoneal lavage Warm water pleural lavage Cardiac bypass	Cold intravenous fluids* Cold water gastric lavage Cold water bladder irrigation Cold water peritoneal lavage Cold water pleural lavage Cardiac bypass

*Able to be easily used in prehospital environment.
†Patient access is poor in full immersion and inappropriate in those with altered GCS.
‡Caution with washout phenomena with return of cold acidotic blood centrally from the peripheries.
§Most powerful and practical technique. Requires water as spray or application direct to skin, with vigorous air flow e.g. fan.
Not as powerful a method as evaporation (7 times less powerful).

Envenomation

Most continents have venomous creatures, with many millions suffering death and disability each year as a result of bites and stings.

It is estimated that worldwide there are 2.5 million envenomings and 125 000 snakebite deaths per year. The health burden of snakebite coupled with reduced production of snake antivenom has seen the World Health Organization list snakebite as a 'neglected tropical disease'. The global distribution of envenomation is shown in Figure 24.3. The two main groups of venomous snakes in the world are vipers (mainly in Americas, Africa, Eurasia) and elapids (mainly southeast Asia, Australia, PNG). It is important to realize that not all people bitten by snakes are envenomed. This explains the frequent reports of homeopathic first aid methods (e.g. black stones or electric shock therapy) resulting in survival from snake bite.

If envenomed, most patients will display a mix of local tissue destruction, paralysis, bleeding disorders and paralysis. Bite sites may be obvious (Figure 24.4) but not always so. First aid revolves mainly around immobilizing the bitten body part and the patient and supportive care. Definitive treatment of envenoming revolves around using antivenom, although adjunct treatments (e.g. neostigmine in management of paralysis due to cobra and death adder envenomings) have proved effective if no antivenom is available. Problems with antivenom include cost, need for refrigeration and a high rate of anaphylaxis. Snake identification can also be difficult making use of specific antivenom problematic.

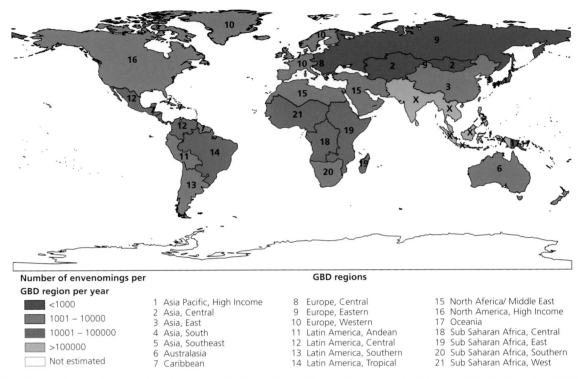

Number of envenomings per GBD region per year

■	<1000
■	1001 – 10000
■	10001 – 100000
■	>100000
□	Not estimated

GBD regions

1 Asia Pacific, High Income	8 Europe, Central	15 North Aferica/ Middle East
2 Asia, Central	9 Europe, Eastern	16 North America, High Income
3 Asia, East	10 Europe, Western	17 Oceania
4 Asia, South	11 Latin America, Andean	18 Sub Saharan Africa, Central
5 Asia, Southeast	12 Latin America, Central	19 Sub Saharan Africa, East
6 Australasia	13 Latin America, Southern	20 Sub Saharan Africa, Southern
7 Caribbean	14 Latin America, Tropical	21 Sub Saharan Africa, West

Figure 24.3 Regional estimates of envenomings due to snakebite (low estimate) (Source: Kasturiratne A, Wickremasinghe AR, de Silva N, Gunawardena NK, Pathmeswaran A, *et al.* (2008). *PLoS Med* **5**(11): e218. doi:10.1371/journal.pmed.0050218).

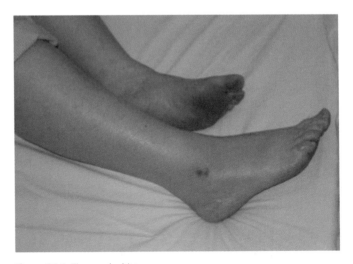

Figure 24.4 Tiger snake bite.

Most spiders are unlikely to cause systemic toxicity other than the *Lactrodectus*, (black widow, red back spider), funnel web and recluse spiders. Usual symptoms are local effects but systemic symptoms require medical attention and may require antivenom. There have been deaths reported from funnel web bites, with pressure immobilization bandaging the required first aid.

Most scorpion stings in the USA and Australia cause local effects only. However, in North Africa, Central and Southern America, and the Middle East stings can result in systemic toxicity resembling a catecholamine surge with a significant number of deaths reported, mainly in children. There is no specific first aid, other than symptomatic care, as the treatment of systemic symptoms requires antivenom.

Many millions of people per year are stung by jellyfish. Few develop significant systemic toxicity. The Portuguese man of war (*Physalia*), Box jellyfish (*Chironex fleckeri*) and other chirodropids in southeast Asia and Irukandji jellyfish can cause significant systemic toxicity and in rare cases death. Antivenom is only available for the Box jellyfish. First aid mainly revolves around using vinegar to neutralize nematocysts, although promising work has been done using heat to reduce the pain of jellyfish stings.

Stings by spiny fish usually result in severe local pain, and heat often provides effective first aid. Regional local anaesthesia blocks may be effective, and antivenom exists for stone fish stings.

Barb injuries from stingrays usually cause local damage, while barbs have venom that can also cause tissue destruction. The major concern is the penetrating injury and the barb should not initially be removed. Infection is another significant issue and wounds should be cleaned and left open.

Preparation is essential, to ensure the ability to care for patients with envenoming injuries and for staff safety. This includes personal knowledge of local wildlife, envenoming risks and clinical management (including first aid), as well as access to expert advice when needed. Access to appropriate antivenoms should be secured and may need a means of maintaining the cold chain during transport. Uniforms should provide appropriate protection for staff (one more reason to wear boots) and care should be taken with arrival at any scene or during patient movement that patients and staff are not exposed to risks of secondary envenomation.

Tips from the field

- Look after yourself – ensure adequate sleep, diet, exercise, PPE and acclimitization
- Look before you leap with regard to the environment you will be working in – don't make yourself an extra patient
- Remember the patient is the one with the illness; if able, ensure the temperature of the transport environment meets their needs not yours
- Patients are not dead until they are warm and dead, unless they are cold and dead in the tropics
- Know your local environment and be prepared – have access to expert toxinology advice organized in advance.

Further reading

Armstrong LE, Casa DJ, Millard-Stafford M, *et al*. American College of Sports Medicine Position Statement: exertional heat illness during training and competition. *Med Sci Sports Exercise* 2007;**39**:556–572.

Kasturiratne A, Wickremasinghe AR, de Silva N, *et al*. () Estimating the global burden of snakebite: A literature analysis and modelling based on regional estimates of envenoming and deaths. *PLoS Med* 2008;**5**:e218.

van der Ploeg GJ. Goslings JC. Walpoth BH. Bierens JJ. Accidental hypothermia: rewarming treatments, complications and outcomes from one university medical centre. *Resuscitation* 2010;**81**:1550–1555.

CHAPTER 25

Environmental: Altitude Injury

Harvey Pynn

Wilderness Medical Training, Kendal, UK

Introduction

High-altitude environments occur on all the world's continents. The highest mountain peaks are accessible to only a few well-equipped climbers, but many people live and travel to areas of very high altitude such as La Paz in Chile, the Tibetan plateau, the Inca Trail as well as more accessible mountains such as Mount Kilimanjaro (summit 5985 metres).

The effects of altitude begin to become apparent over 2500 meters above sea level. Over 5500 meters, the effects of altitude are extreme and the ability of the body to adjust further diminishes. Prolonged time at this elevation will lead to fatigue and degradation. Altitude over 7500 meters is known as the death zone – well-acclimatized climbers can only spend very short periods of time at this altitude.

Physiology at altitude

As one ascends to altitude, the body has to cope with the demands of a lower partial pressure of oxygen. At altitudes of 5500 meters the barometric pressure will be only 50% of that at sea level. Unacclimatized individuals will be breathless and have grossly reduced exercise tolerance. Oxygen saturations will be reduced to as low as 80%.

Acclimatization is the process by which people adjust to altitude hypoxia. Immediate adaptations include an increase in heart rate, respiratory rate and depth of breathing. Following this an increase in haemoglobin concentration will occur, initially from a rapid

Table 25.1 Aids to acclimatization

- Limit ascent to 300–600 m per day (when above 3000 m)
- Incorporate rest days to allow the body to 'catch up'
- Climb high – Sleep low
- Acetazolmide (Diamox) 250 mg bd po (when above 3000 m)

decrease in plasma volume (up to 5%) and later by a slower increase in red cell mass. These changes occur at different rates in different people and there are no predicting factors as to who may perform better at altitude other than previous personal experience. However, if ascent to altitude occurs more quickly than the body can adapt, symptoms of acute mountain sickness (AMS) may develop. Aids to acclimatization are shown in Table 25.1.

Acute mountain sickness

AMS is a common altitude illness affecting 50% of all individuals ascending rapidly to an altitude of 4500 metres. It describes a non-specific collection of symptoms that occur 6–12 hours following arrival at altitude. It is important to recognize AMS as it can progress to life-threatening high-altitude cerebral oedema (HACE) or high-altitude pulmonary oedema (HAPE).

Symptoms and signs of AMS

The cardinal symptom is a throbbing headache. Symptoms are usually worse at night when respiratory drive is depressed. The signs are extremely non-specific (Table 25.2).

Treatment of AMS

Treatment of mild AMS involves symptomatic care with rest, oral fluids, simple analgesia (paracetamol) and antiemetics if required. If symptoms do not settle or indeed worsen, descent should be

Table 25.2 AMS symptoms and signs

AMS Symptoms	AMS Signs
Headache	Peripheral oedema
Anorexia	Tachycardia
Nausea and vomiting	Scattered creps on auscultation
Fatigue	Raised basal temperature
Dizziness	
Sleep disturbance	

ABC of Prehospital Emergency Medicine, First Edition.
Edited by Tim Nutbeam and Matthew Boylan.
© 2013 John Wiley & Sons, Ltd. Published 2013 by John Wiley & Sons, Ltd.

considered. If travelling with a group and AMS symptoms develops in one group member, it is likely that others may be suffering and should be checked.

AMS may be prevented by using prophylactic acetazolamide (Diamox). This is a carbonic anhydrase inhibitor that promotes excretion of HCO_3 leading to a metabolic acidosis, thus increasing respiratory drive and hence oxygenation. This mirrors the effect acclimatization will have on the kidneys but in less time. Side effects include polyuria, paraesthesia and altered taste (of fizzy drinks).

High altitude cerebral oedema

HACE and AMS represent two extremes of the same disease process and, as such, it is unusual for HACE to present without prior warning signs. More commonly the symptoms of mild AMS were ignored. HACE is rare but potentially fatal. Approximately 2–3% of people travelling above 5000 meters will be affected. The exact pathophysiology is yet to be determined but as cerebral blood flow increases with altitude, a combination of capillary leakage due to disruption of the blood–brain barrier and impaired cerebral autoregulation on acute exposure to hypoxia may be responsible.

Symptoms and signs of HACE

HACE is characterized by severe symptoms of AMS plus progressive confusion, disorientation and ataxia. Patients should be assessed for cerebellar signs (e.g. slurring of speech, dysdiadochokinesia, finger-nose incoordination, Romberg's test negative and impaired Heel-Toe walking). If left untreated the patient will become increasingly more lethargic, progressing to coma and ultimately death through brainstem herniation.

Treatment of HACE

The treatment and prevention options for HACE are shown in Table 25.3. Many expeditions to the Great Ranges (Himalayas/High Andes and Rockies) will carry portable hyperbaric chambers (Figure 25.1). These provide an enclosed environment in which the symptomatic casualty can be placed and exposed to greater barometric pressure to represent relative descent. Once the patient has been zipped in to the bag, a foot pump is used to generate pressure. Pumping must continue to enable CO_2 to be expelled while maintaining the internal pressure. It enables the patient to be treated even if descent is not immediately possible. It must not be used instead of descent but as an adjunct. Owing to the enclosed environment, they are unsuitable for patients with a compromised airway.

Dexamethasone is a valuable emergency drug that may be used in cases of suspected HACE to facilitate or buy time for descent.

Table 25.3 HACE prevention and management

HACE Prevention	HACE Management
Adequate acclimatization	Immediate descent (500–1000 m)
Recognition of AMS symptoms	High flow oxygen
Acetazolamide	Dexamethasone 8 mg iv / po
	Portable hyperbaric chamber
	Evacuate to hospital
	Do NOT re-ascend

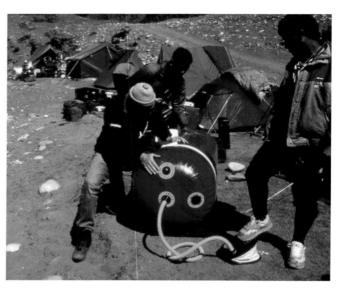

Figure 25.1 Portable hyperbaric chamber (Courtesy of Charles Clarke).

Vascular endothelial growth factor (VEGF) causes angiogenesis and increased permeability in the presence of both hypoxaemia and hypocapnia (causing vasoconstriction and increased hydrostatic pressure) leading to the cerebral oedema. Dexamethasone reverses this process by blocking VEGF.

High-altitude pulmonary oedema

Everybody gets short of breath at altitude but if it is disproportionate to the rest of the group, level of exertion or occurs while resting or lying down it must be treated as HAPE. There is a correlation with sleeping height and an incidence of 2% at 4000 meters. It is associated with rapid ascent and exertion, and AMS is frequently but not always associated. The pulmonary vasculature constricts on exposure to hypoxia. Pulmonary hypertension causes transudative capillary leak and mild alveolar haemorrhage. A degree of pre-ascent evaluation can screen for those at risk of HAPE. HAPE-prone individuals tend to have an abnormal increase in pulmonary artery systolic pressure when exposed to prolonged hypoxia or exercise.

Symptoms and signs of HAPE

HAPE often begins as a dry cough and disproportionate breathlessness at rest (particularly at night) or during minimal exertion. The cough gets progressively more bubbly and wet, and sputum may become blood tinged. Crackles will be audible on chest auscultation. A mild pyrexia is not uncommon and differentiation from pneumonia can be difficult.

Treatment of HAPE

The treatment and prevention options for HAPE are shown in Table 25.4. Nifedipine SR is a valuable emergency drug that may be used in cases of HAPE. It works by reducing the pulmonary artery pressure and has been shown to improve exercise performance and gas exchange. Sildenafil (Viagra) may also have a role by increasing

Table 25.4   HAPE prevention & management

HAPE Prevention	HAPE Management
Adequate acclimatisation	Immediate descent (500–1000 m)
Recognition of AMS symptoms	Portable hyperbaric chamber
Acetazolamide	High flow oxygen
	Sit patient up / head elevated
	Nifedipine SR 20 mg po qds
	CPAP / PEEP (if available)
	Nebulised salbutamol

nitric oxide levels in the pulmonary vasculature causing smooth muscle relaxation and reduction in pulmonary artery pressure.

Essential drugs for altitude emergencies

A summary of the essential drugs used for altitude emergencies is at Table 25.5.

Table 25.5   Essential drugs for high altitude emergencies

Drug	Dose	Indication
Oxygen	High flow	AMS / HAPE / HACE
Acetazolamide	250 mg bd po	Prophylaxis / treatment for AMS
Nifedipine SR	20 mg qds po	Treatment for HAPE
Dexamethasone	8 mg iv then 4 mg po tds	Treatment for HACE
Ofloxacin 0.3% eye drops	Hourly drop	Contact lens related microbial keratitis

Other medical problems associated with altitude

Cold Injury

This may be the presenting medical problem (frostbite/hypothermia) or as a result of another medical problem causing immobility. Patients at altitude must be prevented from becoming more hypothermic with judicious use of commercially available warming blankets during treatment and evacuation.

Venous thromboembolism

At altitude, the air is dry and appetite reduced so maintaining adequate oral intake is difficult. Dehydration is therefore common. Polycythaemia results from dehydration and altitude hypoxia induced erythropoiesis. Polycythaemia increases the risk of venous thromboembolism, e.g. deep vein thrombosis (DVT), pulmonary emboli (PE) and cerebrovascular accidents (CVAs).

Retinal haemorrhage

These are common above 5000 metres because of low barometric pressure (Figure 25.2) and hypoxia and rarely affect the vision unless they involve the macula. Descent is advisable and visual loss exceptional.

Ultravoilet keratitis

The sunlight is more powerful at altitude, and with reflection of the snow can cause significant damage to the cornea if suitable eye protection is not worn. Severe photophobia and lacrimation

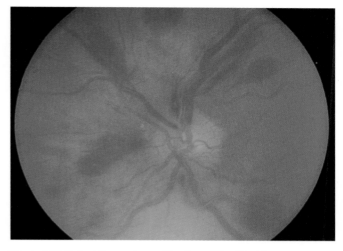

Figure 25.2 Retinal Haemorrhages (Courtesy of Dan Morris).

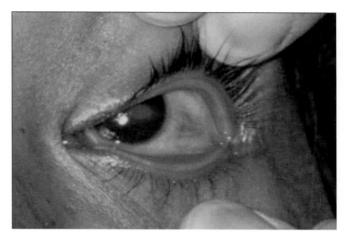

Figure 25.3 UV Keratitis (Courtesy of Dan Morris).

occur (Figure 25.3). Treatment involves rest, topical anaesthesia and antibiotics. Contact lenses, if not kept clean and changed regularly, can cause keratitis and corneal scarring.

Tips from the field

- If you feel unwell at altitude it is altitude illness until proven otherwise
- Never ascend with symptoms of AMS
- If you are getting worse (or have symptoms or signs of HACE or HAPE), go down at once
- DO NOT take sleeping tablets to assist you in sleeping
- DO NOT take narcotics or alcohol at altitude.

Further reading

Johnson C *et al*. *Oxford Handbook of Expedition and Wilderness* Medicine. Oxford: Oxford University Press, 2008.

MEDEX, www.medex.org.uk.

UIAA Medical Commission, www.theuiaa.org/medical_advice.html.

Ward MP, Milledge JS, West JB. *High Altitude Medicine and Physiology*, 3rd edn. Arnold Press.

CHAPTER 26

Environmental: Drowning and Near Drowning

Tim Nutbeam

Derriford Hospital, Plymouth Hospitals NHS Trust, Plymouth, UK

OVERVIEW

By the end of this chapter you should understand:
- Common definitions associated with drowning
- The pathophysiology of drowning
- The prehospital management of drowning and near drowning.

Drowning is the third leading cause of unintentional injury-related death worldwide, accounting for 7% of these cases. There are an estimated 388 000 annual drowning deaths worldwide, of which approximately 400 occur in the UK. A majority of these incidents occur in young adults, with a male to female ratio of 3:1. Alcohol intoxication is considered a factor in up to 20% of deaths. Suicidal intent may account for up to one-third of cases in the developed world.

Definitions related to drowning can be found in Box 26.1, and a summary of the pathophysiology of drowning in Figure 26.1. The temperature of the liquid in which the immersion occurs is important: ice water (associated with rapid and profound cooling) confers a survival benefit over other water temperatures.

Submersion victims are excellent candidates for rapid aggressive prehospital care. It is the treatment delivered at the prehospital stage which gives a majority of the survival benefit.

Box 26.1 **Definitions associated with drowning**

Drowning: Submersion in liquid causing suffocation and death within first 24 hours

Near Drowning: Initial survival beyond 24 hours following submersion in liquid

Immersion Syndrome: Syncope from cardiac dysrhythmias on sudden contact with water that is $\leq 5°C$

Post Immersion Syndrome /Secondary Drowning: Death or serious clinical deterioration following a near-drowning event (latent period of 1–48 hours).

ABC of Prehospital Emergency Medicine, First Edition.
Edited by Tim Nutbeam and Matthew Boylan.
© 2013 John Wiley & Sons, Ltd. Published 2013 by John Wiley & Sons, Ltd.

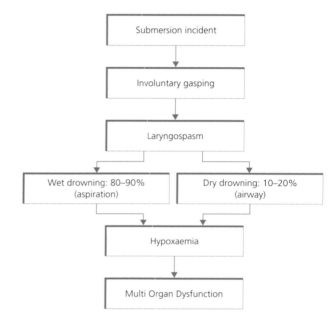

Figure 26.1 Pathophysiology of drowning.

Key points

- Patients should be extracted from water on a long board or using a purpose-designed litter.
- Immobilize cervical spine if mechanism dictates.
- Avoid excessive movement of the patient (body position changes) due to the risk of dysrhythmia.
- Give as much oxygen as possible as soon as possible.
- Traditional resuscitation methods including postural drainage and use of the Heimlich manoeuvre should be avoided.
- Focus should be on oxygen provision; this may mean early intubation (with or without RSI) in the presence of hypoxaemia (e.g. SATS <94%).
- Deliver invasive positive pressure ventilation (IPPV) with high positive end-expiratory pressure (PEEP), e.g. 10–15 cmH_2O. Aim for standard (6–8 mL/kg) tidal volumes with a peak airway pressure of <35 cmH_2O.
- Expect and treat any associated traumatic injuries.
- Consider transportation to a centre offering cardiac bypass and ideally ECMO (extracorporeal membrane oxygenation).

- In non-futile situations and if resources allow continue CPR until "warm and dead" or destination hospital is reached (see Boxes 26.2 and 26.3).

Box 26.2 Predictors of survival

Young age
Submersion of less than 10 minutes
No signs of aspiration
Core body temperature of less than 35°C at admission
Respiratory (versus cardiorespiratory) arrest
Early ROSC (<10 minutes).

Box 26.3 Candidates for aggressive/ prolonged resuscitation attempts

It is appropriate to resuscitate the following groups of patients:

Witnessed submersion time of less than 15 minutes
All those where there is a possibility of their being an air pocket whilst under water
All those submerged for up to an hour in ice water (longer in small children)
Everyone showing signs of life initially on resuce
Those who have been intermittently submerged during their immersion e.g. those wearing a life jacket.

(Adapted from JRCALC Guidelines 2006.)

Tips from the field

- Consider all drowning patients as drowning AND trauma patients
- Prolonged resuscitation is usually appropriate – plan for this and get help early
- Consider the use of automated chest compression devices.

Further reading

Bierens J, van der Velde E, van Berkel M, van Zanten JJ. Submersion in the Netherlands: Prognostic indicators and results of resuscitation. *Ann Emerg Med* 1990;**19**:1390–1395.

Lord SR, Davis PR. Drowning, near drowning and immersion syndrome. *J R Army Med Corps* 2005;**151**:250–255.

National Water Safety Forum: http://www.nationalwatersafety.org.uk.

Quan L. Drowning issues in resuscitation. *Ann Emerg Med* 1993;**22**:2.

The Royal Society for the Prevention of Accidents: http://www.rospa.com.

World Health Organization: http://www.who.int/en.

CHAPTER 27

Environmental: Diving Emergencies

Tudor A. Codreanu

Bunbury and Busselton Hospitals, Bunbury, WA, Australia

OVERVIEW

By the end of this chapter you should:

- Have a basic knowledge of diving physics and physiology
- Understand the common diving emergencies
- Understand how to manage common dive emergencies.

Introduction

Recreational diving is becoming increasingly popular and is not limited to coastal areas. The development of inland diving venues has not only increased the accessibility of the sport but also the distribution of diving incidents. An understanding of dive emergencies and how to manage them is required by all prehospital practitioners wherever they are based.

Dive physics and physiology

Recreational divers use self-contained breathing apparatus (SCUBA) to breath underwater. SCUBA systems consist of a pressurized cylinder containing compressed (up to 300 atm) atmospheric air (78% nitrogen, 21% oxygen) that is delivered to the diver at ambient pressure via a pressure regulator.

Although 60% of the body is represented by incompressible water, the gases contained within air spaces and those dissolved in the blood are subject to the laws of physics as applied to gases.

At sea level a diver is subject to 1 atm (101.32 kPa) of pressure. For each 10 metres of descent, the absolute pressure increases by 1 atm, with the greatest differential pressure occurring between 0 and 10 metres (Figure 27.1).

Dalton's law states that the total pressure exerted by a gaseous mixture is equal to the sum of the partial pressures of each individual component. As pressure increases during descent the partial pressure of the individual component gases (oxygen and nitrogen) also increases.

Henry's law states that the amount of a gas which dissolves in a volume of liquid is proportional to the pressure of the gas

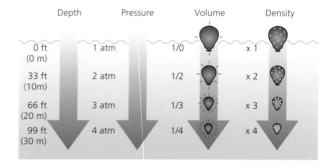

Figure 27.1 Boyle's law.

Solubility of a gas vs. Pressure

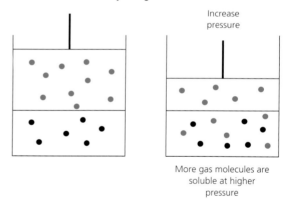

More gas molecules are soluble at higher pressure

Figure 27.2 Henry's Law.

(Figure 27.2). As the partial pressure of each component increases during descent (Dalton's law) the amount of gas dissolved in the diver's blood and lipid tissues increases. During ascent the reverse occurs and dissolved gas (nitrogen and oxygen) re-expands forming bubbles in the blood vessels and tissues. During a controlled, slow ascent these gases move from the tissues into the blood and are eliminated by the lungs. During an uncontrolled, fast ascent to the surface or a rapid ascent to altitude (driving over high hills, flying soon after diving), nitrogen bubbles may form at a rate that exceeds the ability of the body to eliminate them, leading to disruption at cell and organ level.

Boyle's law states that for any gas at a constant temperature, the volume of the gas will vary inversely with the pressure (Figure 27.1).

ABC of Prehospital Emergency Medicine, First Edition.
Edited by Tim Nutbeam and Matthew Boylan.
© 2013 John Wiley & Sons, Ltd. Published 2013 by John Wiley & Sons, Ltd.

A volume of gas will double in volume when ascending from 10 metres depth to the surface. Holding one's breath while ascending or performing too rapid an ascent will lead to rapid increase of the intrathoracic volume and therefore pressure ('reverse squeeze').

Emergencies on descent

Barotrauma

Unbalanced pressures between the surrounding water and air-filled spaces of the face (sinuses, middle ear and dental cavities) can cause severe pain during descent (or ascent). If the pain is ignored, structural damage (e.g. tympanic membrane rupture) may ensue.

Management

Typically the symptoms resolve with aborting the dive and return to the surface. Rupture of the tympanic membrane results in vertigo, nausea, disorientation and hearing loss. ENT follow-up is recommended.

Emergencies at depth

Nitrogen narcosis (rapture of the deep, Martini effect)

Breathing nitrogen at increased partial pressures (usually above 4 atm absolute) may result in a state of euphoria termed nitrogen narcosis. Every 15 metres of depth is said to have the same effect as one Martini alcoholic drink on an empty stomach. Box 27.1 lists the common symptoms of nitrogen narcosis.

Box 27.1 **Symptoms of nitrogen narcosis**

Light-headedness
Poor concentration and attention
Poor judgment, overconfidence
Anxiety
Decreased coordination
Hallucinations
Coma and death.

Management

Typically, the symptoms resolve with ascending to shallower depth; if they fail to resolve after ascent, nitrogen narcosis is not the underlying cause. Alternative aetiology should be sought and its appropriate management should be commenced.

Oxygen toxicity

Oxygen free radicals are formed whenever oxygen is inspired. At normal low oxygen partial pressures the body inactivates these radicals rapidly. At higher oxygen partial pressures such as those which occur at depth, oxygen radicals may accumulate within the body causing cellular disruption, particularly within the brain (CNS toxicity). Box 27.2 lists the common symptoms and signs of oxygen toxicity. Currently, the safe oxygen partial pressure for recreational diving purposes is considered to be 1.4 atm absolute (ATA). This pressure is reached at about 57 metres depth when breathing compressed air, and much shallower if breathing enriched air (higher oxygen concentration in the gas mixture).

Box 27.2 **Symptoms and signs of oxygen toxicity**

Tingling
Focal or generalized seizures
Vertigo, tinnitus
Nausea and vomiting
Tunnel vision
Personality changes, anxiety, confusion
Coma.

Management

Underwater seizures typically result in drowning, which should be managed in the standard manner.

Emergencies on ascent

Decompression illness (DCI) is an umbrella term for the clinical problems that may arise from an uncontrolled ascent. It includes decompression sickness (DCS), pulmonary barotrauma and cerebral artery gas embolism (CAGE).

DCI denial is a real phenomenon among divers who will try to find alternative explanations for their symptoms, leading to delays in diagnosis and treatment. The prehospital physician should have a low threshold to suspect a DCI event and transport any diver with even minor symptoms to a decompression chamber for assessment by a dive medicine specialist.

Decompression sickness

During uncontrolled or rapid ascents, dissolved nitrogen may be released from solution to form small bubbles in blood vessels and tissues. These bubbles can disrupt cells, act as emboli, and can cause mechanical compression and stretching of the blood vessels and nerves. They may also activate the inflammatory and coagulation pathways. Decompression sickness (DCS) is the term used to describe the clinical manifestation of this process and is subdivided into type I (mild) and type II (serious).

Type I (mild) decompression sickness

Symptoms occur within 10–30 minutes of surfacing and involve only the musculoskeletal system, skin or the lymphatic system. If left untreated, type 1 DCS may progress to type 2.

- **Musculoskeletal pain** ('the bends') (70–85%): gradual onset of mild (typically) or excruciating, dull, deep, throbbing, toothache-like pain, usually in a joint (shoulder, elbow, wrist, hand, ankle, knee) or tendon. Usually resolves in 10 minutes. Always present at rest, it may be exacerbated by movement. There may be loss or reduction of movement in the limb (splinting). Many divers will attribute this pain to some form of muscular trauma and therefore delay reporting it.
- Skin itching or burning ('skin bends').
- Lymphatic system: localized pain in lymph nodes and oedema of tributary tissues.

Type II (severe) decompression sickness

Type II decompression sickness is characterized by the involvement of the neurological, pulmonary and/or cardiovascular systems. Symptom onset is usually immediate but may be delayed as long as 36 hours. Pain is a feature in only 30% of cases.

- **Neurological symptoms:** The spinal cord is the most commonly affected area and presents with symptoms akin to a spinal cord injury. Typically, low back pain starts within minutes to hours, followed by a combination of paraesthesia, paresis, paralysis, faecal and urinary incontinence or retention. Any thoracic, abdominal or hip pain should be considered as originating from the spinal cord and treated as type II DCS. Headaches, visual field abnormalities, mental status alteration, and personality changes can also occur.
- **Pulmonary symptoms** ('the chokes'): the patient may present with retrosternal discomfort, haemoptysis, a non-productive cough, and/or tachypnoea. Rapid progression to respiratory failure can occur within 12 hours, which can result in death.
- **Cardiovascular symptoms:** the patient may present with tachycardia, hypotension, hypovolaemic shock or cardiovascular collapse.
- **Skin symptoms:** the skin may appear mottled with a marbled (*cutis marmorata*) or violet discolouration most often seen on the chest and shoulders.
- **Auricular symptoms** ('the staggers'): involvement of the inner ear may cause tinnitus, nystagmus, nausea and vomiting, vertigo and difficulty in walking. Labyrinthine disturbances *not* associated with other symptoms of DCI should be interpreted as secondary to barotrauma.

Pulmonary barotrauma

During rapid ascent (or normal ascent with holding breath) pulmonary overpressurization may occur leading to alveolar rupture with leakage of air into one of the three anatomical spaces (Figure 27.3):

1 The pleural cavity – causing a pneumothorax (chest pain, reduced chest movement, hyperexpansion, hyper-resonance, reduced air entry on the affected side and shortness of breath)
2 The mediastinum – causing a pneumomediastinum (retrosternal pain and subcutaneous emphysema to the base of the neck)
3 The pulmonary arterial system causing arterial gas embolization (see next section).

Arterial gas embolisation (AGE)

The leakage of air into the pulmonary arterial system following alveoli rupture during ascent can lead to the formation of arterial gas emboli which will then distribute themselves around the body. Venous gas emboli are common after recreational dives, but are usually filtered out by the lungs. In the presence of a patent foramen ovale (PFO), an atrial or ventricular septal defect (ASD, VSD) these may bypass the lungs and enter the arterial system

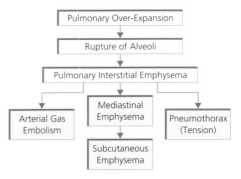

Figure 27.3 Pulmonary barotrauma.

directly. Symptoms of arterial gas embolism occur within 10–30 minutes and are related to the site of embolization, for example:

- Coronary artery embolization can lead to myocardial infarction or dysrrhythmia.
- Cerebral artery emboli can cause stroke, seizures or coma.

Management of decompression illness

Differential diagnosis between type II DCS and AGE is not important as both require recompression.

- Remove from water (Figure 27.4) with trauma precautions if required
- Remove diving gear including wet/dry suit
- Keep supine and horizontal, dry, warm and monitor vital signs
- Use temporary lateral decubitus (recovery position) if vomiting occurs
- Manage ABC
  - give 100% oxygen if DCI is suspected
  - needle decompression if tension pneumothorax suspected
  - commence CPR if required
  - if conscious rehydrate orally with non-alcoholic fluids at 1 L/hour

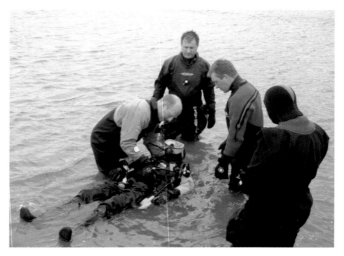

Figure 27.4 Management of DCI – removal from water (Courtesy of BSAC).

- if unconscious administer intravenous crystalloids aiming for a urine output of 1–2 mL/kg/hour
- Evacuate to hyperbaric facility
  - take all the personal diving gear with the patient
  - Ideally take the diving buddy as well, even if asymptomatic
  - flying altitude under 300 metres in unpressurized aircraft
  - cabin pressurized to 1 atm in pressurized aircraft.

Box 27.3 outlines interventions to avoid in the management of DCI. Well-organized dives and diving clubs may supply their members with diving incident pro formas for completion following dive incidents. These documents capture data important for the treating hyperbaric team and should accompany the patient to the chamber where possible. Box 27.4 summarizes the important data captured in such instances.

Box 27.3 **Avoid in DCI**

Avoid the following in the management of DCI:

Trendelenburg position – may increase intracranial pressure

Entonox (50:50 nitrous oxide and oxygen) – may increase bubble size and worsen symptoms

Analgesia, NSAIDS, steroids – may mask the pain that helps localize the site of the problem and helps monitor clinical progress

Dextrose 5% iv – may worsen cerebral oedema

IV fluids if pulmonary DCS – may worsen pulmonary oedema.

Box 27.4 **Diving incident form details**

Dive location and weather conditions

Details of previous dives

Dive details and profile when the incident occurred

Activities during the dive

Gases and equipment used

Type of incident and any other problems

Decompression details

Diver's physical condition before, during, and after the dive

First aid delivered.

Recompression therapy

The hyperbaric chamber is used to repressurize the patient to a depth where the bubbles of nitrogen or air are made smaller and the gas redissolves into the body tissues and fluids. High concentrations of oxygen can be administered during repressurization if required. The pressure is then slowly brought back to surface atmospheric pressure allowing gases to diffuse gradually out of the lungs and body. Treatment tables govern the exact times and depths that the patient will be repressurized to in the hyperbaric chamber.

Tips from the field

- Decompression sickness and arterial gas embolisation can occur during any dive profile (even in swimming pools!)
- Keep all diving gear with diver. Diving gear may provide clues as to why the diver had trouble (e.g. faulty air regulator, hose leak, carbon monoxide contamination of compressed air) and the dive computer will show the dive profile
- Differentiation between severe decompression sickness and arterial gas embolisation is unnecessary in the prehospital phase as both require recompression
- Advice can often be sought from your nearest hyperbaric centre – ensure you have the number in your phone.

Further reading

Bove A.A, Davis J. *Diving Medicine*, 4th ed. Philadelphia: Saunders, 2003.

British Sub Aqua Club. *The Diving Manual*, 3rd ed. Blandford forum: Hinchcliffe Books, 2007.

Naval Sea Systems Command. *US Navy Diving Manual.*, 6th ed. 2008. Washington DC: Direction of commander, naval systems command, superintendent of documents, US Government printing office, Washington DC **20402**, 2008.

Robinson K, Byers, M. *JRAMC* 2005; Vol. **151**(4), pp. 256–63.

CHAPTER 28

Care of Special Groups: The Obstetric Patient

Kristyn Manley[1], Tracy-Louise Appleyard[1], Tim Draycott[1], and Matthew Boylan[2]

[1]Southmead Hospital, Bristol, UK
[2]Royal Centre for Defence Medicine, University Hospitals Birmingham, Birmingham, UK

OVERVIEW

By the end of this chapter you should:

- Understand the relevant anatomical and physiological changes in pregnancy
- Know how to assess the pregnant patient in the prehospital phase
- Recognize and manage common antenatal emergencies
- Understand how to assist with an emergency prehospital delivery
- Recognize and manage common intrapartum emergencies
- Recognize and manage common postpartum emergencies
- Be able to manage the pregnant trauma patient
- Be able to manage the pregnant patient in cardiac arrest
- Know how to perform Neonatal Life support.

Introduction

Caring for pregnant women can be daunting even for the most experienced prehospital practitioner. However a basic understanding of pregnancy related changes in anatomy and physiology and a stepwise approach to care should enable prehospital teams to optimize outcomes for mothers and their babies.

Anatomical and physiological changes in pregnancy

Airway

Several anatomic changes occur during pregnancy that can impact prehospital airway management.

The engorgement and friability of the respiratory tract, mucosal oedema and capillary engorgement of nasal and oropharyngeal mucosa and laryngeal tissues increase the possibility of iatrogenic trauma during airway instrumentation. Pregnancy-induced weight gain and an increase in breast size may obstruct laryngoscope blade insertion when mounted on a standard handle. Unmounted blade insertion or a short-handled 'stubby' laryngoscope handle are useful alternatives.

Delayed gastric emptying, elevated gastric pressure and gastro-oesophageal incompetence all increase the risk of passive regurgitation and aspiration in the obtunded pregnant patient. Early definitive airway management is recommended but a difficult airway should be expected and planned for (expect a failed intubation in about 1 in 250, and a 'can't intubate – can't ventilate' scenario in about 1 in 500).

Breathing

A progressive rise in respiratory rate and tidal volume occurs throughout pregnancy to compensate for increasing oxygen demands. The tidal volume increase occurs at the expense of inspiratory and expiratory reserve volumes resulting in a reduced functional residual capacity and a shortened apnoeic desaturation time.

As the gravid uterus enters the upper abdomen in the third trimester the lower ribs become splayed and relatively fixed, reducing the contribution of the intercostal muscles during forced respiration. There is also elevation of the diaphragm in late pregnancy due to pressure from the compressed abdominal contents and as such it is recommended that thoracostomies are performed one or two intercostal spaces higher than usual.

Circulation

The placental perfusion requirement increases with advancing gestation and is reflected by a gradual increase in cardiac stroke volume and heart rate by 10–20 bpm. By the second trimester, cardiac output has risen by approximately 40%. There is a progressive reduction in blood pressure in the first trimester, followed by a steady increase in the third trimester to pre-pregnancy values. Systemic vascular resistance (SVR) falls by up to 30% placing the pregnant patient at risk of postural hypotension during rapid postural changes.

During the late second and third trimester the gravid uterus compresses the inferior vena cava in the supine position (aorto-caval compression), leading to reduced venous return and syncope (Figure 28.1). This may be prevented by tilting the patient to the left on either an immobilization device or by placing padding under the right buttock. In an emergency the uterus can be manually displaced to the left with the patient supine.

ABC of Prehospital Emergency Medicine, First Edition.
Edited by Tim Nutbeam and Matthew Boylan.
© 2013 John Wiley & Sons, Ltd. Published 2013 by John Wiley & Sons, Ltd.

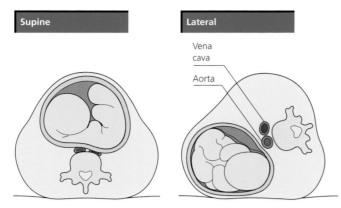

Figure 28.1 Aortocaval compression.

In the event of blood loss the maternal circulation is maintained by diverting blood away from the uterus with only minimal change to the patient vital signs. The pregnant patient may tolerate a loss of up to 20% of their circulating volume without showing clinical signs. The resultant reduction in placental perfusion may lead to foetal hypoxia. With continued blood loss and reduced ability to compensate due to limited cardiorespiratory reserve there will become a point at which rapid decompensation occurs.

Pregnancy causes an increase in clotting factors (VIII, IX, X and fibrinogen) and a decrease in circulating anticoagulants (protein S and antithrombin). This hypercoagulable state increases the risk of deep vein thrombosis and pulmonary embolism.

Uterus

Uterine growth is the most important anatomical change and will clearly affect the presentation of abdominal disease and trauma. The fundus of the uterus lies at the level of the umbilicus from 20 weeks and rises by a centimetre a week (see Figure 28.2). It is then the most anterior presenting organ and therefore the most susceptible

to trauma. The bowels and omentum are displaced which can make the diagnosis of appendicitis or disseminated infection, more difficult.

Assessment of the pregnant patient

In all patients a rapid primary survey should be performed using the <C>ABCDEF approach (Box 28.1). In advanced pregnancy assessment should be performed in the left lateral position to eliminate aortocaval compression. The management of catastrophic obstetric haemorrhage involves immediate transfer to hospital with circulation management en route. In the shocked pregnant patient the uterus should be considered as a fifth source of concealed haemorrhage along with the traditional four sites (chest, abdomen, pelvis, long bones). An assessment of the fundus and fetus forms the final part of the primary survey in the pregnant patient. Make a brief assessment of the fundal height, noting any significant uterine tenderness. A fundal height below the umbilicus suggests that if the fetus is delivered it is unlikely to survive. The introitus should then be inspected for foetal parts, cord prolapse and significant bleeding.

Box 28.1 **Primary Survey in Pregnancy**

<C>	Catastrophic Haemorrhage
A	Airway
B	Breathing
C	Circulation
D	Disability
E	Exposure
F	Fundus / Foetus

In the stable patient a focused history should then be sought. The past medical history and history of illicit drug use is important to determine. An obstetric history is then taken (Box 28.2). The patient will often have hand-held maternity notes which may assist you in identifying potential problems. A more detailed obstetric

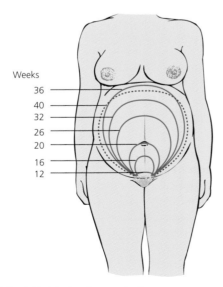

Figure 28.2 Fundal height (weeks gestation).

Box 28.2 **Obstetric history**

Early pregnancy
Last Menstrual Period (LMP)
Normal Period and length
Contraceptive use
Nature of bleeding/pain/discharge
Number of previous pregnancies and deliveries
Complications with previous pregnancies

Established pregnancy
As above plus......
Gestation in weeks
Estimated date of delivery
Which hospital she is booked into
Midwife or obstetric consultant care
Complications in this pregnancy
Nature of bleeding/pain/fluid loss/discharge
Subjective assessment of foetal movements.

examination can then be performed if the patient is stable and the practitioner has the requisite skills. The fundal height can be formally measured and compared with the expected gestational age. The uterus should be palpated for tenderness, rigidity, contractions, foetal parts and movements. If there has been a spontaneous rupture of membranes the colour of the liquor should also be assessed for blood or meconium staining.

Antenatal emergencies

Antepartum haemorrhage

Antepartum haemorrhage is vaginal bleeding after 24 completed weeks of pregnancy. The common causes are placental abruption and placenta praevia (Figure 28.3).

- **Placental abruption** is the partial or complete separation of a normally sited placenta from the uterine wall. The result is bleeding from the maternal sinuses into the space between the placenta and the uterine wall. Blood may remain concealed or track behind the membranes and present per vaginally. Abruption usually presents with severe abdominal pain and a hard, tender uterus. Delay in presentation (up to 48 hours) is not uncommon in post-traumatic abruption.
- **Placenta praevia** is when the placenta implants either completely or partially across the cervical os. If the placenta separates in late pregnancy because of intercourse or contractions the tearing of maternal blood vessels close to the cervical canal leads to blood loss per vaginum. Bleeding is commonly painless, bright red and may be torrential.

Management of antepartum haemorrhage involves urgent transfer to an obstetric unit. Attempts at intravenous/intraosseus access should be made en route and fluid resuscitation commenced.

Severe pre-eclampsia and eclampsia

Pre-eclampsia is a multisystem disorder consisting chiefly of elevated blood pressure (>140/90 mmHg), proteinuria with or without oedema. It usually presents after 20 weeks, but can occur as late as 6 weeks after parturition.

- **Severe pre-eclampsia** is characterized by greatly elevated blood pressure (>170/110 mmHg), proteinuria and one or more of the following symptoms: severe headache, visual disturbance, abdominal pain (epigastric or RUQ), vomiting, or signs of clonus.
- **Eclampsia** is defined as the occurrence of one or more convulsions superimposed on pre-eclampsia. It generally occurs in the third trimester, with 60% of cases reported in the intrapartum period or within 48 hours after parturition. The incidence is higher in developing countries. Convulsions are usually self-limiting lasting 90 seconds or less, but may be severe and recurrent. There is a risk of maternal and foetal hypoxia and placental abruption as a result of the convulsions.

Management of severe pre-eclampsia and eclampsia requires urgent transfer to an obstetric unit. The patient should be placed in the left lateral position for transfer and oxygen applied if SpO_2 <94%. Monitor the blood pressure en route and pre-alert the obstetric unit so that they can prepare drugs and/or theatre. Self-limiting seizures should be managed initially with basic airway adjucts (e.g. NPA) and intravenous/intraosseous access. Further seizures can be prevented by giving magnesium sulphate 4 g intravenously/intraosseously over 15 minutes. If magnesium sulphate is not available *and* the patient has recurrent or prolonged seizures consider parental or rectal benzodiazepines.

Emergency prehospital delivery

Less than 1% of booked hospital deliveries are born before arrival at hospital. Neonatal consequences include a slightly higher perinatal mortality rate (relative risk 5.8) with foetal hypothermia as the commonest morbidity. Maternal consequences can include a prolonged third stage (e.g. retained placenta) with subsequent post-partum haemorrhage (PPH).

First stage of labour

The first stage of labour involves cervical effacement and dilatation to 10 cm. There will be an increase in frequency and intensity of contractions during this stage. In established labour there are three or four contractions every 10 minutes. The membranes can rupture at any stage. The first stage can last from minutes to many hours. Pain can be managed in most cases with entonox alone. Transport to the patient's obstetric unit is indicated.

Second stage of labour

The second stage begins when the cervix is fully dilated and is completed with delivery of the baby. In the absence of a midwife able to perform a vaginal examination, the second stage will usually be recognized when the head becomes visible at the introitus (crowning). At this stage delivery is imminent and an emergency prehospital delivery should be prepared for.

Most babies will delivery spontaneously without assistance. Allow the head to deliver with gentle support to the perineum

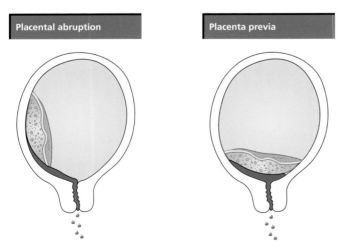

Figure 28.3 Placental abruption and placenta praevia.

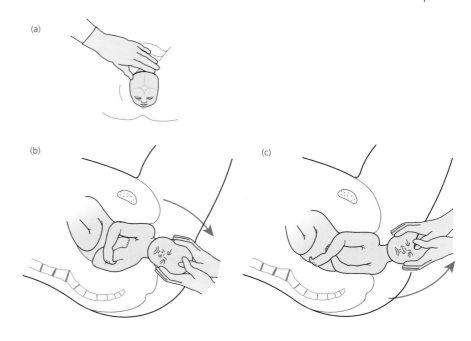

Figure 28.4 The second stage of labour. (a) Controlled delivery of the head. (b) Delivery of anterior shoulder. (c) Delivery of posterior shoulder.

(Figure 28.4a). Encouraging the mother to pant or breathe through her contractions at this stage will also help control the delivery of the head. If cord is seen around the neck it can be left alone as the body will usually deliver through the loops. *Gentle* downward traction may assist delivery of the anterior shoulder (Figure 28.4b) and then upwards traction for the following posterior shoulder (Figure 28.4c). The remainder of the baby should follow rapidly. All babies should be dried immediately post-delivery and placed skin-to-skin, i.e. on the chest under any clothing, with the mother (or occasionally father if mother is incapacitated for any reason).

Third stage of labour

The third stage of labour begins with delivery of the baby and ends once the placenta has been delivered. Following delivery of the baby the cord may be cut after it has finished pulsating (or immediately if resuscitation is required). It should be clamped at 3 cm *and* 6 cm from the baby and divided between the clamps. In most cases the third stage will be physiological unless Syntometrine (1-mL vial intramuscularly/intravenously) is available. Cord lengthening, a rising uterus and a small gush of blood indicate placental separation. Owing to the risk of cord rupture and uterine inversion, prehospital application of cord traction is discouraged unless the practitioner is experienced in this technique. Once delivered the placenta should be kept for inspection by the midwife or obstetrician.

Intrapartum emergencies

Cord prolapse

Cord prolapse is the descent of the umbilical cord through the cervix alongside (occult) or past the presenting part (overt) in the presence of ruptured membranes. It occurs in <1% of deliveries and may lead to foetal hypoxia. Outcome is related to time between diagnosis and delivery.

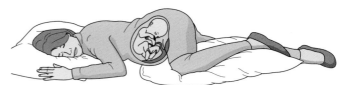

Figure 28.5 Exaggerated Sim's position.

Management should aim to relieve cord compression and facilitate transfer of the mother to a safe place for delivery. The exaggerated Sim's position should be used to transfer the patient with cord prolapse. The mother is laid on her left side with her head flat and her buttocks elevated by pillows (Figure 28.5). The addition of head-down tilt may assist in relieving the pressure of the foetal head on the cord. Use your fingertips to gently push the presenting part upwards and off the cord – this must be maintained during transfer. Alternatively, pass a urinary catheter and fill the bladder with 500 mL of saline via a blood giving set. The increase in bladder size will elevate the presenting part. Any protruding cord should be covered with a large swab soaked in warm saline and handling kept to a minimum.

Breech presentation

This is where the presenting part is the feet or buttocks and occurs in 3–4% of term pregnancies. The safest means of delivering a breech baby is by caesarean section and if labour is not well established the mother should be transferred urgently to hospital. If the presenting part is visible at the introitus a vaginal breech delivery will be required. Urgent midwifery assistance should be requested while preparing for delivery.

The mother should be placed on her back in the lithotomy position and once the breech is visible at the introitus, pushing encouraged. The key is limited intervention – 'hands off the breech'. The breech should rotate spontaneously to the sacroanterior

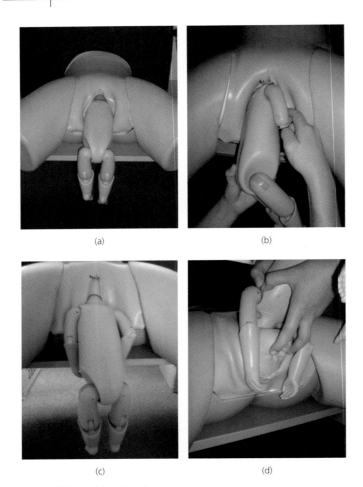

(a)   (b)

(c)   (d)

Figure 28.6 (a–d) Breech delivery.

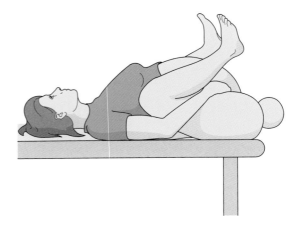

Figure 28.7 McRoberts manoeuvre.

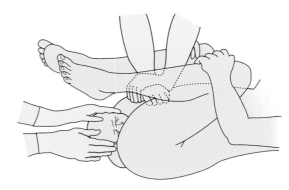

Figure 28.8 Suprapubic pressure.

position. Spontaneous delivery of the limbs and trunk is preferable (Figure 28.6a), but the legs may need to be released by applying pressure to the popliteal fossa (Pinard manoeuvre). Allow spontaneous delivery until the scapulae are seen. Avoid trying to 'pull' the baby out as this can result in the extension and trapping of the baby's arms behind its head, which is difficult to resolve. The arms should be delivered by sweeping them across the baby's face and downwards or by the Lovset manoeuvre – rotation of the baby to facilitate delivery of the arms (Figure 28.6b). Allow the body to hang until the nape of the neck is seen (Figure 28.6c). The Mariceau–Smellie–Veit manoeuvre may be required for delivery of the head (Figure 28.6d). The baby's body should be supported on your arm. The first and third finger of your hand should be placed on the cheekbones. With the other hand, gentle traction should be applied simultaneously to the shoulders, using two fingers to flex the occiput, i.e. keep the chin on the chest. Suprapubic pressure by an assistant can be used to assist flexion of the head during this manoeuvre.

Shoulder dystocia

This is when the anterior shoulder becomes impacted behind the symphysis pubis and it occurs in 1% of deliveries. It is recognized

at delivery when the head retracts back into the vagina (turtle sign) between contractions. Strong continuous traction in an attempt to deliver the head can result in brachial plexus injury and must be avoided. Fortunately, most can be managed with the first two manoeuvres listed.

- **McRoberts manoeuvre** (Figure 28.7) has reported success rates as high as 90%. Lie the mother flat and remove any pillows. Hyperflex her legs against the abdomen. Assess the effectiveness of the manoeuvre with routine traction (one attempt) before moving onto the next manoeuvre.
- **Suprapubic pressure** (Figure 28.8) – an assistant should apply pressure from the side of the foetal back in a downward and lateral direction, just above the maternal symphysis pubis using the heel of the hand (CPR style hand position). This pushes the posterior aspect of the anterior shoulder towards the foetal chest. Again assess the effectiveness of the manoeuvre with routine traction (two attempts).

If each of these measures fails the mother should be asked to assume the 'all fours' position with her head as low as possible and her bottom elevated. Two attempts should be made to deliver the posterior shoulder with gentle downward traction. Failure of delivery at this stage should trigger urgent transfer (in the left lateral position) to the nearest obstetric unit.

Postpartum emergencies

Postpartum haemorrhage

This is defined as a blood loss of more than 500 mL after the second stage of labour is completed and can occur within the first 24 hours (primary) or up to 6 weeks following delivery (secondary). It occurs in up to 10% of deliveries. As around a litre of blood flows to the placental bed every minute at term it can be catastrophic and life threatening. Possible aetiology includes one of the four Ts:

- **tone** – abnormalities of uterine contraction
- **trauma** – to the genital tract
- **tissue** – retained products of conception
- **thrombin** – coagulation abnormalities.

Perform a primary survey including palpation of the uterus (to assess tone) and examination for tears. Estimate the amount of blood loss and then double it to provide a more realistic estimate. Prepare the patient for rapid transfer to an obstetric unit. Early intravenous access and fluid resuscitation is important but should not delay transfer to hospital. Consider the four Ts. Tears can be managed with direct pressure. If the uterus feels atonic (soft and doughy) try massaging the uterine fundus to rub up a contraction. Consider syntometrine early if available. If this doesn't work and bleeding is catastrophic, bimanual (Figure 28.9) or aortic compression (Figure 28.10) may be employed during rapid transfer to hospital. The hospital should be pre-alerted to the patient's condition.

Uterine inversion

Inversion of the uterine fundus may occur spontaneously or more commonly as a result of uncontrolled cord traction during the third stage. It is a potentially life threatening condition which can lead to massive PPH and/or vagally mediated shock. The patient will complain of severe lower abdominal pain and the uterus may not be palpable as expected around the umbilicus. If a bulging mass is visible at or outside the vaginal entrance an immediate attempt should be made to reduce the uterus manually (Figure 28.11). The part of the uterus nearest the vagina should be squeezed and eased back into the vagina and the process repeated until the whole

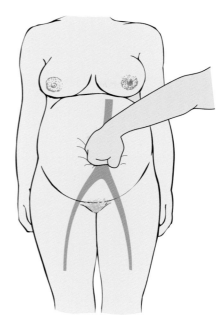

Figure 28.10 Aortic compression. (Source: http://hetv.org/resources /reproductive-health/impac/Symptoms/Vaginal_bleeding_after _S25_S34.html).

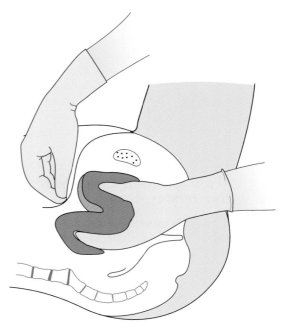

Figure 28.11 Manual reduction of the uterus.

uterus is reduced. The patient should remain flat post-reduction. If reduction fails rapid transfer should be initiated. Shock can be treated with intravenous fluids en route and atropine (500 μg to 3 mg maximum) administered if bradycardic.

Trauma in pregnancy

Domestic violence, road traffic collisions and falls are the commonest causes of blunt traumatic injury in pregnancy. Foetal mortality

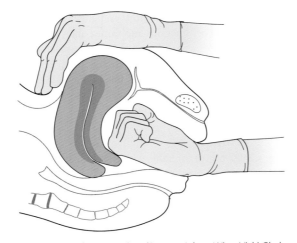

Figure 28.9 Bimanual compression. (Source: Arlene Wise, Vicki Clark. *Anaesthesia & Intensive Care Medicine* 2007; **8**:326–331).

can be as high as 38% due to abruption, uterine rupture or maternal shock (particularly from pelvic fractures). The uterus provides some degree of protection to the mother from penetrating abdominal trauma, at the expense of the fetus.

Initial evaluation is the same as for the non-pregnant patient except the patient should be managed in the left lateral position to prevent compression of the inferior vena cava. Resuscitation of the mother provides resuscitation of the fetus. Fluid therapy should be titrated to a systolic blood pressure of 100 mmHg rather than a radial pulse in this patient group. All pregnant women should be reviewed in hospital after any significant trauma.

Cardiac arrest in pregnancy

Cardiac resuscitation in pregnancy is thankfully rare occurring in only 1 in 30:000 pregnancies. The major causes of maternal death are thromboembolism, cardiac disease, haemorrhage, hypertensive disease of pregnancy, sepsis, exacerbation of other medical disorders in pregnancy and amniotic fluid emboli. Survival rates are the same as for adult resuscitation at 20%.

Resuscitation differs slightly from conventional adult resuscitation in the following ways:

- The uterus must be displaced to the left to prevent aortocaval compression in all unresponsive pregnant patients. Initially manual displacement or a wedge/blanket/knees under the right hip may be used. Preferably the patient should be strapped to a longboard which can then be propped up to a left lateral tilt of 15–30 degrees for transfer and ongoing CPR.
- Early insertion of a cuffed supraglottic device (e.g. LMA) and where possible endotracheal intubation is preferred to minimize the risk of aspiration.
- If the uterus is above the umbilicus, consider prehospital resuscitative hysterotomy.

Prehospital perimortem Caesarean section (resuscitative hysterotomy)

This is a rare, but extremely important procedure that is an essential part of resuscitation and life support after a maternal cardiac arrest. The rationale is that delivery of the foetus makes CPR more effective, aortocaval compression ceases to be a factor and cardiac output increases by as much as 20%. The patient can then be managed in a supine position making resuscitation easier.

- **Indications:** The following conditions should be present before contemplating a perimortem caesarean section:
  ○ pregnancy more than 22 weeks gestation (i.e. uterus above umbilicus)
  ○ mother still in cardiac arrest after 4 minutes of life support
  ○ trained personnel with appropriate equipment available.
- **Timing of procedure:** The best survival rates are reported when caesarean section is performed in under 5 minutes, although there are reports of survivors after up to 20 minutes of cardiac arrest. The decision to deliver the baby should therefore be made after 4 minutes of unsuccessful resuscitation and be completed within 5 minutes.

- **Equipment:** The minimum equipment required for gaining access into the uterus are a 22 blade scalpel and pair of Tuffcut scissors. Universal protection including eye protection should be worn. Assistants wearing sterile gloves can be used as retractors. Large sterile swabs will be required for packing the uterus after delivery. A maternity pack with umbilical clamps should be readied along with equipment for neonatal resuscitation should it be required.
- **Method:** Cardiopulmonary resuscitation should continue during delivery. A midline incision (5 cm below the xiphisterum to 3 cm above the pubis) should be made through the abdominal wall and the peritoneum (Figure 28.12a). Protect the bowel and bladder from injury, remembering that the bladder will not have been emptied. Sterile Tuffcut scissors may be employed to reduce the risk of injury. It will be a relatively bloodless field as there is reduced cardiac output. When making an incision on the uterus, be careful not to cut the baby. Make an initial incision with the scalpel (Figure 28.12b) then extend the incision using the Tuffcut scissors cutting through the placenta if necessary (Figure 28.12c). Deliver the baby by lifting the head out (Figure 28.12d) and pulling downwards until the anterior shoulder is delivered and then upwards. Clamp the cord and cut – pass the baby to a member of the team who can commence neonatal resuscitation. Deliver the placenta with controlled traction on the cord and then wipe any remaining membranes out of the uterus with a swab. Pack the uterus with sterile swabs and transfer. Once the baby has been delivered, the mother can be turned into a supine position to aid resuscitation. Initiate transfer to the nearest obstetric unit immediately, while continuing resuscitation enroute. The mother may require anaesthesia should she regain her cardiac output.
- **Legal considerations:** a perimortem caesarean section is deemed a procedure where consent cannot be obtained and prosecution has not occurred in the case literature thus far. Indeed, prosecution has been sought where this procedure has not been undertaken.

Neonatal life support

The newborn resuscitation algorithm is shown in Figure 28.13.

In babies, resuscitation is nearly always due to a respiratory cause. During the delivery, respiratory exchange is interrupted for up to 75 seconds per contractions and some babies do not tolerate this well. Babies who gasp following delivery are attempting to correct hypoxia and if this doesn't aerate the lungs, breathing will cease. The newborn babies lungs are filled with fluid at birth, so the technique for delivering oxygen is different to an adult. Crying generates PEEP and pushes fluid out

Initial assessment

Babies generally cry or breathe within 90 seconds of delivery. Preventing heat loss is essential, particularly in preterm infants. Drying the baby and then wrapping in a dry towel will keep the baby warm and act as a stimulant. Place the baby in a warm area and minimize draughts. Whilst drying the baby assess the following:

- colour – are they blue or pink centrally
- tone – are they floppy or flexed

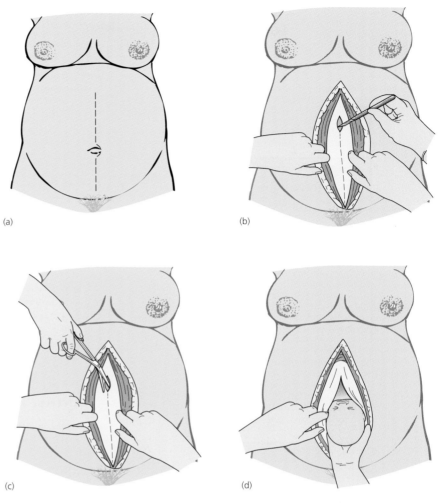

Figure 28.12 (a–d) Perimortem Caesarean section.

- breathing – are they making a good respiratory effort
- heart rate – assess by feeling under the umbilicus or listening over the heart.

Airway

If the baby does not breath spontaneously position the head in a neutral position (Figure 28.13) to open the airway and consider placing a towel under the shoulders. Suction is rarely of benefit and may stimulates a vagal response.

Breathing

If the baby still does not breath spontaneously, deliver five inflation breaths (sustained pressure for 2 seconds) using a paediatric bag–valve–mask (BVM) device and then provide oxygen with ventilation breaths at 30 breaths per minute. A raised heart rate is the first sign of successful resuscitation. 95% will recover within 2 minutes of effective ventilation. Consider tracheal intubation if the heart rate fails to respond to BVM ventilation.

Circulation

This is rarely required but if the heart rate doesn't respond to good ventilation (i.e. remains <60/min) then chest compressions may be

needed. Place your hands around the chest, then place your thumbs on the lower third of the sternum (not ribs) and compress by one third of the depth of the chest. Compression to breathing ratio is 3:1, i.e. 90 compression to 30 breaths per minute.

Drugs

Intraosseous access is the method of choice in gaining venous access in prehospital neonatal resuscitation. A small sample of marrow should be retained to check the blood sugar.

- **Adrenaline** (epinephrine) may be given in the presence of unresponsive bradycardia or cardiac standstill at a dose of 10 μg/kg. Further doses of 10–30 μg/kg may be tried at 3–5-minute intervals if there is no response.
- **Fluid** (e.g. warm normal saline 10 mL/kg) may be required if there is suspected blood loss.
- **Glucose** may be used to treat hypoglycaemia using a slow bolus of 2.5 mL/kg of 10% glucose.
- **Naloxone** 200 μg intramuscularly should be given if opiate induced respiratory depression is suspected.

Meconium aspiration

Meconium aspiration is rare. If the baby is vigorous no treatment is required. If the baby has absent or inadequate respirations, a heart

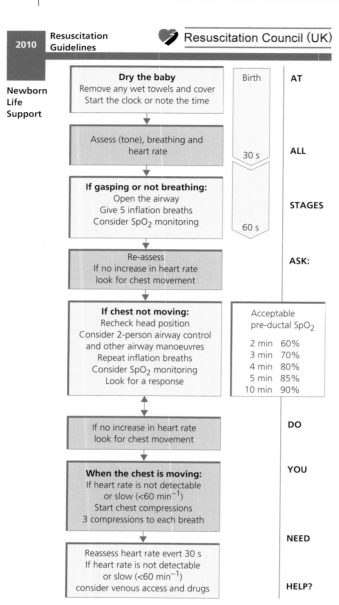

Newborn Life Support

Dry the baby Remove any wet towels and cover Start the clock or note the time	Birth	AT
Assess (tone), breathing and heart rate	30 s	ALL
If gasping or not breathing: Open the airway Give 5 inflation breaths Consider SpO$_2$ monitoring		STAGES
	60 s	
Re-assess If no increase in heart rate look for chest movement		ASK:
If chest not moving: Recheck head position Consider 2-person airway control and other airway manoeuvres Repeat inflation breaths Consider SpO$_2$ monitoring Look for a response	Acceptable pre-ductal SpO$_2$ 2 min 60% 3 min 70% 4 min 80% 5 min 85% 10 min 90%	
If no increase in heart rate look for chest movement		DO
When the chest is moving: If heart rate is not detectable or slow (<60 min^{-1}) Start chest compressions 3 compressions to each breath		YOU
Reassess heart rate evert 30 s If heart rate is not detectable or slow (<60 min^{-1}) consider venous access and drugs		NEED HELP?

Figure 28.13 Newborn life support algorithm (Source: reproduced with kind permission of the Resuscitation Council UK).

rate <60 or hypotonia the oropharynx should be inspected and particulate meconium aspirated. If intubation is possible and the baby remains unresponsive the trachea may be suctioned through the endotracheal tube prior to ventilation breaths being delivered. If intubation is not possible immediately clear the oropharynx and start mask ventilation.

Tips from the field

- Always place the pregnant women in a left lateral position
- When loading pregnant women in the left lateral position onto the ambulance ensure you have access to the face/airway. This may require feet-first loading in ambulances with a side mounted stretcher fit
- McRobert's manoeuvre combined with suprapubic pressure has up to a 90% success rate for shoulder dystocia
- Fluid resuscitation and bimanual compression are holding mechanisms for postpartum haemorrhage
- If considering a perimortem caesarean, undertake within 4 minutes of resuscitation to improve both maternal and foetal outcome
- Keep newborn neonates dry and warm
- Place pre-term infants in a food-grade plastic bag without drying.

Further reading

Bhoopalam P, Watkinson M. Babies born before arrival at hospital. *BJOG* 2005;**98**:57–64.

Draycott T, Winter C, Crofts J, Barnfield S. *PROMPT (PRactical Obstetric MultiProfessional Training) Course Manual*. London: RCOG Press, 2008.

Nelson-Piercy C. *Handbook of Obstetric Medicine*, 3rd edn. London; Informa Healthcare, 2006.

Whitten M, Irvine L. Postmortem and perimortem caesarean section: what are the indications? *J R Soc Med* 2000;**93**: 6–9.

CHAPTER 29

Care of Special Groups: The Paediatric Patient

Fiona Jewkes[1] and Julian Sandell[2]

[1]NHS Pathways Connecting for Health, Leeds, UK
[2]Poole Hospital NHS Foundation Trust, Poole, UK

OVERVIEW

By the end of this chapter you should:

- Understand the key physiological and anatomical differences between children and adults
- Understand how to assess the seriously ill or injured child
- Understand how to manage the seriously ill or injured child.

Why treat children differently?

The principle that 'children should not be simply treated as small adults' has possibly been overstated given that established prehospital 'adult' practices are relatively similar and would often be equally valid if used to assess and manage the sick or injured child or young person. There are, however, important differences, and this chapter aims to highlight these to both improve the child's medical care and also probably make your life easier.

Anatomy and physiology

Key anatomical and physiological differences have a bearing on how we manage the paediatric patient.

Size and weight

Children **sizes** and **weight** vary more than a hundred-fold – from a 500-g preterm baby to a 50-kg (or more) adolescent. This is a crucial consideration when prescribing drugs and fluids, which are typically calculated 'per kilogram'. Formulae may be used to estimate weight (Table 29.1) but are prone to error through miscalculation so must be confirmed by a second practitioner. Alternatively a Broslow or Sandell tape may be used.

Body proportions

Children's **bodily proportions** also vary considerably – a newborn baby's head contributes 20% of their surface area but only 10% of that of a 15 year old. Small children have a relatively large

Table 29.1 Weight estimation formulae

Age	Formula
<12 months	$(0.5 \times \text{age in months}) + 4$
1–5 years	$(2 \times \text{age in years}) + 8$
5–12 years	$(3 \times \text{age in years}) + 7$

surface area to weight ratio and so are more prone to hypothermia (this again decreases with age). Their larger surface area is also an important factor when replacing fluids in situations such as burns.

Airway

The paediatric airway differs from the adult airway in a number of ways (Figure 29.1). The relatively larger tongue and hypertrophic tonsils may cause obstruction and hinder airway management. The shorter, less rigid trachea is prone to compression in both excessive flexion (large occiput) and hyperextension (iatrogenic). The position and structure of the larynx and epiglottis make laryngoscopy more challenging and as a result the Association of Anaesthetists of

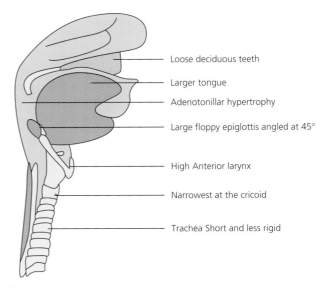

Loose deciduous teeth

Larger tongue

Adenotonillar hypertrophy

Large floppy epiglottis angled at 45°

High Anterior larynx

Narrowest at the cricoid

Trachea Short and less rigid

Child Upper Airway

Figure 29.1 The paediatric airway.

ABC of Prehospital Emergency Medicine, First Edition.
Edited by Tim Nutbeam and Matthew Boylan.
© 2013 John Wiley & Sons, Ltd. Published 2013 by John Wiley & Sons, Ltd.

Great Britain and Ireland (AAGBI) now recommend that prehospital endotracheal intubation should only be performed by those who are already skilled in paediatric anaesthesia in the hospital environment.

The larger occiput of a newborn may force the neck into flexion: be aware of this when positioning their cervical spine in the neutral position.

Breathing

Younger children's ribs (largely cartilaginous) are more flexible and provide less protection to the thoracic and intra-abdominal organs (which are also less well protected by the relatively shallow pelvis), and so thoracic and abdominal contents are more readily damaged. It is worth noting that serious chest injury can occur without rib fractures as a result of their extra compliance.

Circulation

Considering **circulatory differences**, children have more blood *per kilogram* than adults (80–100 mL/kg), although, being significantly lighter than adults, their total circulating volume is significantly smaller, e.g. a 1-year old's total blood volume is only 800 mL.

Paediatric '**vital signs**' differ markedly from adult physiological parameters (Table 29.2).

Table 29.2 'Normal' paediatric vital signs at different ages

Age	Heart rate (bpm)	Respiratory rate (breaths/min)
Under 1 year	110–160	30–40
1–5 years	95–140	25–30
5–12 years	80–120	20–25
>12 years	80–100	15–20

Children typically have healthy hearts that compensate well when stressed and can maintain their systolic blood pressure until advanced states of shock. (Hypotension should be considered a preterminal sign.) Blood pressure increases throughout childhood from a systolic blood pressure of about 70 mmHg in the newborn period, reaching adult levels in late adolescence.

Disability

Electrolyte disturbances, notably hypoglycaemia, are commonly seen in children; especially the young and those stressed by illness or injury. Hypoglycaemia follows exhaustion of glycogen supplies so, importantly, is unlikely to respond well to glucagon.

Psychosocial

Adult-trained practitioners are often anxious about the psychosocial aspects of caring for ill or injured children; clearly children have an age-appropriate understanding of their world and it is vital that they are spoken to in language they can understand and not ignored.

Assessment of the seriously ill or injured child

A rapid **primary assessment** should be performed on any ill child, seeking the early signs of respiratory, circulatory or neurological compromise, using the well-established ABCD (airway, breathing, circulation and disability) approach to life-support. Children are often thought to deteriorate rapidly although this is frequently not the case – rather, early signs are typically more subtle than in adults and often missed.

A and B: airway and breathing

Potential respiratory failure can be identified by assessing the three Es – the effort (or work) of breathing (Table 29.3), the effectiveness of breathing (Table 29.4) and the effect of inadequate respiration on other organs (Table 29.5).

Table 29.3 Signs of increased effort of breathing

Respiratory rate (Table 29.2)
Intercostal, subcostal and sternal recession
Use of additional accessory muscles
Flaring of the alae nasae
Inspiratory and expiratory noises (e.g. stridor, wheeze)
Grunting (a physiological attempt to increase end-expiratory pressure)
'Positioning' (children with croup often sit in a 'tripod' position)

Table 29.4 Assessing the effectiveness of breathing

Chest expansion
Auscultation (assess air entry)
   A SILENT CHEST INDICATES A LIFE-THREATENING STATE
Pulse oximetry
   AN OXYGEN SATURATION < 85% IN AIR INDICATES
   A LIFE-THREATENING STATE

Table 29.5 The effects of respiratory failure on other organs

1. Cardiovascular system:
Tachycardia (see Table 29.2) occurs secondary to hypoxia followed by the development of bradycardia and ultimately asystole
BRADYCARDIA IS A LIFE-THREATENING SIGN

2. Skin colour:
pallor (vasoconstriction as a consequence of hypoxia) and later cyanosis – a sign of very severe respiratory failure
CYANOSIS IS A LIFE-THREATENING SIGN

3. Mental state:
Hypoxia produces agitation ± drowsiness.
EXHAUSTION IS A LIFE-THREATENING SIGN.

C – Circulation

Potential circulatory failure (shock) can be identified following an assessment as detailed in Table 29.6.

In shocked children, blood pressure falls occur later as a result of compensatory mechanisms. In the prehospital setting logistical reasons limit the value of blood pressure measurement, e.g. environmental noise, child agitation, incorrectly sized cuffs, limited personnel and a lack of knowledge of normal child blood pressures ranges. Attempted measurements also delay treatment and transportation.

Table 29.6 Signs of circulatory failure

Heart Rate (see Table 29.2).
  BRADYCARDIA IS A LIFE-THREATENING SIGN

Pulse Volume
Capillary Refill Time (CRT)
  measured centrally on sternum or forehead; this should be < 2seconds

Blood Pressure: Hypotension when SBP < (2 × age) + 65
  HYPOTENSION IS A LIFE-THREATENING SIGN

Circulatory failure produces measurable effects in other organs, reflected by:

- tachypnoea *without* recession (compensating for the metabolic acidosis caused by poor tissue perfusion)
- mottled, cold skin colour
- cerebral agitation followed by drowsiness
  - agitation is seldom noted as such, due to difficulties distinguishing it from the child's general distress.

D – Disability (neurological)

A rapid neurological assessment should be performed and is outlined in Table 29.7.

Any child with a depressed level of consciousness or who is ill enough to need vascular access must have their blood glucose measured.

Table 29.7 Neurological assessment (disability)

Conscious level:
The AVPU score: (A – Alert, V – responds to Voice, P – responds to Pain,
  U – Unresponsive)

Pupils: document size and reactivity
Seizure activity
Posture:
  hypotonia ('the floppy baby'),
  stiffness in the neck and back (meningism) with or without opisthotonus
  decorticate and decerebrate postures

Initial management of the seriously ill or injured child

Abnormalities in the primary survey should generally be treated as they are found. However, very ill children need to be in hospital. Any patient with a significantly abnormal primary survey should be transferred as soon as possible, using blue lights and sirens when necessary. Deciding how much to do before moving a child is always difficult – in general, airway and breathing should be treated at the scene, addressing circulation en route. (Nebulization is a notable exception – this can be prepared and given on the way to hospital.) Any delays transferring a child to hospital must always be clinically justifiable.

Airway

Airway management is crucial and, as in adults, should be managed in a stepwise progression using the simplest interventions first (see Chapter 8). Hypoxia (rather than arrhythmia) is the commonest reason for cardiac arrest in childhood hence the emphasis on oxygenation and the importance of administering high flow oxygen. Laryngeal mask airways (LMAs) are useful and come in the full range of paediatric sizes. When advanced airway management is required, endotracheal intubation has not been found to be superior to bag–valve–mask (BVM) ventilation and, in view of the complexity and skill required, children should not be intubated outside of hospital by 'non-experts' unless there is no alternative. When all other methods have failed to obtain a clear airway in a child, a cricothyroidotomy should be performed. Needle cricothyroidotomy is the technique of choice in children under 12 years.

Breathing

Children with inadequate or absent breathing require ventilation. A paediatric BVM device should be used with a two-person technique where possible. Careful mask size selection is essential and an appropriate mask is one that does not cover the patient's eyes and does not extend beyond the chin. A circular mask may be more suitable in infants. Most BVM devices have a pressure-limiting valve set at 4 kPa (45 mmHg) to prevent barotrauma and stomach insufflation with high ventilation pressures. In some cases (e.g. life-threatening asthma) higher than normal airway pressures may be required and in these cases the valve may be overridden and closed.

High-flow oxygen via a non-rebreather mask should be provided for all seriously ill or injured children who are breathing. If the child is fully stabilized before arrival *and* it is possible to measure oxygen saturations continuously, it is reasonable to reduce the oxygen to maintain oxygen saturations of 95–98%. If there are any doubts or if the saturation monitoring does not appear to be reliable (e.g. hypovolaemia causing poor signal, severe anaemia, sickle cell, etc.) continue high-flow oxygen.

Circulation

Vascular access is required to treat shock and to give antibiotics or analgesia. Generally the equipment for this can be prepared on the way to hospital. If it is not possible to gain intravenous access after two attempts (or immediately in cardiac arrest in young children), the intraosseous route should be used. Intraosseous access is a very useful prehospital technique providing reliable rapid central vascular access and is skill worth learning. Intravenous fluid should be used to treat shock (circulatory failure). In medical conditions fluid boluses of 20 mL/kg are recommended whereas in trauma 5 mL/kg aliquots are recommended. Repeated aliquots reassessing vital signs after each one should be given until the child has made a very significant improvement; the aim is *not* to normalize vital signs. Current, adult, 'hypotensive resuscitation' practices cannot be safely used in children as hypotension is a late and preterminal sign.

Management of paediatric medical emergencies

Table 29.8 provides an overview of some of the commoner paediatric medical conditions, highlighting where treatments are significantly different from adults.

Table 29.8 Common childhood illnesses and the differences in their management

Condition (common causes)	Principle treatments which may vary from adult practice	Comments
Stridor: Croup Epiglottitis Foreign body	If stridor thought to be due to croup give oral dexamethasone (0.15 mg kg). In severe cases give nebulised adrenaline 5 mL 1:1000 once only.	Do not examine throat Do not upset the child (no needles, nebs, etc.) Do not attempt to remove foreign body if child is breathing
Wheezing: Asthma Anaphylaxis Bronchiolitis	Give 8–10 puffs of salbutamol MDI via spacer device. Repeat Salbutamol dose every 20 minutes or give continuously if necessary. Give Ipratropium if severe or poor response IM adrenaline (10 μg/kg 1:1000) may be tried in asthma or anaphylaxis if wheeze is not responding and is considered life-threatening. Oxygen MUST be given concurrently if adrenaline used.	In childhood asthma, spacers are at least as, and are sometimes more effective, than nebulisers. Salbutamol and ipratropium may both be tried as one may work better. Use nebulised salbutamol if requiring oxygen Salbutamol: 2.5 mg (<5 years) or 5 mg (>5 years) Ipratropium: 125 μg (<2 years) or 250 μg (>2 years) Children under 1 year old may not respond well to bronchodilators. Do not repeat if they do not respond. Consider bronchiolitis or heart failure.
Presumed meningococcal sepsis (Figure 29.2)	Benzyl penicillin – preferably IV or IO but can be IM rather than delay treatment Treat shock with 20 mL/kg fluid boluses Check the blood glucose	Give benzylpenicillin early <1 year 300 mg 1-8 year 600 mg >8 year 1200 mg Do not give if no rash. (NICE 2010)
Presumed meningitis (without septicaemic rash)	Do not give antibiotics Transfer using blue lights and sirens	NICE (2010) advise NO antibiotics without a septicaemic Rash (if rapid access to hospital)
Seizure: Febrile convulsion Epilepsy Hypoglycaemia	Rectal diazepam(0.5 mg/kg) or buccal midazolam (0.5 mg/kg) if no IV or IO access. Subsequent IV lorazepam (0.1 mg/kg) or diazemuls (0.4 mg/kg) if ongoing seizure. Repeat × 1 if required Check the blood glucose	Do not delay treatment to gain vascular access Some children may have febrile convulsions in response to a rapid rise in temperature. These are usually self limiting
Hypoglycaemia (BM <3 mmol/L)	Oral glucose or glucose gel if possible 10% glucose (2 mL/kg) IV/IO if necessary Consider glucagon IM only if diabetic: <1 month -Not recommended <6 years 0.5 mg >6 years 1 mg	Do NOT use concentration of >20% glucose in children Glucagon may not work in hypoglycaemia not due to excess insulin (i.e. non-diabetics)
Diabetic ketoacidosis	Do not give any IV fluids unless shock is severe. If required give 10 mL/kg slowly	Greater risk of cerebral oedema than in adults

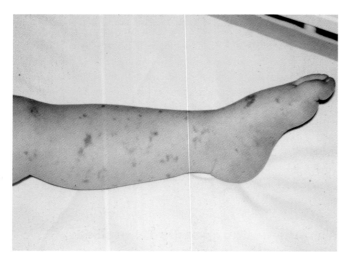

Figure 29.2 The purpuric rash of meningococcal septicaemia (Source: with permission from the Meningitis Research Foundation).

Additional interventions may also be required (see Chapter 23 on medical emergencies).

Management of paediatric trauma emergencies

Scene assessment

The differences in scene assessment and management when children are involved include the following:

- Children or babies may be overlooked – especially if they are in the footwell of a car or have been ejected from an open car window. Look for clues as to the presence of a child – toys, nappies or a baby's bottle. Do not be afraid to mention concerns that a child involved in an accident may not have been found.
- Emotions cloud judgement when children are involved. Do not be tempted to compromise your own or others' safety just because it is a child. Pressure from bystanders can be a problem.

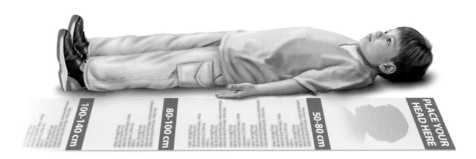

Figure 29.3 The paediatric triage tape (Reproduced with permission of Advanced Life Support Group).

- Triage can be difficult when children are involved as their vital signs change with age. Where possible, use the Paediatric Triage Tape (Figure 29.3) rather than the adult triage sieve and try not to over-triage children to the detriment of adult patients.
- Parents may be very demanding. Do not allow them to endanger themselves. It is best to involve them in the child's care where possible by carrying out some simple task such as holding the oxygen mask.

Primary survey in trauma

The initial assessment of the traumatized child follows a **structured approach** in the same airway, breathing and circulation order as the medical assessment but with two caveats. Firstly, *catastrophic haemorrhage* is treated immediately and, secondly, the **cervical spine** must be immobilized (where indicated) at the same time as the airway. Any clinical deterioration should prompt a return to the beginning of the primary survey.

Head and neck injury

In children, the aims of head injury management are much the same as for adults – preventing secondary brain injury. Hypoglycaemia may be a feature and requires prompt treatment. The cerebral perfusion pressure must be adequate and body temperature kept normal. Cervical spine injuries are rare but if present are often high and may be devastating. When immobilizing a child on a spinal board it may be necessary to pad the shoulders to obtain neutral alignment of the head and neck if not using a paediatric board. Adult long leg vacuum or box splints provide ideal immobilization devices for infants and small toddlers. Combative children are difficult to manage. They must not be forcibly restrained but should receive manual immobilization of the head and neck along with reassurance and adequate analgesia. Parental involvement may help.

Chest injury

The compliant rib cage of a child means forces can be transmitted internally causing severe internal injury without apparent external injury.

Abdominal injury

Children are prone to certain patterns of abdominal injury as their liver and spleen are more exposed and the bladder sits higher out of the pelvis than in an adult.

Burns

Because of their smaller airways, children with facial and upper airway burns are more likely to develop airway obstruction earlier than adults and so early intubation (usually in hospital) would be recommended where airway burns are suspected. Where journey times are prolonged (e.g. more than 1 hour before hospital arrival) 10 mL/kg fluid should be commenced. A Lund–Browder chart is the most reliable way of assessing the size of a burn, as it takes into account the child's age. The rule of nines (used in adults) is not accurate. When estimating small burns (e.g. <15% TBSA) the child's palmar surface (the area of their closed palm, including fingers is approximately 1% of their body surface area) and can be used.

Analgesia

Analgesia is mandatory for children of all ages who are in pain. Additionally, non-pharmacological approaches such as splinting, distraction and a child-friendly environment should be employed. Pharmacological methods are similar to adults.

Oral medications (e.g. paracetamol, ibuprofen or oral morphine) are used in minor injuries with stronger analgesia employed for moderate and severe pain (Figure 29.4). Entonox can be used in any child old enough to understand how to use it. Intranasal diamorphine is particularly effective in children and increasingly used in emergency practice, acting rapidly and avoiding venepuncture. Intravenous morphine continues to be the 'gold standard' and should not be withheld when required. It may also be given intraosseously if necessary.

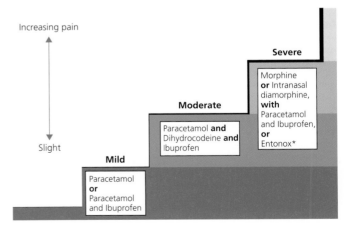

Figure 29.4 The analgesia ladder (Source: with permission Sandell Medical Images © 2006).

Making life easier

Paediatric doses are usually prescribed per kilogram but a child's weight is difficult to predict accurately in the prehospital environment. In addition, attempting to memorize every paediatric drug dose and vital sign for children across all the age groups is impossible and potentially dangerous. To minimize drug and equipment errors and overcome these difficulties, various charts, tapes and even mobile phone 'Apps' have been developed and their use is recommended. Common examples include the Oakley Chart or tapes such as the Sandell Tape and Broselow Tape. The latter take advantage of the relationship between a child's length and their weight and/or age. By laying the child alongside these tapes their weight/drug doses/vital signs/equipment sizes can be read off according to their length (Figure 29.5). Tapes and charts are preferred over mathematical calculations (Table 29.1) as mistakes can easily occur. Many healthcare professionals prefer to make their own note books or charts and so it is worth looking at the spectrum of aides-memoires and choosing the one most suited to your needs or even creating your own!

Safeguarding

All healthcare professionals have a duty of care to protect children from abuse and must report suspicions as per their child protection procedures or to social services. Prehospital personnel have an unrivalled opportunity to see the child's normal environment usually denied those working in hospital. If there are suspicions of abuse of any kind, handover at the hospital should be to a senior member of staff and detailed notes should be given and a copy kept. Deliberate injury must always be borne in mind and certain injury patterns such as finger tip bruising, bruising in an unusual place such as the pinna of the ear or abdomen, marks of objects such as that caused by a belt buckle etc. should be considered as non-accidental unless a very good explanation exists. Any injury that is inconsistent with the history or where there has been an inexplicable delay in presentation should raise major concerns. Evidence of neglect must be acted upon without delay. Safeguarding issues are really beyond the scope of this chapter, but if in doubt, they must be reported and the child must be kept safe. In an emergency, any police officer has the power to take a child into a 'place of safety'.

> **Tips from the field**
>
> - Pre-prepare paediatric drug and equipment cards – avoid doing calculations on scene
> - In extremis use an adult BVM and mask – invert mask and ventilate to chest movements
> - Use IO as primary means of access in all seriously unwell/traumatized children
> - Use a long leg box or vacuum splint to immobilize an infant/small child
> - If a stable child is restrained in a portable child seat, leave them in it for onward transportation (with additional head padding and tape as required)
> - Transport a parent with the child where possible to provide further medical details and consent for procedures.

Further reading

AAGBI Safety Guideline. *Prehospital Anaesthesia.*. Association of Anaesthetists of Great Britain and Ireland: London, 2009.

Advanced Life Support Group. *Prehospital Paediatric Life Support (PHPLS)*, 2nd edn. Oxford: Blackwell Publishing, 2005.

Sandall J. Accidents and Emergencies. In: Gardiner M, Eisen S, Murphy C (eds) *Training in Paediatrics. The Essential Curriculum*. Chapter 2. Oxford: Oxford University Press, 2009: Chapter 2.

Sandell JM, Maconochie IK, Jewkes F. Prehospital paediatric emergency care: paediatric triage. *EMJ* 2009;**26**:767–768.

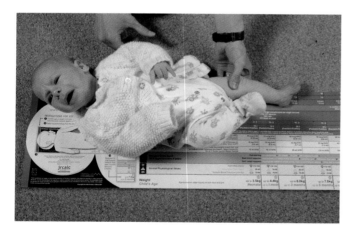

Figure 29.5 Length-based assessment demonstrated using the Sandell Tape (Source: with permission from TSG Associates).

CHAPTER 30

Care of Special Groups: The Elderly Patient

Tim Nutbeam

Derriford Hospital, Plymouth Hospitals NHS Trust, Plymouth, UK

OVERVIEW

By the end of this chapter you should know:

- The challenges of providing care to elderly patients
- The physiological changes which occur with old age
- The confounding factors which may mask symptoms and signs
- Symptoms and signs which must be thoroughly investigated in elderly patients.

9 A knowledge of baseline functional status is essential for evaluating new complaints
10 Health problems must be evaluated for associated psychosocial adjustment
11 The emergency department encounter is an opportunity to assess important conditions in the patient's personal life.

Introduction

The elderly population in the developed world is growing and will continue to grow: the 'over 85' age group is increasing at a rate of four times that of the general population. Elderly people consume approximately one-third of healthcare resources. The use of prehospital services by the elderly is four times that of younger patients. Elderly people can be challenging emergency patients (Box 30.1): they are more difficult to diagnose, take longer to treat and often require more investigations and tests.

Box 30.1 The Society for Academic Emergency Medicines Geriatric Taskforce: Principles of Geriatric Emergency Medicine

1 The patient's presentation is frequently complex
2 Common diseases present atypically in this age group
3 The confounding effects of co-morbid diseases must be considered
4 Polypharmacy is common and may be a factor in presentation, diagnosis, and management
5 Recognition of the possibility for cognitive impairment is important
6 Some diagnostic tests may have different normal values
7 The likelihood of decreased functional reserve must be anticipated
8 Social support systems may not be adequate, and patients may need to rely on caregivers

---

Despite elderly people being the most frequently encountered patient group in prehospital emergency medicine, education about their care takes up a disproportionately small amount of postgraduate and continued professional developed curriculums. Additionally, they are infrequently the subject of emergency research, and it has been shown emergency physicians prefer to care for younger patients.

This chapter will discuss the challenges of managing elderly patients in the prehospital environment.

Physiology

Ageing in itself is not a disease process. Both physiological and biological ageing have characteristics which mean that the body's ability to respond to challenges such as infection and trauma is compromised (Box 30.2).

Box 30.2 Characteristic features of ageing

1 Ageing is universal: it affects all living organisms
2 Ageing is progressive: the ageing process is continuous
3 The changes associated with ageing are detrimental
4 Ageing by itself is not a disease
5 Ageing makes the individual more vulnerable to disease.

A patient's physiological age can be very different from their biological or chronological age: indeed many younger people may be 'elderly' physiologically. It is the physiological age and not the biological age that is important when assessing and managing patients.

Every body system is affected by the ageing process, leading to overall decreased physiological reserve. It is important to be aware that this is a heterogeneous non-linear process: the physiological

ABC of Prehospital Emergency Medicine, First Edition.
Edited by Tim Nutbeam and Matthew Boylan.
© 2013 John Wiley & Sons, Ltd. Published 2013 by John Wiley & Sons, Ltd.

Table 30.1 Physiological changes with age

System	Physiological change	Implications
Respiratory	Decreased compliance of both lungs and chest wall Decreased functional alveoli and alveolar surface area Decreased number of cilia	Decreased vital capacity with increased residual volume Decreased gas transfer, increased gas trapping Increased susceptibility to infections and aspiration
Cardiovascular	Increased stiffness/decreased elasticity of the arterial system Decreased number of atrial pacemaker cells Decreased response to catecholamines	Increased blood pressure Left ventricular hypertrophy Decrease in intrinsic heart rate Reduced heart rate response to physiological stress
Musculoskeletal	Loss of muscle mass and coordination Loss of bone mass	Decreased mobility, increased risk of falling Increasingly prone to fracture

age of individual organs and systems within a patient may be dramatically different.

The key physiological changes of age relevant to emergency management are those which affect the cardiovascular, respiratory and musculoskeletal systems (Table 30.1). It is important to note that these changes are in addition to and must be considered alongside those related to chronic diseases common in elderly people, e.g. coronary artery disease.

Presentation

The patient's presentation is frequently complex with a wide array of vague, ambiguous, multisystem symptoms. Common conditions will often present atypically, without 'classic' symptoms or signs. This is due to a number of causes.

1 Confounding effects of disease and heterogeneous system decline

The heterogeneous physiological changes with increasing age are confounded and complicated by the presence of chronic disease, e.g. the presence of hypertension may temporarily mask depletion in intravascular volume. Not all elderly people have chronic diseases, but a directed past medical history and collaborating evidence (relatives, medication list, etc.) may indicate those that do.

Note that not all chronic confounding disease will have been diagnosed prior to your assessment: a high index of suspicion is vital.

2 Confounding effects of medications, especially polypharmacy

- The average elderly person in the developed world takes 4.5 prescribed medications daily with an additional two over-the-counter (OTC) medicines.
- The risk of adverse drug-related events (ADREs) rises exponentially with the number of medicines used – with seven medicines

the risk of adverse interaction is greater than 80%: up to 25% of hospital admissions in elderly people can be attributed to ADREs.
- Patients and their relatives may not report OTC medicine use, but the interactions can be significant, e.g. ginseng and warfarin.
- Non-linear physiological changes that can alter drug action include drug bioavailability, distribution, metabolism and clearance.
- Poor compliance with medication is common. Contributing factors include poor hearing and eyesight, multiple caregivers, poor memory and cognition. Many people will choose to omit and adjust medication themselves based on side effects and other factors.
- Warfarin, NSAIDs, beta-blockers and antipsychotics are particularly high-risk medications.

3 Cognitive impairment

Cognitive impairment is rarely due to old age alone: sudden changes in levels of cognition and function need to be taken seriously and investigated acutely.

Conditions such as Alzheimer's disease may mean that symptoms go unreported, histories are unclear and recent interactions are forgotten.

4 Healthcare professional attribution error

Healthcare professionals are repeatedly guilty of attribution error when assessing elderly people. Multiple complaints, symptoms and signs are ignored and attributed to the 'natural aging process'. It is rare in an emergency situation for the healthcare professional to have a thorough understanding of the patient, their medication, any confounding past medical history and their 'normal' level of function and cognition: do not make assumptions.

Any acute change needs investigation: decrease in power, falls, decline in functional ability, incontinence and confusion are not normal deteriorations with age. These conditions need to be aggressively worked up and treated.

When evaluating the elderly patient consider what you may be missing (Box 30.3).

Box 30.3 **Considerations when evaluating an elderly patient**

Does this symptom complex represent myocardial Ischaemia?
Does this represent acute cerebral vascular disease?
Does this represent an infectious process e.g. sepsis?
Does this represent an acute abdominal condition?
Are the symptoms related to the patient's medications?
Are the symptoms an exacerbation of a pre-existing disease?
Do the symptoms fit a new disease process?

Aggressive therapy

Healthcare professionals are guilty of denying elderly people the aggressive interventions and care which they may give a younger patient. Judgements about a patient's quality of life, and their true physiological age cannot and should not be made in the prehospital environment. Data on high impact interventions such as thrombolysis in myocardial infarction does not support reserving these treatment for the (relatively) young – in fact in some cases the opposite is true and the treatments are more efficacious in the elderly population.

Appropriate drug doses

The doses of all medications (including oxygen and fluids) should be calculated taking into account the patients weight, likely physiological age and potential impairment.

Trauma in elderly people

Falls are the most common cause of trauma in elderly people, with approximately 10% of these leading to serious injury. Closed head and blunt chest injuries predominate in the elderly trauma population. Motor vehicle accidents, interpersonal violence and burns are other common causes of trauma in this age group.

In significant trauma, decreased functional reserve must be anticipated. Elderly patients with multisystem trauma often do not

Table 30.2 The primary survey in the elderly people

Assessment/ management	Complicated by
Airway	Dentures, loose teeth, etc.
Breathing	Decrease sympathetic response to stimulus Low physiological reserve Significantly obtunded by spinal board immobilization
Circulation	Effects of beta-blockers and other cardiac medications Risk of pulmonary oedema with fluid boluses High chance of occult bleeding/shock Unreliable abdominal examination
Disability/neurological	Unknown previous level of cognition Other factors causing neurological signs (beware attribution error) Late presentation of significant head injury
Exposure	High risk of hypothermia

manifest classic signs and symptoms of shock such as tachycardia (Table 30.2).

Occult shock is common in elderly people: point of care lactate monitors may have a role in detecting this.

Elder abuse

Elder abuse is often unrecognized and less than 10% of cases are appropriately reported. Historically it has not received the same level of attention as paediatric abuse and many services/departments do not have specific protocols to apply in suspected cases. Elderly patients are most often abused by their care giver.

All healthcare professionals need to be aware of the potential for abuse, document their findings accurately and ensure that all concerns are reported to the appropriate authorities.

Tips from the field

- Distinguish physiological age from the biological age of your patient
- Elderly people are physiologically heterogeneous: one organ/system may have significantly less reserve than another
- Aggressive resuscitation strategies may be appropriate and mandatory to improve trauma outcomes in this age group
- Take any acute change seriously: falls, declines in functional ability and confusion, etc., are not 'normal'
- Check the names and date on medications you presume the patient may be taking. Try to gather collaborating evidence (this may be the only chance)
- Elderly skin is extremely delicate – take care when handling/moving patients.

Further reading

Gallo J, Bogner H, Fulmer T, Paveza G (eds). *Handbook of Geriatric Assessment*. Sudbury, MA: Jones and Bartlett Publishers, 2006.

Medlon S, MA OJ. Woolward R. *Geriatric Emergency Medicine*. New York: Mcgraw-Hill, 2004

The Society for Academic Emergency Medicine: Geriatric Taskforce: http://www.saem.org/SAEMDNN/Default.aspx?tabid=627

CHAPTER 31

Care of Special Groups: The Bariatric Patient

Lynn Gerber Smith[1], Suzanne Sherwood[1], Anna Fergusson[2], and Dennis Jones[3]

[1] University of Maryland Medical Center, Baltimore, MD, USA
[2] Birmingham School of Anaesthesia, Birmingham, UK
[3] The Johns Hopkins Hospital, Baltimore, MD, USA

OVERVIEW

By the end of this chapter, you should know:

- The physiological changes that occur with obesity
- The specific challenges related to the clinical management and transportation of the bariatric patient
- How to dose common medications in the bariatric patient.

Table 31.1 Body mass index chart

Body mass index (BMI): is the standard measure for determining obesity.
$BMI = weight (kg)/ height^2 (m^2)$

BMI	Category
Below 18.5	Underweight
18.5–24.9	Normal
25.0–29.9	Overweight
30.0–39.9	Obese
Over 40	Morbidly obese

Introduction

Obesity is a global epidemic affecting one-quarter of the UK population and one-third of the US population. Morbid obesity, defined as a body mass index (BMI) of $>40\,kg/m^2$ (Table 31.1), has a UK prevalence of 1.9%. This figure is expected to rise considerably in the coming years. Obesity should be considered as a multisystem disorder and presents numerous challenges in the prehospital environment. The purpose of this chapter is to review the clinical and practical challenges faced by the prehospital provider caring for morbidly obese patients.

Physiological changes in morbid obesity

Numerous physiological changes occur in the morbidly obese, affecting all systems. The most relevant of these involve the respiratory and cardiovascular systems.

Respiratory

Functional residual capacity (FRC) of the lungs is significantly reduced in obesity; because of small airway collapse, reduction in chest wall compliance, displacement of abdominal contents into the thorax and increased thoracic blood volume. Closing volumes can encroach on functional residual capacity (FRC) during normal respiration, causing airway closure with associated V/Q mismatch and intrapulmonary shunting. Supine positioning exacerbates these problems resulting in further hypoxia.

The incidence of obstructive sleep apnoea (apnoeic episodes secondary to pharynhgeal collapse during sleep) and obesity

ABC of Prehospital Emergency Medicine, First Edition.
Edited by Tim Nutbeam and Matthew Boylan.
© 2013 John Wiley & Sons, Ltd. Published 2013 by John Wiley & Sons, Ltd.

hypoventilation syndrome (Pickwickian syndrome) are high in obese patients and often unrecognized. Long-term effects include desensitization of the respiratory centre and reliance on hypoxia to drive respiration. This results in chronic type 2 respiratory failure.

Cardiovascular

Stroke volume, cardiac output, ventricular workload and blood volume are all increased in the obese patient. This can lead to systemic and pulmonary hypertension, left ventricular hypertrophy and dilatation. Eventually right ventricular hypertrophy and dilatation will develop resulting in cor pulmonale.

Oxygen consumption and carbon dioxide production are also increased due to the metabolic demands of excess adipose tissue.

Comorbidities

The prevalence of comorbidities in the morbidly obese patient increases as the BMI increases; however, BMI alone is a poor predictor of comorbidity. In general, gynaecoid obesity ('pear-shaped body') is associated with fewer comorbidities than android obesity ('apple-shaped body'). Patients with morbid obesity have a median survival 8–10 years less than those with normal body weight.

Obesity is associated with a number of cardiovascular comorbidities including hypertension, ischaemic heart disease, arrhythmias, cardiomyopathies and cardiac failure.

Common respiratory comorbidities include asthma, obstructive sleep apnoea and obesity hypoventilation syndrome. It is important to note that patients may not experience the symptoms of their comorbidities due to their sedentary lifestyle. Symptoms may therefore only manifest when the patient experiences a traumatic event or physiological stress.

Other relevant conditions associated with obesity include diabetes (40× increased risk compared with non-obese population) and gastro oesophageal reflux disease.

Management

Management of the morbidly obese patient should begin with the ABC approach.

Airway

Airway management in the morbidly obese patient can be problematic. Airway compromise can occur with less impairment of consciousness compared with non-obese patients.

Contributors to the high incidence of difficult airways amongst this population include excess tissue around the neck, a large tongue and increased adipose tissue in the pharyngeal wall. The ideal 'sniffing the morning air' position may be difficult to achieve due to the large soft tissue mass of the neck and chest wall. In addition the patient is likely to be hypoxic (especially when supine) and will rapidly desaturate during even a brief period of hypoventilation or apnoea. BMI alone does not necessarily predict a difficult intubation and patients should be carefully assessed for other indicators of a difficult airway (see Chapters 6 and 9). Conversely, BMI can predict difficulty with face mask ventilation.

The decision to perform prehospital RSI and advanced airway management should not be taken lightly. If the circumstances allow, timely transfer of the patient to a facility with experienced anaesthetic personnel and advanced difficult airway equipment is preferable. If advanced airway management is necessary, meticulous preparation and patient positioning should minimize unsuccessful attempts. Prolonged pre-oxygenation should be performed using high flow oxygen with a tight fitting mask. Correct patient positioning may include the reverse Trendelenburg position or an elevation of the head and shoulders using wedges, blankets and pillows. The ideal position is having the sternum level with the tragus of the ear (Figure 31.1), this aids laryngoscopy and improves ventilatory function as well as reducing the risk of aspiration. Technologies such

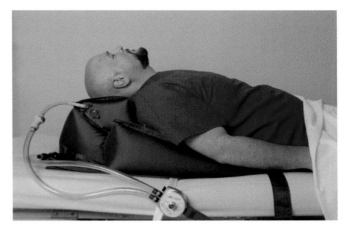

Figure 31.2 Patient on Rapid Airway Management Positioning (RAMP) device.

as the portable Rapid Airway Management Positioning (RAMP) system (Figure 31.2) are available to aid patient positioning.

Laryngoscopy can be easier with a 'stubby' or polio handle and a long blade; these should be considered for the first attempt. Difficult airway equipment should be readily available; this should include basic equipment such as bougies and LMAs as well as more advanced equipment such as the Airtrach or glidescope according to local policies and practitioner expertise. If bag valve ventilation is required, a four-handed technique will often be necessary.

Once endotracheal intubation has been secured, the ramped position should be maintained, as it will aid ventilation mechanics. Careful attention should be paid to airway pressures and tidal volumes.

Spinal immobilization

Care should be taken when choosing the appropriate size of neck collar the largest size available may not fit the largest of patients. A towel roll could be used instead of a collar but is not ideal as it will only limit extension, not flexion. Not all patients will safely fit onto a standard spinal board; an adjustable scoop stretcher should be suitable for some obese patients (maximum load approximately 150 kg). Specially designed bariatric rescue stretchers are available for immobilization and patient movement and should be used where available.

Breathing

Assessment of breathing, in particular auscultation, is often difficult in morbidly obese patients due to their body habitus. Excellent clinical acumen and a high index of suspicion are therefore necessary. Specialized equipment is available including stethoscopes with increased sound amplification and ambient noise reduction as well as Doppler stethoscopes. Measurement of peripheral oxygen saturations may not always be accurate due to excess adipose tissue: probes should ideally be placed on an ear lobe.

Aspiration of pulmonary contents is a considerable risk in morbidly obese patients due to abnormal positioning of the diaphragm,

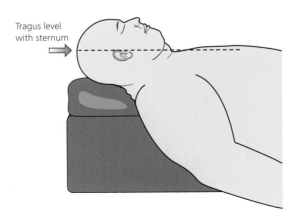

Tragus level with sternum

Figure 31.1 Ideal positioning for airway management.

larger volume of gastric fluid, increased intra-abdominal pressure and increased incidence of gastro-oesophageal reflex disease (GORD). The patient's risk is escalated if they are positioned supine, sedated or paralysed.

Circulation

Thorough cardiovascular examination is difficult due to excess adipose tissue. An appropriate size blood pressure cuff should be used; a cuff too small may lead to falsely elevated blood pressures. Obese patients often have hypertension and ischaemic heart disease (IHD): a normal blood pressure in these patients may be indicative of shock.

Vascular access can be challenging in this patient population. Intraosseous access should be considered early if attempts to gain peripheral access fail. The yellow 45 mm EZ-IO needle set would be most appropriate; consideration of less commonly used insertion sites such as the distal tibia may be necessary. If available and time allows, the use of ultrasound-guided intravenous catheters may be beneficial.

Disability and exposure

Exposure of all areas may be difficult due to the patients weight; log-rolling, etc., should only be attempted when adequate numbers of trained staff are available to minimize risk to staff. Wounds may be concealed by skin folds, so vigilance is essential.

Drugs

The pharmacokinetics of many drugs are affected by the mass of adipose tissue resulting in a potentially less predictable response. This can make calculations of appropriate doses difficult. As a general rule, drugs which are hydrophilic should be dosed according to ideal body weight and those which are lipophilic should be dosed according to total body weight. The Broca formula can be used to estimate the ideal body weight (Table 31.2). Whenever possible doses should be carefully titrated to response.

Suxamethonium dosing should always be calculated using total body weight and given at a dose of 1 mg/kg (up to 2 mg/kg in children) to optimize intubating conditions during rapid sequence induction.

Table 31.3 shows some commonly used Prehospital drugs and the weight that should be used to calculate the required dose.

Communications

Communicating between the prehospital providers and the receiving facility is essential to provide the safest care for the morbidly obese patient. This can allow the receiving hospital to prepare suitable trolleys, equipment and manpower.

Table 31.2 Broca formula to calculate ideal body weight (in kg)

| Men | Height in centimetres minus 100 |
| Women | Height in centimetres minus 105 |

Table 31.3 Drug dosing in obesity

Ideal body weight (IBW) (Broca formula)	Corrected body weight (CBW = IBW + 40% of excess weight)	Total body weight TBW
Propofol	Fentanyl	Suxamethonium
Thiopentone	Sugammadex	Midazolam bolus
Ketamine	Local anaesthetics	Atracurium
Rocuronium	Antibiotics	
Vecuronium		
Morphine		

Equipment, transport and manual handling

Equipment to care for and safely transfer the morbidly obese patient is both essential and expensive; prehospital providers may need to share this equipment.

Helicopter transport may not always be possible; aircraft weight limits will depend on a number of factors including the type of aircraft, space within aircraft, weight of the crew, weather conditions and the fuel status. Specially adapted ground ambulances should be available and should contain all the necessary bariatric equipment. This will include expandable, double width stretchers capable of carrying 318 kg (50 stone), compared to the 191 kg (30 stone) limit of standard stretchers (Table 31.4, Figure 31.3). Additionally, they can be equipped with stronger tail lifts, capable of taking weights up to 476 kg (75 stone), hoists, winches and inflatable lifting cushions which can be used to lift people from the floor (Figure 31.4).

Correct manual handling techniques are essential when dealing with morbidly obese patients. Back injuries are the number one injury for all prehospital staff. All staff should receive adequate training and should not attempt to move patients unless sufficient

Table 31.4 Examples of prehospital equipment weight limits

Product	Limits	Other information
Ferno Model 65 Scoop Stretcher	Load limit: 350 lbs (159 kg)	
Stryker Power-pro Powered Ambulance Cot Equipment Hook – Model 6500-147-000	Weight capacity: 700 lbs (318 kg)	Battery powered hydraulic lift system
Ferno Kendrick Extrication Device (K.E.D)	Load capacity: 500 lbs (227 kg)	

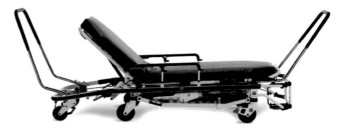

Figure 31.3 Stryker bariatric stretcher.

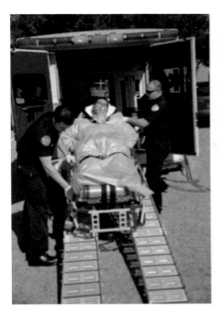

Figure 31.4 Specially adapted bariatric ambulance.

numbers of trained staff are present; in the prehospital environment this can often include members of the fire service.

Extrication from the scene of an accident or even from the patients home can be complex. In extreme cases, firefighters have been required to remove doors and even house walls to enable safe removal of the patient.

Summary

Morbid obesity is becoming increasingly common in the developed world and presents a variety of complex challenges to prehospital providers. Every prehospital service should have specific protocols for the care of morbidly obese patients to ensure that they receive the same standard of care as the rest of the population. This should include the purchase of specialized equipment as well as adequate training of their personnel.

Tips from the field

- Get help early. These are complex patients and require a multidisciplinary approach
- Always assume multiple comorbidities, particularly those affecting the cardiovascular and respiratory systems
- Although tracheal intubation is not necessarily more difficult than in non obese patients, rescue techniques (such as bag valve mask ventilation) are, and patients can rapidly desaturate and decompensate. Fully optimize conditions for your first intubation attempt
- Correct patient positioning is of paramount importance, as are correct manual handling techniques to achieve this positioning!
- Thorough communication with the receiving hospital is essential.

Further reading

Dargin J, Medzon R. Emergency department management of the airway in obese adults. *Ann Emerg Med* 2010;**56**:95–104.
Lotia S, Bellamy MC. Anaesthesia and morbid obesity. *Contin Educ Anaesth Crit Care Pain* 2008;**8**:151–156.
The Society for Obesity and Bariatric Anaesthesia. www.sobauk.com.
World Health Organization. www.who.int/topics/obesity/en.

CHAPTER 32

Retrieval and Transport

Peter Aitken[1], Mark Elcock[1,2], Neil Ballard[1], and Matt Hooper[1]

[1]James Cook University, Townsville, QLD, Australia
[2]Retrieval Services Queensland, Brisbane, QLD, Australia

OVERVIEW

By the end of this chapter you should know

- The importance and purpose of retrieval and transport
- The different types of retrieval
- The advantages and disadvantages of different transport modes
- The factors affecting the choice of transport
- The factors affecting the ability to provide care in transit.

Introduction

Retrieval and transport is an essential element of quality patient care. To be most effective there should be seamless transition between care in the prehospital, transport and hospital environments.

The usual operating paradigm in patient transport has been to 'bring the patient to care' and enable access to higher levels of care or definitive management. The concept of 'bringing care to the patient' is increasingly important. Highly trained retrieval teams can optimize patient outcomes by earlier introduction of critical care management.

This mandates the deployment of appropriately trained staff with essential equipment, and liaison between referring, transporting and receiving staff. Clinical management during transport must aim to at least equal care at the referral point and also prepare the patient for admission to the receiving service. The risk of transport should not exceed any potential benefit the patient may obtain from the receiving centre.

Definitions and terminology

Patient retrieval can be defined as the use of clinicians (medical, nursing, paramedic, other) to facilitate clinical management and safe transport of a patient(s) from one location to another.

Retrievals are classified as primary or secondary. Primary retrievals are from a prehospital site to a health facility. Secondary retrievals are from one health facility to another and are also referred to as interfacility transfers. Patient movement between

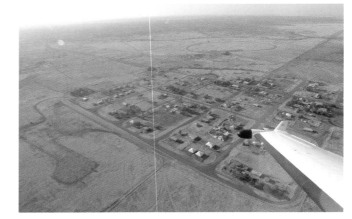

Figure 32.1 Transport from isolated rural centres.

large centres usually for subspecialty services are sometimes called 'tertiary' retrievals.

Primary retrievals may be further categorized as 'land on' or 'winch', depending on whether site access is possible. The term 'modified primary' has also emerged and involves an interfacility transfer where the referring centre has only rudimentary facilities. For all intents this becomes a primary retrieval with shelter and power. The characteristics of primary and secondary retrievals are described in Table 32.1. This has important resource implications (transport frame, equipment, staff), and helps define retrieval services roles.

Retrieval services are extremely varied. Some are purely prehospital, some offer neonatal services, while others are mixed (all ages, 'medical' and trauma). Distances may range from inner-city responses, to decentralized rural populations where long fixed-wing flight times may be needed (Figure 32.1). Casemix and geography are integral in determining the structure of retrieval services including selection of crewmix, platform and equipment.

Crewmix

Physicians, paramedics, nurses and other personnel are all used as transport and retrieval crew. System variances are determined mainly by historical difference in prehospital care models. Regardless of discipline, crew should be adequately trained and equipped for both the prehospital and retrieval environment.

ABC of Prehospital Emergency Medicine, First Edition.
Edited by Tim Nutbeam and Matthew Boylan.
© 2013 John Wiley & Sons, Ltd. Published 2013 by John Wiley & Sons, Ltd.

Table 32.1 Characteristics of primary and secondary retrievals

		Primary	Secondary
Pre-tasking clinical information		Limited May be from member of public	Detailed Received from referring clinician
Response coordination		Rapid Scene response reliant on integrated emergency medical system, e.g. 000/999	Graded response Generally more complex and time consuming. Multiple clinician involvement and critical care bed finding
Patient priority		Immediate Response	Graded, triaged response Dependant on patient condition and service capability of referring facility
Patient severity		Criticality Inferred	Variable Dependency Ability to tailor clinical crewing
Platform crewing		Paramedic ± physician	Paramedic/nurse ± physician
Platform		Dependant on scene characteristics and distance	Dependant on distance and platform availability
Equipment	Scene	Fluid and unpredictable Multiagency management presence of media and bystanders	Controlled Multidisciplinary Management Interface with unfamiliar clinical staff
	Lighting	Variable	Controlled
	Temperature	Variable (hot/cold)	Controlled
	Humidity	Variable	Controlled
	Power	Dependant on scene response	Mains source
	Suction/oxygen	Portable and finite	Fixed and reliable
Personal protective equipment		Highly specific for scene response	In general; normal standard precautions
Clinical equipment		Familiar Limited to that carried in standardized retrieval packs	May be unfamiliar Access to enhanced capabilities and resources; e.g. pathology, radiology
Clinical support		Limited to responding clinical crew mix	Enhanced access dependant on service capability of referring facility
Clinical interventions		Life/limb saving	Potential for advanced critical care procedures and interventions
On scene time		Rapid turnaround Minimal patient packaging	Time may be less crucial More scope for enhanced packaging

Modes of retrieval

Patient retrieval and transport may occur using any transport means available but usually involves road, air (rotary or fixed wing) and marine platforms (Figures 32.2, 32.3 and 32.4). Each has advantages and disadvantages which need to be understood by retrieval services,

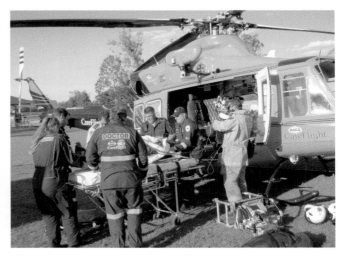

Figure 32.3 Rotary wing task.

tasking agencies and referral and receiving centres. These issues are summarized in Table 32.2 and can be classified as system (cost, availability), logistics (site access, space, range) and patient care (patient access, effects of transport).

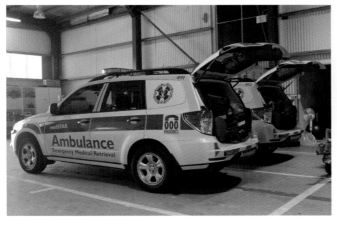

Figure 32.2 Road ambulance support vehicle.

Table 32.2 Comparison of transport platforms

	Road	Rotary wing	Fixed wing
Distance	Best <100 km	Best 100–350 km	Best >350 km
Access	Allows 'point to point' transfer thus minimizes double handling of patient	Allows 'point to point' transfer thus minimizes double handling of patient	Needs secondary road transfer
Special access	Limited to road Can be supplemented by off road vehicles	May be the only option for some geographic or rescue situations	Needs landing strip
Speed	60–120 km/hour depending on roads/traffic	240–300 km/hour	500 km/hour propeller 750 km/hour jet
Equipment	Usually well equipped – stretcher/oxygen/suction	Often well equipped for patient transport if dedicated platform	Dedicated aeromedical aircraft are very well equipped
Capacity	Usually one or two patients	Usually one or two patients	Usually one or two patients but larger aircraft available
Response times	Usually rapid Able to stop or divert if patient deteriorates	Can be rapid depending on system Limited diversion and ability set down	Often slower Very limited diversion
Limitations	Limited by road conditions and traffic Less limited by weather	Limited by weather	Limited by weather (less than rotary wing)
Transport effects	Motion effects (including acceleration and deceleration)	Noise/vibration effects particularly problematic	Effects of altitude–allayed by ability to pressurize cabin
Altitude	Sea level	0–10 000 feet (non pressurized)	0–35000 feet (pressurized)
Cost	Low cost	Very high cost	High cost
Availability	Widespread	Less common	Less common

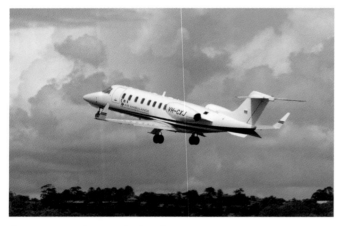

Figure 32.4 Fixed wing task take off.

Tasking and coordination

Tasking and coordination of patient retrieval is summarized by the adage 'getting the right patient to the right place in the right time using the right platform and with the right level of care'. Increasingly in health care we need to add 'at the right cost'.

Clinical coordination serves to align the response (urgency, platform and crew) to a specific clinical task. Under-triage may result in delayed transport with possible adverse patient outcomes. Over-triage may increase resource utilization with associated costs, exposure of transport risks for crew and patients and risk that services are not available for others in need.

Tasking is a risk–benefit analysis, balancing potential patient benefit with safety and optimal resource utilization. Decision-making processes should consider issues such as logistics (distance, platform range, remoteness, availability, access), patient needs (diagnosis, urgency, specific needs), crew skill mix and safety issues (hours worked, weather and night flight). Efforts should be made to reconcile all factors in the tasking decision.

Computer-assisted dispatch systems offer consistency and data integrity while clinician-based systems offer clinical acumen and local knowledge. Both systems are used with the best approach probably a combination of the two.

While the outcomes of tasking decisions may be different for an injured swimmer and a sick child on a remote property (Figures 32.5 and 32.6) the process used should be the same. While safety and patient outcomes are the primary considerations these are not mutually exclusive. A process of formal recognition of risk factors aids decision making. One example of a coordination risk matrix is displayed in Table 32.3.

Effects of transport

Patient transport is not without risk even in perfect weather. The transport environment has its own unique characteristics that influence patient care and the ability of staff to provide this.

The range of transport effects are detailed in Table 32.4. Some are common to both road and airframes such as noise, vibration, lighting, temperature and effects of acceleration/deceleration. These affect both patient care and crew wellbeing. Fatigue management is important as anyone who has spent time in the back of a transport frame will be aware. It requires significant awareness, and forward planning to maintain concentration when it is cold and dark, and you are hungry and tired with a full bladder.

Table 32.3 Risk matrix for tasking and coordination

Patient priority score → Aviation risk score ↓	1	2	3	4	5
Critical safety decision (10+)	Mandatory consultation between Senior Medical Coordinator and Senior Pilot	X	X	X	X
Extreme caution (8–9)	✓	Consultation within aeromedical crew required	Consultation within aeromedical crew required	X	X
Caution (5–7)	✓	✓	✓	Consultation within aeromedical crew required	X
Normal operations (0–4)	✓	✓	✓	✓	✓

This matrix combines scoring systems used to assess patient priority and aviation risk in an effort to recognize both safety and patient outcome. (Further details of scoring systems are available on request from Retrieval Services Queensland)

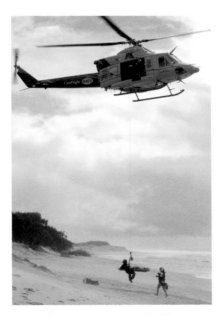

Figure 32.5 Rotary wing winch job – either off cliff/in trees/over water.

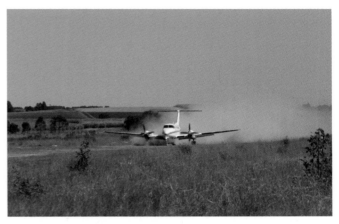

Figure 32.6 Fixed wing task (Royal Flying Doctor Service) in Australian outback.

Air transport involves the effects of altitude as outlined in Table 32.5. A simplified summary is that with increasing altitude it is colder, with less oxygen and gas volumes expand. All of these have implications for patient care.

Preparation for transport and care en route

The ability to provide care is further compromised by space, access to patient and equipment, ability to move secondary to safety restraints and visibility. This mandates a high degree of planning addressing seating/stretcher configurations and access to packs, drugs, monitors and supplemental oxygen. Platform configurations are shown in Figures 32.7, 32.8 and 32.9.

All patients being transported should be reviewed carefully before loading. Table 32.6 outlines the factors to be considered in optimally preparing a patient for transport.

Table 32.4 Effects of transport and clinical implications

Effects of Transport	Clinical Implications
Vestibular dysfunction/spatial disorientation	Fatigue; nausea
Temperature – cold	Coagulopathy; shivering; fatigue
Temperature – heat	Fatigue
Linear accelerations	Haemodynamic instability (especially if hypovolaemic) Positioning of patient
Vibration	Clot disruption; interference BP, ECG; fatigue
Turbulence	Nausea; fatigue; safety
Noise	Communication; alarm systems; fatigue
Confined space	Access to patient and equipment
Often poor ambient lighting	Ability to visualize patient, monitors, equipment and documentation
Psychological effects of transport	Especially flight – anxiety, increased oxygen use, safety

Table 32.5 Flight physiology

Physiology Issue	Clinical Implications
Risk of hypoxia with increasing altitude Total barometric pressure is the sum of partial pressures (Daltons Law) The percentage of oxygen is constant but partial pressure decreases	Borderline gas exchange may be compromised (acute illness/injury or chronic lung conditions) *Always use supplemental oxygen on patients being transported*
Gas volume increases with altitude due to decreasing pressure P1V1 = P2V2 Boyle's	Gas-filled cavities middle ear, sinuses, lungs especially with air trapping disorders, pneumothorax, bowel obstruction, cranium and eye with penetrating injuries Equipment cuffed endotracheal tubes, pneumatic lung splints, vacuum mattress, gravity controlled IV giving sets, MAST suits, Sengstaken tubes *Consider decompression of gas filled cavities or equipment prior to flight*

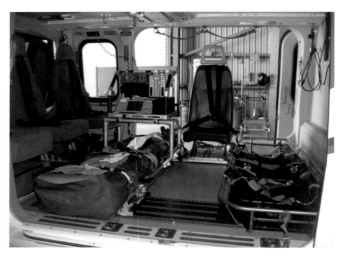

Figure 32.8 Space and configuration inside a rotary wing aircraft.

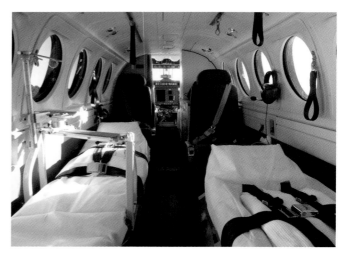

Figure 32.9 Space and configuration inside a fixed wing aircraft.

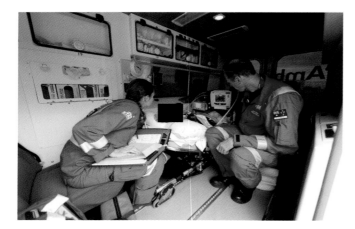

Figure 32.7 Space and configuration inside a road vehicle.

Equipment

Equipment selection should consider transport specific and general issues as well as anticipated care needs and the limitations of the transport environment (Table 32.7). You cannot have everything normally present in a hospital. Equipment should be essential for roles and be light, small, robust and easy to use.

Packs need to be organized and compartmentalized with division into sections such as 'Airway', 'Drugs' or 'Procedures'. A cluttered pack decreases the ability to locate equipment. Fragile items should be secured and protected. Use of padding or elastic loops for ampoules is one approach with plastic ampoules also preferred. Pack lists should be standardized with a daily 'pack check' followed by sign off and bag seal. Team members should not add items to the pack without formal approval otherwise pack weights and volumes progressively increase ('pack creep').

The ability to secure equipment, while maintaining ready access is important. This is addressed by using stretcher bridges (Figure 32.10) which can accommodate ventilators, monitors and pumps. These need to withstand considerable acceleration/deceleration and rotational forces and require endorsement by regulatory bodies before use.

Monitors and ventilators have additional issues. Screens should be visible in both darkness and bright daylight. Viewing angle should be considered in relation to the stretcher configuration. Alarms may not be audible and vibration may affect functions such as blood pressure recording and ECG trace. Planning should also ensure access to power (and power type) to minimize battery drain during longer transports or delays. There needs to be sufficient oxygen for transport tasks and the ability to access and swap systems during transport for longer tasks and replenish afterward. Oxygen cylinders have been associated with aircraft critical incidents and need to be properly secured. The amount of oxygen to have on board, and knowing whether you have enough, often causes debate. The overall amount should be determined by standard

Table 32.6 Preparation of a patient for transport

Decision phase	Considerations
Initial care decisions Determine if transport critical vs treatment critical	What care does the patient need? Where can they get this care? How urgently is the care needed?
Decisions about management Determine what care is/may be needed before and during transport	What care is needed to improve the patients condition? What might change en route due to the patients condition or the effects of transport? What can I do en route? What can't I do en route? What do I need to do before loading? What might I need to be prepared to do during transport?
Preparation for transport Making sure that everything is done so able to provide care en route	Remember oxygen IV access ± fluids Adequate monitoring 'Prophylactic' interventions – do it before you leave! Consider antiemetics Draw up drugs in advance if likely to be needed (or have readily available) Decompression of gas filled cavities and equipment when going to altitude Restraint – patient and equipment Access to important equipment Be conscious of effects of the flight environment on the patient and their injury/illness Communicate with team, referral and tasking agency Don't forget your documentation

Table 32.7 Key considerations in equipment selection

Transport issues	General Issues
Use (essential? non essential?) Does it offer flexibility or redundancy? Ease of use? Size and space? Weight? Battery life and alternative power source? Robustness? (consider drop test) Vibration effects? Noise (including audible alarms)? Ability to be secured?	Cost? Training needed? Compatibility with other equipment? Reliability? Warranty? Service requirements? (frequency, cost, location) Spare/replacement parts and consumables? (cost and availability)

tasking arrangements and transport durations. Retrieval staff should know the size of oxygen cylinders on board (there are varying international classification systems), whether they have 'spares' and how to access these. Table 32.8 illustrates a simple approach to anticipated oxygen use for a task.

Portable ultrasound has recently secured its place as core equipment for retrieval services. The decrease in size of these devices, accompanied by improved picture resolution and utility has contributed to this.

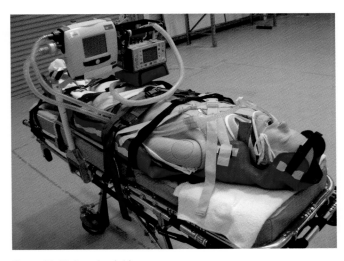

Figure 32.10 Stretcher bridge.

Table 32.8 Simple oxygen calculations using one example of cylinder size

Anticipated oxygen use for a single task:
'Minute volume × transport time (site to site allowing for handover)'
Add 50% for safety buffer (delays/diversion/leaks)

Worked Example	Cylinder type	Capacity (L)
Respiratory rate 10 and tidal volume 600 mL *Transport time 30 minutes* *Minute volume = 10 × 0.6 = 6.0 L* *Minute volume × transport time = 6.0 L × 30 = 180 L* *Add safety buffer = 180 L + 90 L = 270 L* *This would mean one C size oxygen cylinder may be adequate if no delays. A safe approach would mean access to either a second C size cylinder or a larger cylinder*	A B C D E	113 164 255 425 680

An additional point is the impact of body fluids on aircraft. Blood, urine, vomitus and amniotic fluid can damage avionic wiring which may be located underfloor. Cleaning may take an aircraft 'off line' for hours. This can be prevented by avoidance of fluid spills and use of 'spill sheets'.

Specialized additions

A number of specialized additions (equipment or people), may need to be considered. This is often dictated by retrieval service role or specific needs of an individual patient.

Equipment may include blood products, antivenoms and specific drugs (e.g. antidotes). Consideration should be given to ready access of blood products from retrieval bases if blood is used frequently, as well as preparation of 'massive transfusion packs'.

Larger items such as neonatal transport cots (Figure 32.11) or balloon pumps may also need to be considered. This implies preplanning given the weight, size and ability to safely secure these items which some platforms will not be able to accommodate. Patient loading systems, while contributing to improved safety (securing patients and minimization of lifting injury) add weight to transport platforms.

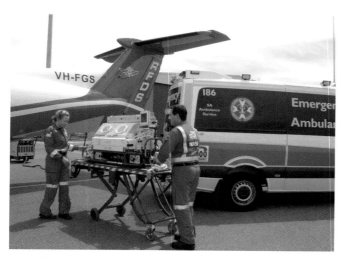

Figure 32.11 Rotary wing loading with stretcher bridge visible on ground.

Additional equipment may not always relate to patient care. Additional fuel may be needed for long-range transports, life rafts for over water missions and a winch for search and rescue operations.

There is often a fixed weight and space available for health personnel on board any transport platform. The addition of any equipment, particularly large items, may mean leaving something behind. This reinforces the need for retrieval and transport services to compartmentalize equipment, minimize weight and space, ensure flexibility and remember they are part of a team.

Personnel added to transport and retrieval services, if not part of the regular service, need additional support to ensure both their safety and ability to provide patient care.

Communication and handover

The most common reason for complaints in health care relate to communication. Patient retrieval and transport is no different. Communication and handover needs to occur at multiple points across a number of organizations. This includes, as a minimum: at the site or referring centre to the retrieval team, during transport to the coordinating agency and then on arrival at the receiving centre. The use of a concise structured handover is recommended to address major problems and avoid omitting information. This

helps minimize the period of inactivity in care that may accompany handover and allows the retrieval team to return to service. For interfacility transfers it is essential that documentation is brought by the retrieval team.

Key points

- Retrieval is about the balance between 'risk versus gain'.
- Remember that safety of the retrieval team is paramount.
- Always check your gear at the start of a shift.
- Think about what might go wrong during transport and act to prevent it or prepare for it.
- Use a structured handover process and practice it.

Tips from the field

- Try to keep families together during transport if possible (or at least to the same destination). Failure to do this leads to increased angst for all parties and consent issues for those caring for an unaccompanied child
- Don't leave home without money and identification. You may not come back by the same transport means, or if adverse weather may be stranded overnight
- You have pockets – use them for essential items and think about basic survival gear
- Be able to find items in your pack blindfolded (literally)
- For retrievals from remote centres the quality of food offered to the team is usually inversely proportional to the quality of care able to be provided (Ballard's rule).

Further reading

Baker SP, Grabowski JG, Dodd RS, *et al*. EMS helicopter crashes: what influences fatal outcome? *Ann Emerg Med* 2006;**47**:351–356.

Ellis D, Hooper M. *Cases in Pre-Hospital and Retrieval Medicine*, 1st edition. Chatswood, Australia: Churchill Livingstone, 2010, ISBN 978-0-7295-3848-8. Churchill Livingstone, Elsevier. Australia.

Shirley PJ, Hearns S. Retrieval medicine: a review and guide for UK practitioners. Part 1: clinical guidelines and evidence base. *Emerg Med J* 2006; **23**: 937–942.

Thomas SH. Controversies in prehospital care: air medical response. *Emerg Med Pract* 2005;**7**:1–26.

CHAPTER 33

Emergency Preparedness: Major Incident Management

Damian Keene[1], Tim Nutbeam[2], and Claire Scanlon[3]

[1]University Hospitals Birmingham, Birmingham, UK
[2]Derriford Hospital, Plymouth Hospitals NHS Trust, Plymouth, UK
[3]City Hospital Birmingham, Birmingham, UK

OVERVIEW

By the end of this chapter you should know:

- The initial principles of mass casualty management
- The principles and application of triage
- Key roles at the scene of a mass casualty incident.

Introduction

This chapter covers the responsibilities of the first clinician on scene and the responsibilities of other medical personnel attending a major incident. The strategic management of an incident is beyond the scope of this text.

Definitions

The terminology describing incidents where a large number of people are injured varies across the globe. The terms 'major incident' and 'mass casualty incident' have been used interchangeably, though mass casualty incident (MCI) is the preferred international standard. However, this term is also used to describe an uncompensated major incident.

There is no internationally accepted definition of what constitutes a MCI, the overall theme remains the same; it is a situation where the local health resources are initially unable to cope with the number, severity or type of live casualties or where the location requires extraordinary resources.

For example; a car accident involving four participants with severe injuries may overwhelm local resources in an undeveloped area, whereas in a large city this casualty load would be unlikely to strain local resources. However, if the casualties were all children or had severe burns this may overwhelm larger/non-specialist hospitals because of the need for specialist intervention.

Some countries such as the UK have specified the number of predicted casualties as the differentiating factor with a major incident being tens and a MCI involving hundreds.

ABC of Prehospital Emergency Medicine, First Edition.
Edited by Tim Nutbeam and Matthew Boylan.
© 2013 John Wiley & Sons, Ltd. Published 2013 by John Wiley & Sons, Ltd.

Table 33.1 Examples of mass casualty incidents

Type	Location	Deaths	Injured
Tsunami	Japan	15534	5364
Attack on World Trade Centre	United States	2993	8700
Night club bomb	Bali	202	300
Train bombings	Madrid	191	1900
Theatre siege	Moscow	168	unclear
Multiple bombings	London	52	650
Shooting	Norway	77	153
Sarin gas	Japan	13	1100

Overall the aim of MCI response should be to maximize the positive casualty outcomes in an overwhelmed medical system (to do the most for the most). Ultimately this will lead to some less injured patients receiving care preferentially.

Mass casualty incidents can be natural or man-made. The casualties may be trauma victims but incidents requiring mass medical treatment need to be considered such as the Tokyo Underground Sarin attack (Table 33.1).

Identifying a MCI

It is likely the first responder to a MCI will not have encountered or declared one before. There is a reluctance to inappropriately 'call' an MCI as it leads to a large resource commitment. If unsure, those on scene should seek immediate senior advice through their chain of command. As the key to maximizing success is the effective and timely delivery of extra resources it is extremely important to recognize and communicate a likely MCI as soon as possible.

A structured approach

The basic principles for dealing with a major incident or an MCI are the same.

Either, by definition is going to present the initial responders with an overwhelming situation. In order to maximize the effectiveness of the medical response it is important to have a framework upon which to start initial casualty management. An example of this can be seen in Table 33.2.

CSCATT can be applied at all stages, whether it is the first responder or the most senior medical practitioner to arrive on scene.

Table 33.2 CSCATT

C	Command and control
S	Safety
C	Communication
A	Assessment
T	Triage
T	Treatment

First on scene

On arrival the first vehicle should be parked conspicuously with the lights on, at a safe location, as close to the scene as possible. In the UK the only vehicle with its emergency lights on should be that of the scene commander; this makes it easily identifiable for arriving personnel. PPE should be worn as available, as with any prehospital scenario.

The first priority is to take command of the scene. In this instance, where no other personnel are present this may just involve clearing the scene of ambulant survivors to prevent further casualties. It is best not to enter the scene itself unless relieved by a more senior clinician and instructed to do so.

Survivors are best served by an informed and coordinated response rather than by the immediate treatment of one or two.

A fast initial scene assessment is required to allow further emergency personnel to be tasked. This may be limited to information on type of incident and suspected number of casualties. This information needs to be communicated in a clear and logical manner. Poor communication is the most common failing at an MCI. It is recommended to use the NATO phonetic alphabet alongside tools such as METHANE or CHALETS (Table 33.3). This communication tool can be used repeatedly to update information previously provided.

A method of communication needs to be established (e.g. mobile phone, radio channel or runners) and call signs designated. Familiarity with radio communications is desirable and messages should be kept as short as possible. If using a radio it is likely responders will be asked to switch to a second reserved MCI frequency/channel so familiarity with equipment is essential.

Scene safety needs to be assessed, this should consider firstly the responders own safety, that of the response team and survivors.

Table 33.3 METHANE and CHALETS mnemonics

M	My name/call sign/reference. Major incident standby or declared
E	Exact location – grid reference if possible
T	Type of incident – chemical, transport, radiation
H	Hazards
A	Access/egress
N	Number of casualties and severity
E	Emergency services on scene or required
C	Casualties- number, type, severity
H	Hazards present
A	Access routes that are safe to use.
L	Location
E	Emergency services present and required
T	Type of incident, e.g. explosion and fire in a tall building, release of gas in the underground system
S	Safety

Table 33.4 Incident types and safety considerations

Incident type	Considerations
Road Traffic	Controlling Traffic, Stopping running engines, Contents of vehicles/Tankers, Airbags, HAZCHEM label
Train Derailment	Unstable carriages, Stopping other trains, Live overhead or third rail
Flood	Submerged debris, unsafe buildings/bridges, flow and current of water
Chemical	Wind Direction, Type of Chemical, Required safe distance, specialist protective equipment
Explosion	Secondary devices, 'Dirty' bombs, safety of surrounding structures, Fires

Each scene will provide unique safety concerns dependant on the initiating event and structures or vehicles present at the time (Table 33.4) (refer to Chapter 4).

Depending on the type or location of the incident, further assistance maybe required before proceeding any further, for instance the fire service for a building collapse.

A log of action timings should be started and an inner cordon should be established. Those wishing to enter the inner cordon should have the permission of the scene commander. This is to stop injury to other personnel on the scene and to allow control of activity within the inner cordon. Once the other emergency services arrive the responsibility of maintaining the inner cordon may fall to them (in the UK this will be the fire service).

As more personnel arrive it will be the duty of the first clinical responder to act as the medical/ambulance commander, they will be responsible for briefing and tasking personnel (until relieved by more senior personnel). All information to ambulance control should ideally be relayed through the designated medical/ambulance commander to limit confusion.

Once the area is deemed safe triage must commence. Prehospital personnel should be directed into the inner cordon to triage all casualties. This information should then be collated and relayed to the ambulance service to guide the further allocation of prehospital assets.

It is important to remember that excessive medical intervention should be avoided at this stage, but life saving intervention should occur. Allowable interventions (though situation specific) would include: insertion of a Guedel airway, placing a casualty in the recovery position or applying a CAT tourniquet.

In these situations, if treatment is not delivered, by the time scene triage is complete they may well have died from their injuries. This was highlighted by the coroner as a specific failure on review of the London bombings in 2005.

Access/egress

The emergency services will need to get to and from the site. Ideally there should be a one-way system of traffic flow with a designated holding area for vehicles to park and a second area for loading of casualties. One of the most pressing matters will be to advise of the best approach to the scene. The best route may soon become obstructed if there is only single lane access. Where helicopter evacuation is likely overhead obstructions should be considered.

Attending after MCI declared

If not first on scene:

- listen to any briefing prior to arrival
- ensure appropriate personal protective equipment is donned
- consider the unique hazards of each incident.

'Control' is a fluid situation with responsibility passing to senior personnel as they arrive at scene. At handover consider the possible loss of vital information; a robust handover is key. The most senior medical practitioner will normally assume the role of overall scene medical command. Additional roles include medical command of the inner cordon or control of the casualty clearing station (CCS).

The CCS is a safe area, outside of the inner cordon to hold, triage and in some cases treat casualties awaiting evacuation (Figure 33.1). The responsibility of the CCS officer is to ensure adequate flow of casualties through the CCS. Casualties should be evacuated in order of triage category, within each category the order of evacuation is decided by the senior clinician present based on the relative urgency of further interventions required that are not possible at scene.

It is important to monitor use of equipment within the CCS to ensure timely and adequate resupply. It may be necessary to restrict use of oxygen in particular, as this is likely to be in limited supply.

Type of incident

Chemicals that may have caused an incident or have been released by an incident may dictate that decontamination is required. This may require specialist HazMat (Hazardous materials) teams. Clues of actual or potential chemical release may come from objects on or around the scene, toxidromes of casualties or most likely vehicle labelling.

Triage

Casualty distribution at MCIs is typically described according to triage categories. The term comes from the French verb *trier*, meaning to separate, sift or select. Triage in this context is a method of allocation of limited medical and transport resources.

Application of a triage system requires a quick, reproducible method of assessing a casualty to determine the most appropriate level of care and medical intervention. There are many triage systems in use across the world: they all share the common application of utilitarian ethics. To this end the application of the triage process is designed to do more good than harm while accepting that some individuals, who would normally have been salvageable if resources were infinite, will not survive.

Triage is a way to take out subjective opinions on the severity and importance of a particularly injury and instead replace it with a means of assessing the physiological effects on the individual of the injuries. This is why it is important that triage is repeated, as the natural course of injuries is not static. A casualty for example who is walking initially may eventually collapse once blood loss from internal injuries leads to a significant degree of shock.

Triage is a dynamic process as casualty needs and medical resources are likely to be fluid.

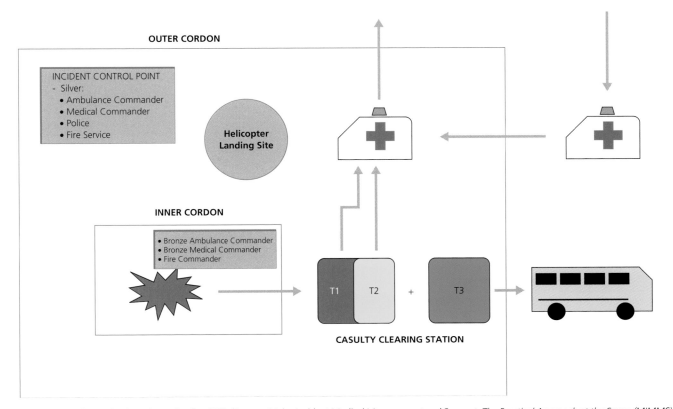

Figure 33.1 Typical organization schematic of an MCI. (Source: *Major Incident Medical Management and Support: The Practical Approach at the Scene (MIMMS)*, 3rd Edition. BMJ Books. John Wiley & Sons).

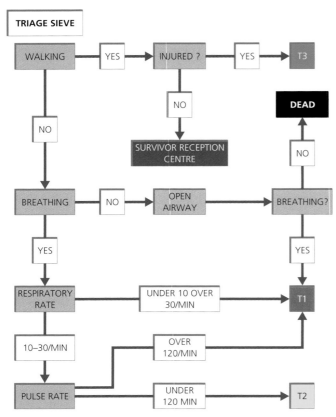

Figure 33.2 Triage sieve. (Source: *Major Incident Medical Management and Support: The Practical Approach at the Scene (MIMMS)*, 3rd Edition. BMJ Books. John Wiley & Sons).

Table 33.5 Categories

US Military	UK Military	Civilian	
Descriptive	**Treatment**	**Descriptive (START)**	**Colour Code**
Immediate	T1	Immediate	Red
Delayed	T2	Delayed	Yellow
Minimal	T3	Minor	Green
Expectant	T4	Expectant	Blue
Dead	Dead	Deceased	Black

gives the outcome. The system should not be deviated from, as the principle of triage is to apply the same rule to all.

Casualties are allocated into one of four or five categories, each given a descriptive/colour code. Despite the different physical labels the attributes of each category are similar across the systems (Table 33.5). It should be noted that even countries whose primary language is not English still attach the same colour code to each of their categories.

The one exception to this is the category of T4 or expectant; this is not universal to all systems. It is not always associated with blue colour code or specific card, some systems identify T4 casualties by the folding over of a corner of a red label.

Categories

As the colour coding of T1–T3 and dead is universal we will look at it in these terms, each one is best thought of as urgency of treatment and evacuation needed.

Red

These are casualties who require immediate medical treatment and evacuation, within minutes to the first hour, who will not survive if not treated soon. For example those with airway obstruction or catastrophic haemorrhage.

The assessment process varies between triage systems, as do the exact definitions of the individual categories. However, many common features exist across the most widely triage systems.

As you can see from Figures 33.2 and 33.3, both are from different systems but both follow a set sequence laid out as a flow chart that

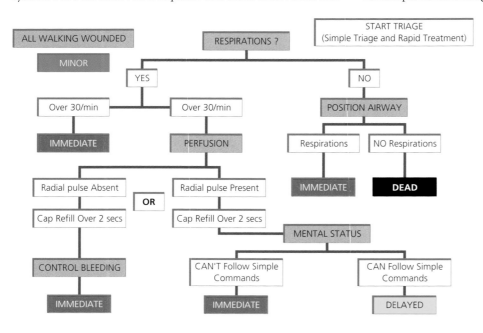

Figure 33.3 START triage. (Source: *Major Incident Medical Management and Support: The Practical Approach at the Scene (MIMMS)*, 3rd Edition. BMJ Books. John Wiley & Sons).

Yellow

These are patients who are likely to deteriorate without further treatment in the first few hours. Long delays in treatment may result in death or serious morbidity. Although these patients can wait they will still eventually require treatment and transfer to hospital. In a majority of triage sieves these patients are non-ambulant.

Green

This group is often described as 'walking wounded' as in the majority of triage sieves they are ambulant; they do not usually require stabilization or monitoring. Their outcome is unlikely to be affected by delayed treatment.

Black

Casualties who fail to breathe despite an open airway are categorized as dead. There is no role for cardiopulmonary resuscitation in the MCI scenario. Death will need to be formally certified at a later stage.

Expectant or T4

Only used when the number/severity of casualties is so great that allocating resources to an individual who is unlikely to survive would compromise the care of other casualties who have a chance of survival. It is instigated at the discretion of the senior medical commander.

Special Circumstances

There are variances on this system for CBRN (Chemical Biological Radiological and Nuclear) incidents and paediatric cases. These systems still follow the same ordered principle and result in casualties being allocated into the categories previously described. The differences in structure allow for the different normal physiological ranges in children, and the timely identification of exposed individuals in a CBRN incident who require decontamination and specific treatment (Figures 33.4 and 33.5).

Triage Sort

Once more personnel are available it may be possible to use secondary triage systems such as the Triage sort, which in the UK would occur within the CCS. This is based on the Triage-Revised Trauma Score (TRTS). It considers Glasgow Coma Score (GCS), Respiratory Rate (RR) and systolic blood pressure. It also allows for upgrading of the triage category at the discretion of a senior clinician dependant on the injury/diagnosis.

Treatment

Actual treatments and techniques are far beyond the scope of this chapter. The most important factor to consider here is where treatment should be delivered (Casualty clearing station CCS).

It is not safe practice to deliver anything other than immediate life saving treatment in close proximity to the scene. A safe area to allow treatment, further triage and transport of casualties needs to be identified.

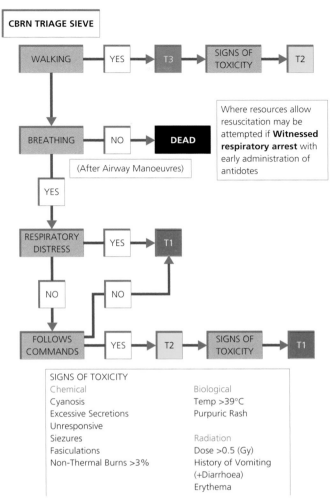

Figure 33.4 CBRN triage sieve British military. (Source: https://www.gov.uk/government/publications/jsp-999-clinical-guidelines-for-operations).

The ideal area would be on hard standing with overhead cover. It should be safe and free from any further hazards but also close enough to allow easy transfer of casualties on stretchers. There should be vehicle access to avoid repeat movement of casualties. Ideally different areas should be allocated to casualties' dependant on triage category to allow allocation of resources more easily. Initially treatment should be directed at the T1/T2 casualties. It may be that with the arrival of further personnel you become responsible for running the casualty clearing station.

Transport

Not only do casualties need to be triaged for initial treatment they also need to be triaged for transfer. This is where the triage sort can become more useful. A casualty who was initially T1 with a tension pneumothorax that has been treated with initial decompression will require less urgent hospital intervention than a shocked casualty with internal bleeding. This will be down to the discretion of the senior clinician within the CCS. Thought should also be given to which receiving hospitals are most appropriate for the casualty, e.g. transport to a burns or neurosurgical unit.

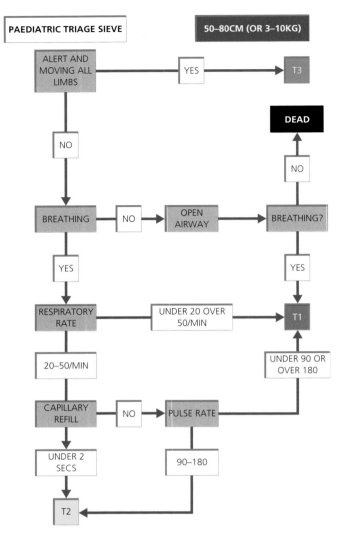

Figure 33.5 Paediatric triage sieve. (Source: Hodgetts T & Porter C, *Major Incident Management System,* 2002. John Wiley & Sons Ltd.)

Certifying death

Death can only be certified by the pathologist performing a post mortem after the event. Death can be pronounced at the scene by a doctor, but in the UK, must be in the presence of a police officer. Death can be diagnosed following triage with the application of the dead label.

Summary

Major incidents are, by their very nature, complex and evolving situations. Dependant on when you arrive your role can be very variable; if you arrive first it is important to try to remain as detached as possible from casualty treatment and not forget the basics of any prehospital scene; remain safe at all times. Decisions may be very hard but by remaining within the initial confines of triage this should minimize difficult choices and maximize the successful outcomes.

> **Tips from the field**
>
> - Keep safe – your personal safety must be your number one priority, heroes are potential additional casualties!
> - Ensure you are adequately fed and watered. Ensure regular rest breaks
> - Do what your told: the command and control structure relies on people doing the task allocated to them
> - Communicate well (but don't over communicate). This fine balance is difficult to achieve but can make all the difference at an MCI
> - Triage is Dynamic: if a patients condition changes or the resources available change re-triage the patient
> - If doing initial scene assessment be the 'triage butterfly', maximum of 30 seconds per patient
> - When triaging – minimal life saving interventions. Limited to: Airway opening / positioning/simple adjunct. Decompress tension pneumothorax. CAT (or equivalent tourniquet). Bystander haemorrhage control.

Further reading

Champion HR, Sacco WJ, Copes WS, Gann D, Gennarelli T, Flanagan ME. A revision of the trauma score. *J Trauma* 1989; **29**: 623–629.

Coroner's Inquests into the London Bombings of 7 July 2005 Government response to the Report under Rule 43 of the Coroner's Rules 1984.

Department of Health. Mass Casualties Incidents – A Framework for Planning. Published Mar 2007,

Hodgetts T, Mackway-Jones K. *Major Incident Medical Management and Support: the practical approach.* London: BMJ Publishing, 1995, BMJ Publishing.

Hodgetts T, Porter C. *Major Incident Management System The scene aide memoire for Major Incident Medical Management and Support.* London 2004: BMJ Publishing, 2004.

Hodgetts T. Triage: a position Statement. T Hodgetts. May 2001.

http://www.nrk.no/nyheter/norge/1.7734595 Accessed (accessed Nov 25 February 20102013).

http://www.wpro.who.int/sites/eha/disasters/2011/jpn_earthquake/ (accessed November 2010).

Joint Defence Publications 4-03.1 Clinical Guidelines for Operations. https://www.gov.uk/government/publications/jdp-4-03-1-clinical-guidelines-for-operations (accessed 25 February 2013).

Phillips SJ, Knebel A, Johnson K, (eds.) *Mass Medical Care With Scarce Resources: The Essentials. AHRQ Publication No. 09–0016.* Rockville, MD: Agency for Healthcare Research and Quality: 2009.

CHAPTER 34

Emergency Preparedness: Chemical, Biological, Radiation and Nuclear Incidents

Christopher A. Kahn[1], Kristi L. Koenig[2], and Matthew Boylan[3]

[1]University of California, San Diego, CA, USA
[2]University of California at Irvine, Orange, CA, USA
[3]Royal Centre for Defence Medicine, University Hospitals Birmingham, Birmingham, UK

OVERVIEW

By the end of this chapter you should:

• Understand how to recognize a CBRN incident
• Understand the basic principles of managing a CBRN incident
• Understand the importance of rescuer protection
• Understand the importance of decontamination
• Understand how to identify and manage CBRN casualties.

Introduction

Chemical, biological, radiologic and nuclear (CBRN) events present unique challenges that complicate the management of prehospital casualties. These can be successfully managed with careful planning, training in use of protective gear and decontamination techniques, and exquisite attention to provider and facility safety. Good communication between all response entities will facilitate safe and effective management.

This chapter will assist prehospital personnel in the basic management of a CBRN incident.

Scene management

CBRN scenes should be managed using an incident command system (ICS). ICS provides a universally understood framework which delineates authority, responsibility and expectations of each responder. Personnel who may be responding to CBRN or other disaster scenes should have training in ICS or the local equivalent.

Assessment and safety

As with all incidents involving hazardous materials, a rapid but thorough assessment of the scene to ensure that it is safe to approach the victims is necessary. Failure to ensure scene safety prior to initiating rescue and medical aid can cause prehospital personnel to become additional victims.

ABC of Prehospital Emergency Medicine, First Edition.
Edited by Tim Nutbeam and Matthew Boylan.
© 2013 John Wiley & Sons, Ltd. Published 2013 by John Wiley & Sons, Ltd.

In addition to standard scene safety assessment techniques, CBRN responders should be aware of the following:

• Not all CBRN agents can be easily seen, smelled or otherwise sensed.
• In some scenarios (such as an aerosolized release of a biological agent), there may not be a discrete scene that can be readily identified by prehospital personnel.
• In terrorist incidents, a small primary release or explosion may be followed by a larger, secondary one designed to harm rescuers (the so-called 'secondary device').

It is often not immediately obvious that a CBRN event has occurred. While concern may be raised due to specific threats or observation of suspicious powders, many CBRN events will only be properly identified through toxidrome recognition after treatment of initial casualties has begun or through assessment by a CBRN team. The 'Safety Triggers for Emergency Personnel (STEP) 1-2-3' approach is a useful method to use when approaching an incident of unclear etiology (Figure 34.1).

Scene organization

Although terminology may vary, most systems organize the CBRN scene into zones (Figure 34.2). The area containing the toxic hazard is known as the hot zone. The warm zone is where casualties

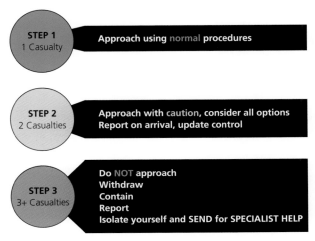

Figure 34.1 The STEP 1–2–3 approach.

CBRN Incident Layout

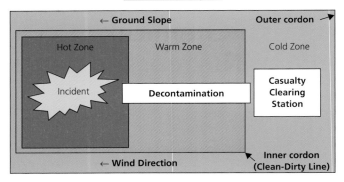

Figure 34.2 Chemical, biological, radiation and nuclear (CBRN) incident layout.

undergo decontamination and the cold zone is where casualties undergo conventional medical assessment, treatment and onward evacuation. The warm zone and cold zone are separated from each other by the 'clean–dirty line'.

There have been recent moves in some countries to push life-saving clinical interventions (e.g. tourniquet application, airway positioning), therapies (e.g. nerve agent antidotes) and clinical judgement (e.g. CBRN triage) forward into the hot zone using specially trained CBRN medical teams.

Provider protection

Several types of protective clothing exist, offering various levels of protection. In general, rescuers working within the hot zone will be hazmat specialists with dedicated training and experience using extended duration breathing apparatus and gas tight suits (Figure 34.3). Those rescuers working within the warm zone to provide emergency medical care and decontamination will require chemical-resistant suits with respiratory protection to protect against chemical splash and off-gassing (Figure 34.4). Rescuers in the cold zone should not need this level of equipment but should use standard precautions universal precautions (including gloves, gown, mask and eye shielding).

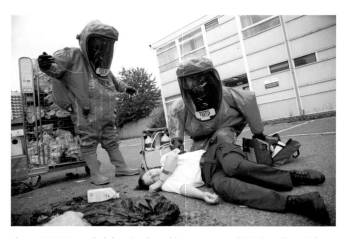

Figure 34.3 Extended duration breathing apparatus (EDBA) and gas tight suits. (Courtesy of www.justinedesmondphotography.co.uk).

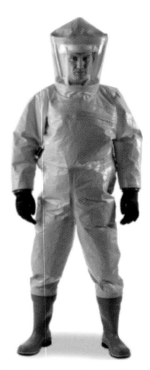

Figure 34.4 Powered respirator protective suit. (Courtesy of Respirex International Ltd).

Some countries issue electronic personal dosimeters to prehospital medical responders. These devices alarm when the wearer is exposed to dangerous levels of ionising radiation and also measure cumulative radiation exposure.

Patient decontamination

All patients suspected of being exposed to a CBRN agent should undergo decontamination unless agent identification has occurred and decontamination is deemed unnecessary (e.g. asymptomatic after cyanide gas exposure).

Clothing removal is the first and most important phase of decontamination as the clothes hold 90% of the contaminant load (liquid chemical or radioactive material). Removed clothing should be placed in a sealed container marked with the patient's name for evidence collection and possible repatriation.

Once clothes are removed any remaining surface contaminants are removed using the RINSE–WIPE–RINSE method of decontamination (Figure 34.5). For ambulatory patients this will usually be

RINSE – WIPE – RINSE Decontamination technique	
Step 1 RINSE	**Gently wash affected areas with soapy water (0.9% saline for open wounds and eyes)** this dilutes the contaminant and removes particles and water based chemicals
Step 2 WIPE	**Wipe affected areas gently but thoroughly with sponge or soft brush or washcloth:** this removes organic chemicals and petrochemicals
Step 3 RINSE	**Gently rinse affected areas**

Figure 34.5 Decontamination – 'Rinse–Wipe–Rinse'.

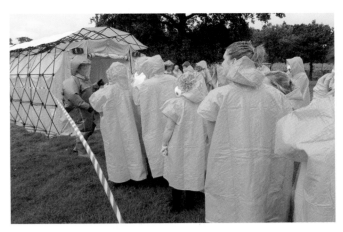

Figure 34.6 Mass decontamination (Courtesy Mr David Broomfield of Hampshire Fire and Rescue Service).

undertaken in a formal decontamination shower tent (Figure 34.6), except when numbers are large when improvised mass decontamination may be employed using standard fire service equipment. Non-ambulatory casualties should be decontaminated by decontamination teams in formal decontamination tents. Roller systems may be employed to improve casualty flow though such a system. Water from decontamination procedures should be collected, but may be directed to storm drains if no other option is available. Rescuers that have been operating within the warm or hot zones will also require decontamination (Figure 34.7).

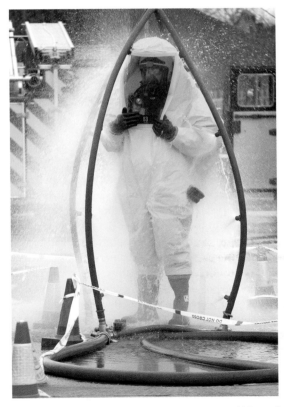

Figure 34.7 Decontamination of rescuers (Courtesy Mr David Broomfield of Hampshire Fire and Rescue Service).

Chemical casualties

Chemical casualties generally present shortly after exposure, making it easier to determine that a release has occurred. Latency of symptoms ranges from seconds to about a day. Agent detection equipment may assist in early identification of some chemical agents. Chemical agents fall into four major classes: nerve agents, cyanides, vesicants and pulmonary agents.

Nerve agents (e.g. Sarin, VX) inhibit the enzyme acetylcholinesterase, which breaks down the neurotransmitter acetylcholine leading to overstimulation of the parasympathetic nervous system and progressive motor paralysis. Mild exposure leads to eye irritation, pain and miosis. Moderate exposure is characterized by parasympathetic cholinergic symptoms : salivation, lacrimation, urination, defecation, gastrointestinal distress and emesis (SLUDGE). Bronchospasm and sweating are also seen at this stage. Severe exposure is characterized by progressive paralysis of the respiratory muscles, seizures and death. Treatment is with atropine, and oxime (e.g. pralidoxime/obidoxime) antidote kits along with supportive care for seizures (e.g. diazepam) and respiratory failure (e.g. ventilation). Atropine and pralidoxime are available in autoinjectors that can be deployed forward in the hot or warm zone if required (Figure 34.8). After decontamination atropine should be titrated to relief of symptoms (e.g. drying of secretions), not to heart rate or amount of pupillary dilation. Large amounts may be required.

Cyanides are chemical asphyxiants that inhibit mitochondrial enzymes within cells and prevent normal aerobic respiration. Severe exposure can cause death within minutes, with victims experiencing dyspnoea, hypotension and syncope, followed by cardiorespiratory arrest. These patients are likely to die before the prehospital responders arrive. Moderate exposure may lead to confusion and hyperventilation. These patients have a significant metabolic acidosis due to excessive anaerobic cellular respiration. Patients with milder exposures present with nausea, dizziness and agitation. Cyanide antidote kits (e.g. dicobalt edetate or sodium/amyl nitrite and sodium thiosulphate) must be rapidly administered after

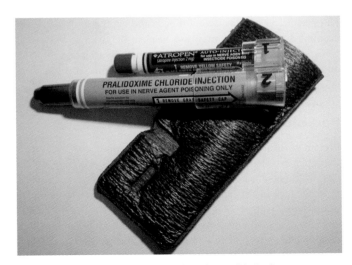

Figure 34.8 Nerve agent autoinjector (atropine/pralidoxime).

decontamination in severe or moderate exposures (long before laboratory verification of the agent will be available) to be effective. Near-patient lactate testing may help identify this patient set. All cyanide casualties should be given high-flow oxygen.

Vesicants such as mustard or Lewisite damage DNA, resulting in cell death within exposed tissue of the skin and airways. Symptoms develop over minutes to hours, with ocular involvement (pain, irritation) being followed by respiratory symptoms (irritation, inhalational burns, acute lung injury) and then by skin blistering. Decontamination and symptomatic burn management are required.

Pulmonary agents such as chlorine and phosgene damage the cell membranes within the respiratory tract and lungs leading to progressive airway irritation, pulmonary oedema and in severe exposures death. Symptoms can present rapidly, although some may be delayed by hours. Mild exposure causes eye irritation alone. Supportive care is appropriate with oxygen and ventilatory support if required.

Biological casualties

Delayed presentation often complicates the presentation of biological casualties, and it can be difficult to initially discriminate between a few sick patients and a group of victims intentionally exposed to a biological agent. Additionally, many biological agents that are considered to be possible components of biowarfare or bioterrorism plots are also endemic to certain areas of the world (e.g. anthrax), further complicating the identification of a biological release. Consequently, a high index of suspicion regarding unusual clusters of disease or presentations of a disease unusual to the area or in the wrong season is key to identifying a biological agent exposure and initiating the investigative process.

Although diseases caused by bioterror agents have a wide range of presentations, courses and treatments, they are similar in that they do not require specific prehospital therapy. Supportive care, along with attention paid to appropriate standard precautions, constitute the mainstay of prehospital management. If a patient is known or strongly suspected to suffer from a contagious illness, the local medical director may consider instituting a destination system that takes resources such as isolation beds and ventilator capacity into account. Consideration may also need to be given to designated transport teams and equipment (e.g. patient isolation unit) in an effort to minimize contamination of non-infected individuals (Figure 34.9).

Radiological and nuclear casualties

Presentation of radiological casualties can occur any time, from immediately after an exposure to weeks later depending on the dose and type of radiation source. Delayed presentations can lead to challenges in establishing the correct diagnosis. These radiation exposed patients may have disorders of several organ systems, including the integumentary (skin), gastrointestinal, nervous, cardiac, and haematopoietic systems. Nuclear casualties, in contrast, are promptly exposed to high levels of radiation, and if they are in the area of the detonation are also exposed to typical explosive/blast

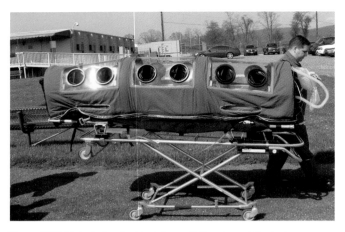

Figure 34.9 Biological patient isolation unit (Courtesy of Gentex).

effects such as pressure waves, thermal exposure, and debris-related injuries including shrapnel.

Once stabilized from potentially life-threatening traumatic injuries, patients exposed to radiation should undergo prompt decontamination to avoid spreading particles of radioactive material; once decontaminated, there is minimal risk to healthcare providers (who should still, as a matter of course, observe standard precautions). Pure radiation exposure without contact with any material does not cause a patient to become radioactively dangerous to others. Patients who have ingested radioactive material may receive decorporation therapy at the hospital, but are not likely to be a significant source of exposure to prehospital personnel. A few specific types of radiation sources, when ingested, are amenable to particular antidotal therapies; however, these are not sufficiently time critical to require field antidote treatment unless the event is of sufficient magnitude to overwhelm local transportation and hospital resources. Radioisotopes that have specific antidotes include ^{131}I and ^{137}Cs.

Dirty bomb

A dirty bomb, or radiological dispersion device (RDD), consists of radioactive material incorporated into a conventional explosive device. When detonated, there is not a nuclear event, but radioactive material is dispersed into the area in addition to the typical sequelae of an explosion. In these events, the victims are at much higher immediate risk from explosion-related trauma than the radiation exposure, and should be treated as trauma patients. When possible, after immediate life-stabilizing treatment, decontamination can then be performed to minimize spread of radiation and risk to healthcare personnel. Additional debridement and decorporation therapy will probably be provided in the hospital setting. As with any radiation exposure, the principle of 'time–distance–shielding' is paramount, i.e. providers should minimize the amount of time of exposure to contaminated patients or radioactive sources, increase the distance between themselves and the source(s) and separate themselves by physical barriers when possible (e.g., lead shields, buildings). Personal dosimeters can help identify and monitor ongoing radiological hazards.

Summary

- CBRN events require special consideration beyond typical pre-hospital responses.
- Providers and facilities may need to delay patient care to assure their own safety
- Standard precautions are the most basic standard for provider protection; specially trained providers working closer to the actual incident sites may require higher-level protection.
- Clothing removal, followed by washing with mild soap and water is the most widely applicable and effective decontamination method.
- Some chemicals have specific antidotes that need to be used rapidly to be effective.

Tips from the field

- If a CBRN event is suspected do not proceed into the scene, remain uphill and upwind and inform control immediately
- As it may be difficult to identify CBRN events, standard precautions are advisable for all multiple casualty responses
- Use basic decontamination measures on all patients with suspected exposures
- Be suspicious of odd presentations of patients, such as clusters of unusual disease, events following a terror warning or witnessed exposure to unknown powders, fumes or liquids followed by onset of symptoms.

Further reading

Cone DC, Koenig KL. Mass casualty triage in the chemical, biological, radiological, or nuclear environment. *Eur J Emerg Med* 2005;**12**:287–302.

Darling RG, Woods JB, Dembek ZF, *et al.* (eds) *USAMRIID's Medical Management of Biological Casualties Handbook*, 5th edn. Fort Detrick, Frederick, MD: U.S. Army Medical Research Institute of Infectious Diseases, 2004.

Emergency Medical Services Authority. *Hospital Incident Command System Guidebook*. Sacramento: California Emergency Medical Services Authority, 2006.

Hurst CG. Decontamination. In: Zajtchuk R, Bellamy RF, Sidell FR, *et al.* (eds) *Medical Aspects of Chemical and Biological Warfare*. Washington, DC: Office of the Surgeon General, Department of the Army, USA, 1997:351–360.

Koenig KL. Strip and shower: the duck and cover for the 21st century. *Ann Emerg Med* 2003;**42**:391–394.

Koenig KL, Schultz CH (eds) *Koenig and Schultz's Disaster Medicine: Comprehensive Principles and Practices*. Cambridge: Cambridge University Press, 2010.

Koenig KL, Boatright CJ, Hancock JA, *et al.* Health care facilities' 'war on terrorism': a deliberate process for recommending personal protective equipment. *Am J Emerg Med* 2007;**25**:185–195.

Koenig KL, Goans RE, Hatchett RJ, *et al.* Medical treatment of radiological casualties: current concepts. *Ann Emerg Med* 2005;**45**:643–652.

Koenig KL, Kahn CA, Schultz CH. Medical strategies to handle mass casualties from the use of biological weapons. *Clin Lab Med* 2006;**26**:313–327, viii.

CHAPTER 35

Emergency Preparedness: Mass Gatherings

Lee Wallis and Wayne Smith

University of Cape Town, Cape Town, South Africa

OVERVIEW

At the end of this section, the reader will:

- Understand that mass gathering have a higher rate of illness and injuries
- Know that planning for mass gathering requires a thorough risk analysis
- Understand that the risk profile is dependent on many different factors
- Appreciate that medical planning for a mass gathering requires an integrated approach with the input of all relevant role players.

Introduction

Mass gatherings, although a common occurrence worldwide, do not have a universally accepted definition. Most of the definitions, as cited in the literature, are based on the number of persons attending the event. Some authors have opted to define it as any event with more than 1000 persons in attendance, while others use the definition of a crowd size exceeding 25 000 attendees. Whichever of the definitions we choose to use, mass gatherings have been shown to have a higher rate of illness and injuries than that of the general population. Wherever a large number of people gather in one defined area, there is an increased risk of a mass casualty incident.

A number of disasters or mass casualty incidents have occurred at mass gatherings throughout the world. Football matches seem to be of particular concern as many documented disasters having occurred over a relatively short period of time (Table 35.1).

Despite these alarming statistics, it is not just football events that carry the risk of developing into a mass casualty incident. Rock concerts, political gatherings and even religious meetings have been shown to lead to an increase in the number of persons that present to medical facilities. The presence of alcohol as well as recreational drugs further complicates matters for event organizers and medical planners of mass gatherings. Medical planning for a mass gathering is not as simple as just deploying medical personnel on the basis of

Table 35.1 Mass casualty Incidents at soccer events over the last 60 years

Year	Country	Cause	Injured	Dead
1946	UK	Stampede	400	33
1964	Peru	Riot	500	300
1967	Turkey	Stampede	600	44
1968	Argentina	Stampede	150	70
1971	Scotland	Crush	140	66
1978	Ghana	Collapse	35	15
1979	Nigeria	Stampede	27	24
1981	Greece	Stampede	54	21
1982	Moscow	Crush	?	340
1982	Algeria	Collapse	600	8
1982	Columbia	Stampede	250	26
1885	UK	Fire	200	56
1985	Mexico	Stampede	27	10
1985	Belgium	Riot	240	39
1988	Nepal	Stampede	100	93
1989	UK	Crush	200	95
1991	South Africa	Crush	50	40
1991	Kenya	Stampede	24	1
1992	Corsica	Collapse	?	15
1992	Brazil	Collapse	50	0
1995	Sierra	Collapse	40	0
1996	Zambia	Stampede	42	15
1996	Guatemala	Crush	147	82
1996	Liberia	Riot	39	8
1996	Nigeria	Crush	?	5
1999	Egypt	Stampede	?	11
2000	Zimbabwe	Crush	100	13
2001	Iran	Collapse	150	2
2001	South Africa	Crush	160	43
2001	Congo	Stampede	50	10
2001	Ghana	Stampede	150	130

the expected number of people that will attend the event. Instead, a thorough risk and vulnerability analysis needs to be undertaken. To achieve this, medical planning needs to be done in conjunction with the event organizer and other relevant safety and security role players. Many risk factors have been described which have a direct impact on the number of persons requiring medical intervention at a mass gathering. Commonly described factors that determine the potential number of patients that may present and the ability to deal with these patients at a mass gathering are listed below:

- nature of the event
- nature of the venue

ABC of Prehospital Emergency Medicine, First Edition.
Edited by Tim Nutbeam and Matthew Boylan.
© 2013 John Wiley & Sons, Ltd. Published 2013 by John Wiley & Sons, Ltd.

- seated or unseated
- spectator profile
- past history of similar events
- expected number of spectators
- event duration
- seasonal considerations
- proximity to hospitals
- profile of hospitals
- additional hazards.

Nature of the event

The nature of the event being hosted has been identified as being just as an important risk factor as the number of spectators when predicting likely medical requirements. For example: a rock concert with the potential of a younger spectator profile and increased potential of alcohol and/or drug abuse is likely to result in more patients than a classical musical concert.

Nature of the venue

Is the event being hosted in a purpose built stadium or does the venue consist of temporary structures which may elevate the risk profile? Indoor events have been shown to produce lower patient numbers than similar events held outdoors where exposure to the elements may have a detrimental effect on the spectators.

Seated or unseated

An event that allows only for a seated audience, as seen in Figure 35.1, is more likely to have a lower risk profile than one that allows for unseated spectators. More often than not, the capacity of the venue will be exceeded when unseated spectators are catered for, and this has its own inherent problems.

Spectator profile

The importance of profiling the potential spectators cannot be over emphasized. An event attracting mainly family groups is unlikely

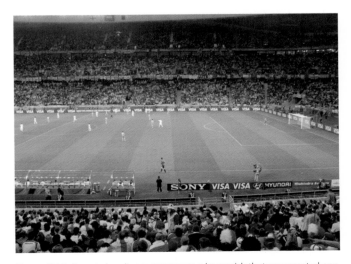

Figure 35.1 A seated audience represents a lower risk that an unseated one.

to be associated with the same risk as one such as a rock concert, with a predominantly younger audience. Although the literature describes events that have an audience younger than 35 years of age as being associated with a greater number of patient presentations, one must not forget that events that attracts predominantly elderly people can likewise result in large patient numbers. This has been documented in many descriptive studies, particularly large religious gathering such as Papal visits.

Past history of similar events

The history of previous events of a similar nature, with particular reference to the type of incidents that occurred and the medical problems that arose, is an important piece of information to be considered when planning the medical coverage for an event. Every mass gathering should add to a database which in turn can aid in evidenced based planning for similar events worldwide. It is thus the responsibility of all medical planners to adequately document such events in terms of the risks as well as the associated patient presentation rates.

Expected number of spectators

The number of spectators may be one of the easier parameters to quantify. Early consultation and planning in conjunction with the event organizers will aid in determining the expected numbers of persons that will be attending. Pre-booked tickets will further confirm the numbers.

Event duration

The duration of the event is an important determinant of the number of medical staff that will be required to provide cover at a mass gathering. Events of an extended duration add a number of additional risks that need to be considered. Medical staff may need to be deployed in a shift system so as to adhere to legislation that covers the maximum hours that a medical staff member can be deployed at any one time. It is also likely that the number of patients presenting for medical attention is likely to increase the longer the event continues. This is especially relevant where alcohol is sold at the venue as well as when the spectators are exposed to environmental elements. The length of time that people are expected to queue to enter a venue should be included in the determining the duration of the event

Seasonal consideration

Weather is noted to be an important but all too often neglected factor that determines patient presentation rates at mass gatherings. This is especially relevant when the event is being hosted in an outdoor venue. Hot and humid conditions are noted to be associated with a higher patient presentation rate. Be aware that medical staff deployed at these events are also potentially exposed and thus the planning should also include suitable shelter from where the medical staff can operate. (Figure 35.2).

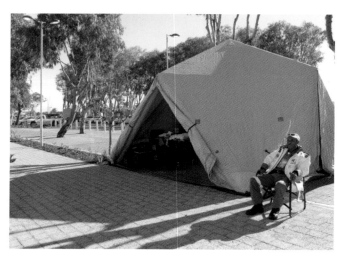

Figure 35.2 Temporary medical post is vital to ensure adequate shelter for staff and patients.

Hospitals

The distance between the event venue and suitable hospitals has a direct impact on the number of medical resources that need to be deployed. A longer distance to hospital relates to longer transport times and thus the longer the period of time that a resource, such as an ambulance, may not be available to the event. It may also necessitate the need to ensure that suitably qualified medical staff are deployed at the event to ensure that patients can be stabilized prior to transportation. If a helicopter emergency medical service is available, then consideration may be given to incorporating it into the medical plan and ensuring that a suitable landing zone is identified and the relevant aviation approvals are obtained to operate out of such a landing zone (Figure 35.3).

On-site medical facilities can be a mitigating factor. Such a facility is often present at stadia, and allows for small uncomplicated medical procedures to be performed without the need to transport the patient to hospital.

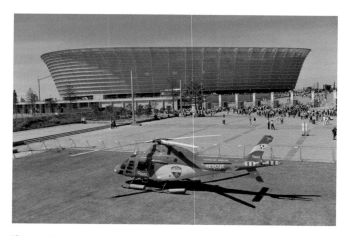

Figure 35.3 A helicopter emergency medical service may be included into medical planning provided all safety and legislative requirements are met.

Staffing models

There are no universally accepted standards to determine the number of medical staff that should be provided at mass gatherings. A guide often quoted is *A Guide to health, safety and welfare at music and similar events*, which was developed by the UK Health Services Executive. This guide provides a way in which to quantify the risk profile of an event based on the factors listed earlier in this chapter (Tables 35.2–35.13).

Table 35.2 Risk score for nature of the event

Nature of event		
	Classical performance	2
	Public exhibition	3
	Pop/rock concert	5
	Dance event (Rave / Disco)	8
	Agricultural/country show	2
	Marine	3
	Motorcycle display	3
	Aviation	3
	Motor sport	4
	State occasions	2
	VIP visits/summit	3
	Music festival	3
	International Event	3
	Bonfire/pyrotechnic display	4
	New Year celebrations	7
	Demonstrations/marches	
	With Low risk of disorder	2
	with Medium risk of disorder	5
	With High risk of disorder	7
	Opposing factions involved	9

Table 35.3 Risk score for venue

Nature of venue		
	Indoor	1
	Stadium	2
	Outdoor in confined location, e.g. park.	2
	Other outdoor, e.g. festival	3
	Widespread public location in streets	4
	Temporary outdoor structures	4
	Includes overnight camping	5

Table 35.4 Risk score – seated and standing

Seated or unseated		
	Seated	1
	Mixed	2
	Standing	3

Table 35.5 Risk score for spectator profile

Spectator profile		
	Full mix, in family groups	2
	Full mix, not in family groups	3
	Predominately young adults	3
	Predominately children and teenagers	4
	Predominately elderly	4
	Full mix, rival factions	5

Table 35.6 Risk score for past history of similar events

Past history	Good data, low casualty rate previously (less than 1%)	−1
	Good data, medium casualty rate previously (1%-2%)	1
	Good data, high casualty rate previously (more than 2%)	2
	First event, no data	3

Table 35.7 Risk score per expected attendance numbers

Expected numbers	<1000	1
	<3000	2
	<5000	8
	<10 000	12
	<20 000	16
	<30 000	20
	<40 000	24
	<60 000	28
	<80 000	34
	<100 000	42
	<200 000	50
	<300 000	58

Table 35.8 Risk score per event duration

Expected event duration (including queuing from gate open time)	Less than 4 hours	1
	More than 4 less than 12 hours	2
	More than 12 hours	3

Table 35.9 Risk score as affected by the seasons

Seasons (outdoor events)	Summer	2
	Autumn	1
	Winter	2
	Spring	1

Table 35.10 Proximity to hospital as a risk determinant

| Proximity to definitive care (nearest suitable A&E facility) | Less than 30 min by road | 0 |
| | More than 30 min by road | 2 |

Table 35.11 Risk score as affected by hospital profile

Profile of hospitals	Choice of A&E departments	1
	Large A&E department	2
	Small A&E department	3

Table 35.12 Risk score for additional hazards

Additional hazards	Carnival	1
	Helicopters	1
	Motor sport	1
	Parachute display	1
	Street theatre	1

To calculate the risk score for an event, the following calculation, referring to the categories described above, is done:

Event risk score = (the sum of the scores of Tables 35.2–35.12) minus the score of Table 35.13

Table 35.13 Risk score for onsite medical facilities

Additional on-site facilities	Suturing	−2
	X-ray	−2
	Minor Surgery	−2
	Plastering	−2
	Psychiatric / GP facilities	−2

Table 35.14 Medical staff resource model

Score	Ambulance	BLS	ILS	ALS	Ambulance crew	Doctor	Nurse	Coordinator
<20	0	2			0	0	0	0
21–25	0	4			0	0	0	0
26–30	1	4	1	0	2	0	0	0
31–35	1	6	1	1	2	0	0	visit
36–40	1	8	1	1	2	0	0	visit
41–45	2	12	1	1	4	1	0	1
46–50	2	16	2	2	4	1	1	1
51–55	3	20	3	3	6	2	1	1
56–60	3	24	3	3	6	2	2	1
61–65	4	32	4	4	8	2	2	1
66–70	5	40	5	5	10	3	3	1
71–75	6	48	6	6	12	3	3	1
76–80	8	64	8	8	16	4	4	1
81–85	10	80	10	10	20	5	5	2
86+	15	120	15	15	30	6	6	2

ALS, advanced life support; BLS, basic life support; ILS, immediate life support.

The resultant risk score obtained is then referenced against the medical resource matrix as defined in Table 35.14, so as to determine the medical resources that should be deployed at the event.

This resource model is a useful guide to determine the medical resources that may be required at an event. The resource has been developed, based on the level of care as well as resource availability of a particular country. It does however serve as a basis for medical resource planning, which could be modified to meet the particular requirements of any an organisation or country.

Of importance, it highlights that a risk assessment must be done when doing the medical planning for a mass gatherings and that early and continuous communication with all role players is critical.

Tips from the field

- Planning is essential. In order to plan effectively you need high quality, pertinent information regarding the events location, demographics and previous history
- In high-risk sporting events remember it is easy to plan for the competitors and forget about the medical needs of the large crowd
- Inform local hospitals and establish relationships with key personnel in the early stages of event planning
- Remember most mass gatherings are only a small step away from a mass casualty incident – be prepared.

Further reading

Arbon P. Mass-gathering medicine: a review of the evidence and future directions for research. *Prehosp Disaster Med* 2007;**22**:131–135.

Arbon P., Bridgewater FH, Smith C. Mass gathering medicine: a predictive model for patient presentation and transport rates. *Prehosp Disaster Med* 2001;**16**:150–158.

Darby P, Johnes, M, Mellor G (eds) *Soccer and Disasters: International Perspectives*. Abingdon: Routledge, 2005.

Health & Safety Executive. *A Guide to Health, Safety and Welfare at Music and Similar Events (HSG)*, 2nd edn. Guidance Booklets, 1999.

Milsten AM, Maguire BJ, Bissell RA, Seaman KG. Mass-gathering medical care: a review of the literature. *Prehosp Disaster Med* 2002;**17**:151–162.

CHAPTER 36

Clinical Governance

Assiah Mahmood[1] and Rod Mackenzie[2]

[1]Magpas Helimedix, St. Ives, UK
[2]Cambridge University Hospitals NHS Foundation Trust, Cambridge, UK

OVERVIEW

By the end of this chapter you should:

- Understand the principles of clinical governance
- Understand the key challenges to provision of a high functioning clinical governance structure within a prehospital system
- Understand personal responsibilities within a clinical governance system.

Introduction

Prehospital clinical care is undertaken in an environment that is often characterized by being hazard rich, resource limited and technically and environmentally challenging. Critically unwell patients are often at greater risk, with a lower physiological reserve and a requirement for more complex prehospital care. It was historically considered that these difficult circumstances made it impractical to attempt to apply rigorous performance, quality or patient safety standards – providing access to prehospital care was often seen as the measure of performance and the mere presence of a prehospital clinical response was considered synonymous with high standards of care.

This implicit notion that clinical presence equates to quality, not just in prehospital care but across all aspects of health care, has been formally challenged in many countries across the globe. As a result, almost all health organizations, including ambulance services, are mandated to develop clinical governance processes. Many international insurance, indemnity and accreditation bodies have incorporated clinical governance within their standards.

Although there are many definitions, clinical governance is best thought of as an umbrella term which encompasses a range of structured and managed processes, often referred to as the 'pillars' of clinical governance (Figure 36.1). They include:

- service user involvement
- human resource management
- personal and professional development
- clinical effectiveness

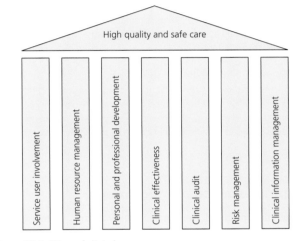

Figure 36.1 Pillars of clinical governance.

- clinical audit
- risk management
- clinical information management.

Many aspects of these processes were in place prior to 1999 but there was no clear accountability framework, little appreciation of their role in supporting high-quality clinical care and a limited understanding of how they could be applied to the prehospital clinical environment.

Service user involvement

Prehospital services are part of a wider emergency medical service (EMS) system and are provided for the benefit of the public. Service user involvement therefore relates to processes to ensure that the public, patients and operational partners have the opportunity to interact with, understand and shape the service. Although prehospital clinical activity is often focused on a very narrow spectrum of immediately life-threatening acute medical and traumatic emergencies, there is still opportunity to engage patients and other service users through:

- providing public access to information about the service and mechanisms for providing feedback (e.g. through websites, leaflets in hospitals or patient follow-up letters)

ABC of Prehospital Emergency Medicine, First Edition.
Edited by Tim Nutbeam and Matthew Boylan.
© 2013 John Wiley & Sons, Ltd. Published 2013 by John Wiley & Sons, Ltd.

- undertaking formal patient surveys (usually conducted in partnership with ambulance and hospital services)
- actively liaising with health oversight and scrutiny bodies, patient groups, ambulance services, local emergency departments and other emergency services.

There are many ways to engage with all of those involved in a prehospital service – from volunteers and staff, through to emergency services and hospital personnel as well as patients and the wider public (Box 36.1). Involvement of all service users should be seen as central to good governance.

Box 36.1 Service user involvement

A prehospital care service developed a process for electronically distributing short clinical incident summaries a few days after every serious case treated by the service's medical teams. These anonymized summaries provided the basic details of the incident, the initial clinical findings, the patient's immediate care needs, major interventions, clinical progress in hospital and key learning/discussion points. The summaries were sent to the relevant ambulance, rescue and hospital personnel and feedback was invited. There was an extremely positive response from all those involved with the service who felt much more included, engaged and involved in the work the service undertook.

Human resource management

Clinical staff often fail to appreciate how human resource management strategies can limit clinical risk, support the development of positive organizational cultures and contribute to effective clinical governance. These wider corporate functions often seem far removed from front line clinical care but without them it is easy to appreciate how safeguards, systems and services may fail. They include:

- Workforce planning – developing staffing strategies that take into account the wider emergency medical system and developments in other professional groups.
- Recruitment – attracting and appointing staff and volunteers with the appropriate knowledge, skills and attitudes required to engage in effective prehospital work.
- Pre-appointment screening – ensuring compliance with legal and regulatory requirements for employees and personnel who work with vulnerable people (e.g. identity, right to work, professional registration, qualification, references and criminal records checks).
- Occupational health support – applying standards for physical fitness and functional capability required to undertake the role, identifying limitations related to pre-existing health matters at recruitment and supporting personnel health and well-being in terms of ongoing access to physical and psychosocial health support.
- Personnel management – providing the framework for maintenance of good working conditions, mechanisms for appraisal and personnel development and the management of grievances and misconduct.
- Talent and performance management – developing and retaining personnel and providing a transparent framework for addressing concerns about poor clinical performance.

Prehospital care organizations vary from state-funded services with thousands of employees and complex management structures to charity organizations with a handful of volunteer clinicians. It is usually possible for the smaller organizations to outsource many of these human resource functions to larger affiliated hospitals and services. Being small and/or charity funded and/or volunteer based does not, however, absolve the service of its regulatory or legal responsibilities.

Personal and professional development

All healthcare organizations should value, encourage and support the concept of relevant, focused and effective lifelong learning and professional development. If the human resource functions have been effective in recruiting the right personnel, it is beholden on the organization's personal and professional development processes to ensure that they are properly inducted, trained and kept up to date. Mechanisms to achieve this include:

- Regular training needs analysed to assess whether training program are fit for purpose. This typically involves a survey of personnel to ascertain, based on their operational experience, the extent to which their training fulfills their needs.
- Formal programmes of induction and orientation training. As with safety critical in-hospital practice (in surgery and anaesthesia for example), many prehospital organizations conduct a summative assessment to ensure that the necessary underpinning knowledge and technical skills have been assimilated.
- Structured continuing education and training which includes regular case review and clinical update meetings and attendance at wider educational meetings and conferences.
- Access to educational resources. All personnel should be able to access a clinical library and all that it offers in terms of textbooks, journals and librarian resources.
- On-line resources can be particularly useful for services with personnel spread over a large geographical area or who undertake remote and rural practice. These can include an on-line virtual learning environment that provides more focused and relevant resources (e.g. a digital library), a means to complete assessments and greater interactivity with peers, mentors and supervisors.
- Requirements for recency and currency. Many organizations apply time or activity-based thresholds as triggers for refresher training. These can apply to duty periods, case exposure and operational activity.
- Supervision, mentorship and an appraisal process that provides opportunity for focusing on personal development.
- Support with accreditation and examination processes, e.g. the Diploma in Immediate Medical Care of the Royal College of Surgeons of Edinburgh. Development programmes to support individuals undertaking these are often highly valued.

Clinical effectiveness

Clinical effectiveness is a term used to describe the process by which an organization ensures that 'best practice' is applied across the spectrum of clinical services. To be an effective clinical service means to be applying care which is tailored to the needs of the patient: doing 'the right thing to the right person at the right time' and using 'the right transport platform, with the right in-transit care, to get the patient to the right hospital in the right timeframe'.

What 'right' means may be different in different emergency medical systems with differing geography and constraints. What is important is that 'right' is defined and is included in induction and training programmes. Many organizations make use of written documents that guide practice (DtGP) such as organizational policies, clinical guidelines, standard operating procedures or protocols (SOPs), aides-memoires and checklists to articulate their expectation of 'right' for clinicians operating with the service.

Organizational polices are written documents which provide an authoritative framework within which the service works. They combine the views, experience and values of the organization with any relevant legal, ethical or regulatory requirements. Examples of important prehospital clinical policies include a medicines management policy which ensures compliance with controlled drugs legislation and may also include the rationale for a restrictive prehospital formulary, and a resuscitation policy which ensures compliance with legislation and guidance related to advanced directives and end-of-life decision making.

Published clinical practice guidelines for prehospital care, such as those produced by the International Liaison Committee on Resuscitation (ilcor.org), professional bodies such as the National Association of EMS Physicians (naemsp.org) and the Faculty of Prehospital Care (rcsed.ac.uk) and guideline development groups such as the National Institute for Health and Clinical Excellence (nice.org.uk) and the Joint Royal Colleges Ambulance Liaison Committee (jrcalc.org.uk) should be interpreted in the context of the prehospital service and, where appropriate, incorporated into organizational policies or SOPs.

SOPs provide operational detail, instructions and advice on implementing specific clinical care or operational tasks. SOPs are commonly used for safety critical and essential operational activities within many prehospital and hospital services. Guidance on many prehospital processes can be provided by a comprehensive suite of DtGP (Box 36.2).

Box 36.2 **Clinical effectiveness**

1 Example of a suite of clinical and non-clinical DtGP in a prehospital service

Non-clinical policies
Development and approval of policies
Risk management policy
Scheduling and currency policy
Significant event reporting and investigation policy
Staff appraisal and development policy
Volunteer policy
Dignity and work and volunteering policy
Equal opportunities policy
Grievance policy
Health and safety policy
Clinical governance policy
Consent policy
Disciplinary policy
Leaving policy
Media handling policy
Recruitment of individuals with previous convictions policy
Patient privacy and dignity policy
Records management policy

Clinical policies
Resuscitation policy
Infection control policy
Medical gases policy
Medicines management policy
Moving and handling policy
Protection of children and vulnerable adults policy

Non-clinical standard operating procedures
Team composition and responsibilities
Personal protective equipment
Operating base daily routine
Activation and call-out
Emergency driving
Documentation and record keeping
Statements to the police and coroner
Photography at the scene
Observers
Interaction with the media
Equipment maintenance and resupply
Major incident medical support procedures
Hospital triage
Helicopter operations
Water rescue
High angle rescue
Confined space rescue
Working on the motorway
Working on the railway
Manual handling
Working near electricity

Clinical standard operating procedures
Medicines management
Infection control
Discharge from the scene
Emergency airway management
Traumatic brain injury
Maxillofacial injuries
Spinal injuries
Chest injuries
Abdominal injuries
Pelvic injuries
Limb injuries
Thermal burns
Fluid replacement
Near drowning
Electrocution

Life-threatening asthma
Life-threatening sepsis
Recurrent seizures
End-of-life decisions
Emergency amputation
Resuscitative thoracotomy
Focused abdominal ultrasound
Central venous access
Managing myocardial infarction
Management of open fractures
Paediatric life support
Emergency childbirth
Children with respiratory distress
Children with seizures
Children in coma
Emergencies in pregnancy
Management of suspected abuse of children or vulnerable
    adults
Acute behavioural disturbance
Regional nerve blockade
Procedural sedation
Induction of anaesthesia
Extrication
Packaging and transporting patients
Chemical incidents
White powder incidents
CBRN incidents
Firearms incidents
Public order incidents.

Procedural aides-memoires (PAMs) are a form of DtGP intended to aid rapid recall of an essential or critical clinical or operational procedure. They assume prior knowledge of the relevant underpinning polices and procedures and are intended to be very easy to refer to in an operational setting. The most common example of a PAM in clinical practice is a pocket sized cardiac arrest resuscitation algorithm.

Emergency action checklists (EACs) are another form of DtGP. They are intended to provide an immediate emergency reference for the rapid and safe management of life-threatening complications of treatment or interventions. Mirroring aviation systems, they are intended to be easy to read by an assistant to allow the operator to problem solve in a systematic way. Examples include ventilator associated emergencies and sudden physiological deterioration (e.g. hypotension, hypo/hypercarbia and hypoxia).

Clinical effectiveness programmes ensure that their DtGP are up to date and accessible and incorporate mission or case review meetings, journal clubs, clinical topic reviews, local expert opinion and feedback from audit, incidents, staff and service users to achieve this. Key to success is the connection between these often disparate sources of information the processes for maintaining the range of integrated DtGP (Table 36.1).

Clinical audit

Clinical audit is a detailed examination of clinical practice to ensure quality by identifying (and explaining) variances from agreed

Table 36.1 Illustration of integrated documents that guide practice

Overarching clinical policy	SOP	PAM	EAC
1. Prehospital emergency anaesthesia	S1.1 Induction of anaesthesia S1.2 Difficult airway management	P1.1 Difficult airway management	E1.1 Post-induction desaturation E1.2 Post-induction hypotension E1.3 Post induction hyper/hypocapnia E1.4 Ventilator associated alarms

EAC, Emergency action checklist; PAM, procedural aide-memoire; SOP, standard operating procedure.

explicit standards of care. All healthcare professionals should engage in clinical audit – particularly in relation to their own practice. For an individual, this might involve submitting a series of case notes for analysis of documentation or clinical peer review, conducting a detailed analysis of all aspects of the care of a single case (sometimes referred to as longitudinal audit) or undertaking a formal structured audit of several cases of a specific clinical intervention (e.g. procedural sedation) or the management of a specific condition (e.g. seizures). Prehospital organizations should also conduct audit at the organizational or service level and coordinate the activity of personnel to ensure that audit is appropriately resourced and that the recommendations are disseminated and acted on.

Appropriate prioritization is often the greatest challenge for many practitioners and organizations – it simply isn't practical to attempt to audit everything across the spectrum of prehospital care. Impact on patients, potential to influence change and the existence of evidence based guidelines are arguably the most important criteria to consider when selecting topics for audit. However, other factors to consider include the relationship to organizational priorities, risk, cost, frequency, relation to complaints or incidents and evidence of wide variation in practice. In all cases, a well-governed service should articulate an audit strategy and the rationale for inclusion (or exclusion) of topics (Box 36.3).

Box 36.3 **Clinical audit**

- An outline audit strategy
- Significant event audit – triggered by adverse incidents or excellent outcomes and audited against relevant standards appropriate to the case
- Continuous (rolling) audit with monthly or quarterly reports:
  - Prehospital deaths
  - Prehospital emergency anaesthetics
  - Prehospital procedural sedation
  - Unexpected outcomes (unexpected survivors or deaths based on injury severity score and probability of survival – an unexpected outcome being a patient who died with a probability of survival of, for example, > 75% or a patient who survived with a probability of death of > 75%)
- Continuous (rolling) audit with annual reports:
  - Controlled drugs management
  - Documentation and record keeping

- ∘ Activation and call-out of resources (including stand-downs)
- ∘ Helicopter operations (in all aircraft types)
- Focused audit activity undertaken in relation to local and national priorities, published guidelines and operational exposure (e.g. management of open fractures, cardiac arrest or prehospital fluid administration).

Risk management

Provision of emergency care in the prehospital environment is inherently high risk and risk management means having robust systems in place to understand, monitor and minimize these risks in order to protect patients and personnel. The two key elements to implementing effective risk management for prehospital care are:

(**a**) developing and sustaining a safety culture and
(**b**) maintaining generic and dynamic risk management strategies.

A safety culture results when accountability and learning are balanced (Figure 36.2). It relies on an underpinning reporting culture, a learning culture and a just culture – personnel need to feel confident about reporting actual and potential adverse events, no matter how trivial, and the organization should be actively seeking to learn from mistakes. In many healthcare systems, such a culture is conspicuously absent – only the most serious incidents are reported and investigated and subsequent actions tend to be punitive and person focused rather than system focused.

In addition to risks identified by reporting systems, a number of risks may be considered 'generic' such as those associated with common incident scenes (e.g. high-speed roads or railway lines), transport platforms (e.g. response cars, ambulances and helicopters) and the operational environment (e.g. mountain rescue or combat operations). Generic risks can be controlled to a large extent by planning and training. Generic risk assessments identify the control

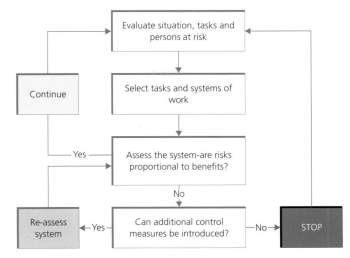

Figure 36.3 Dynamic risk assessment.

measures, be they protective equipment, operational procedures or restrictions on practice, and ensure that training is specific for the purpose.

Other sources of risk information include clinical audit, complaints and the statutory reporting systems in place for medicines, medical devices, aviation and other aspects of healthcare provision.

Generic risk assessments do not, by definition, cover every incident scene or clinical challenge. Prehospital care is, by definition, a dynamic and continuously changing activity. Dynamic risk assessment is the term used to describe the continuous assessment of risk carried out in such a rapidly changing environment (Figure 36.3). It relies on the existence of generic risk assessments, DtGP and training. It also requires effective leadership, communication, situational monitoring and mutual support – all 'learnable' skills. Risk management is therefore essential to the maintenance of high-quality safe care.

Clinical information management

Accurate and timely information, which by necessity often includes confidential and sensitive personal and organizational information, underpins all clinical governance processes. In many countries, there are professional, ethical, regulatory and legal requirements related to how clinical information is captured, maintained and disclosed. The challenge for healthcare providers is how to balance these requirements in terms of confidentiality, integrity and availability (Figure 36.4).

The International Standards Organisation (iso.org) provides a range of standards relevant to records management and information security (e.g. ISO 27000). From a practical clinical perspective, compliance with these standards ensures that:

- patient information is accurate and up to date
- there is compliance with the law
- confidentiality is respected
- clinical and operational information is used to monitor, plan and improve the quality of patient care
- full and appropriate use of the data is made to support clinical governance processes.

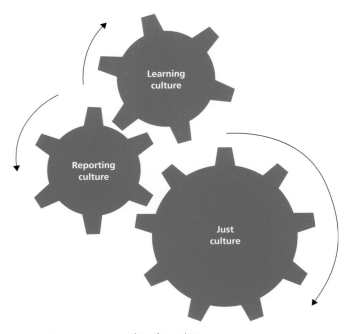

Figure 36.2 Components of a safety culture.

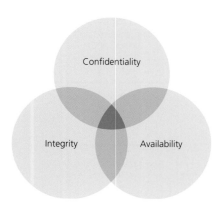

Figure 36.4 Balancing clinical information requirements.

Confidentiality and data protection can often be perceived as barriers to information access and analysis. In fact, compliance with information governance and medical record standards often allows greater access and use! (Box 36.4).

Box 36.4 **Clinical information management**

A specialist prehospital care charity developed detailed inter-agency information sharing protocols with receiving hospitals which allowed its staff, in a formal, structured and organized way, to directly access detailed patient follow up information within a few days of the incident, analyse this and provide feedback to the medical teams and the wider organization. In return, the hospital could access detailed prehospital information for its trauma register.

Summary

Clinical governance was originally defined (in the UK) as: 'A framework through which NHS organizations are accountable for continually improving the quality of their services and safeguarding high standards of care by creating an environment in which excellence in clinical care will flourish.' It should be clearer how the 'pillars' of clinical governance support such a framework and can be applied to all healthcare organizations irrespective of operational environment. The pillars of clinical governance, properly managed and resourced, will ensure that clinical services are provided, organized and managed in a manner which reliably supports the delivery of high-quality and safe care no matter what the circumstances.

The ideal of a 'high-reliability organization' – a term describing an organization operating in complex, hazardous, dynamic and time-pressured conditions but with an extremely low incidence of adverse events – is one that all prehospital services should aspire to. The most striking feature of high-reliability organizations is their collective preoccupation with the possibility of failure – at individual and system level. They maintain a mindset of 'intelligent wariness', expecting errors to happen and training their personnel to recognize and recover them. An effective clinical governance framework should be seen as one component in maintaining that 'intelligent wariness'. Another component is the individual practitioner. Many aspects of the pillars of clinical governance described here relate to organizational processes rather than individual attributes. In the pursuit of clinical excellence, clinicians should consider how they might both support organizational governance and apply these principles to their own clinical practice.

Tips from the field

- An effective clinical governance system is an essential part and process of any prehospital system – try to address this within your own system
- Ensure dedicated, protected time is set aside within rotas/on calls to ensure clinical governance requirements are fulfilled
- Share knowledge: if a problem, equipment failure or similar has occurred it is unlikely to be unique. Sharing knowledge can prevent future morbidity and mortality.

Further reading

Dekker S. *Just culture: Balancing safety and accountability*. Farnham: Ashgate Publishing Ltd, 2007.

Dekker S. *Patient Safety: A Human Factors Approach*. Oxford: CRC Press, 2011.

Halligan A, Donaldson L. Implementing clinical governance: turning vision into reality. *BMJ* 2001;**322**:1413–1417.

Keyser T, Dainty C. *The Information Governance Toolkit*. Oxford: Radcliffe Publishing Ltd, 2005.

Narinder K. On the pursuit of clinical excellence. *Clin Govern Int J* 2009;**14**: 24–37.

Reason J. *Human Error*. Cambridge: Cambridge University Press, 1990.

Robertson-Steel I, Edwards S, Gough M. Clinical governance in pre-hospital care. *J R Soc Med* 2001;**94**:38–42.

Scally G, Donaldson LJ. Clinical governance and the drive for quality improvement in the new NHS in England. *BMJ* 1998;**317**:61–65.

CHAPTER 37

Medicolegal and Ethical Aspects of Prehospital Emergency Medicine

Craig M. Klugman[1] and Jennifer Bard[2]

[1]DePaul University, Chicago, IL, USA
[2]Texas Tech University School of Law, Lubbock, TX, USA

OVERVIEW

By the end of this chapter, you should know:

- The difference between morals, ethics and law
- A method for applied ethical decision-making
- Duties to treat
- How and when to request consent
- The rules for privacy and confidentiality
- When to disclose patient information
- How to approach patient's end of life decision-making.

Table 37.1 Values of prehospital emergency medicine

Altruism	putting the concerns of others before yourself
Communication	being transparent and open in sharing with others
Compassion	understanding the vulnerability of humans and treating them with kindness
Competence	being excellent in one's skills; continuing to improve one's knowledge and proficiency
Empathy	able to appreciate the feelings and pain of others
Honour	having integrity and pride
Humility	being humble in one's interactions.
Justice	being fair and equitable
Resilience	having the quality of hardiness; ability to be tough and bounce back
Respect	positive feeling of esteem for oneself and others
Teamwork	working with others toward common goals
Wisdom	holding deep understanding of people, events and situations
Tolerance	having a fair, objective and permissive attitude toward others who may be different than oneself
Trustworthy	being reliable; deserving of another's confidence

Ethics, morals and law

Everyone comes to their profession with their own personal beliefs regarding right and wrong. These ideas are based on a lifetime of learning, experience and exposure to people and values. These beliefs are called 'morals'. When you enter a profession, you must be aware that your morals may sometimes be challenged by law and professional ethics. In fact, in addition, to your clinical skills and knowledge you are obligated to know health-related laws and ethical standards of your community. This chapter aims to help you to refine your skills and understanding in making professional ethical decisions.

Laws are rules which specific societies impose upon themselves and which are enforced by the government. Laws establish the rules of behaviour which all citizens and visitors to that jurisdiction are obligated to follow and are enforced by the state through criminal penalties including fines and prison terms. Think of law as stating what you absolutely cannot do and the minimum that you are required to do.

Ethics is a social and applied skill where one looks at the right and wrong of a situation and makes well-reasoned, rational choices. In addition to being a process, professions and groups can create codes of ethics, which are a list of *dos* and *don'ts* that members are expected to follow. Ethics introduces you to the skills you need to make critical evaluations of complex problems and to be effective

when you may not have a clear answer. Good ethics draws on the values important to a profession (Table 37.1).

Ethical decision-making

As a healthcare provider, you must know the legal requirements under which prehospital emergency personnel function. Laws concerning the delivery of health care vary significantly from country to country and even from city to city. You are responsible for knowing the law where you work. In general, there are three areas of law that you need to know:

1 *Criminal law* – offences against the state. Charges are usually brought against an individual or a service by public prosecutors and can result in being imprisoned.
2 *Licenses* – privileges to treat patients are granted by governments and may be revoked at any time. The state delegates self-governance to professionals including the authority to certify those qualified to practice and the authority to revoke a license for violations of professional standards.
3 *Negligence* – Refers to lawsuits brought by individuals, not the state, asserting that there has been a deviation from an accepted standard of care which caused further injury to a patient.

ABC of Prehospital Emergency Medicine, First Edition.
Edited by Tim Nutbeam and Matthew Boylan.
© 2013 John Wiley & Sons, Ltd. Published 2013 by John Wiley & Sons, Ltd.

Negligence actions are often referred to as 'Torts.' An injured person seeking monetary compensation must prove that:

- he/she has been harmed by a person who had a duty to act with reasonable care towards him/her
- the person did not act with reasonable care, and
- the failure to act with reasonable care resulted in his/her injury. The injury can be physical or psychological in nature.

Ethics is a tool to help you make decisions when faced with an ethical dilemma – a situation in which two or more values conflict. Different health professions rely on different tools when making choices, a situation that can often lead to misunderstanding between the professions. For example, nursing ethics is based on the feminist ethics of care which states that all action should aim toward nurturing and caring for individuals. Public health ethics follows utilitarianism, which states any action should produce the greatest good for the greatest number. Medical ethics is based on deontology (the idea that what is right is strictly following the rule) and casuistry (what is right is what has worked in similar situations in the past). Prehospital emergency medicine is based on a variety of these philosophical theories.

When dealing with an ethical dilemma in a prehospital emergency situation, you should consider four principles to guide your thought process:

1 *safety* or preventing harm to yourself or others
2 *virtue* or goodness and excellence of character
3 *dignity* or caring for all individuals with respect
4 *fairness* or treating all people fairly and justly.

Using the guiding questions in Table 37.2, you would then assess the situation according to the four principles. When you have completed that task, you can ask which of these principles is the primary one at issue in this case. Which principle is really behind the dilemma? Then you can use the identified principle to guide you in making your choice.

Duties to treat

In general, on-duty prehospital emergency medical personnel have an obligation to treat patients who are in need of their services. If you are off-duty then you may have an ethical duty to provide care if no one else is around, or if help is not available in a reasonable period of time and you have the appropriate training. If a person is in imminent harm (i.e. high likelihood of dying or suffering irreversible physical/psychology damage in the next few hours) then you may have an ethical imperative to provide assistance even if you lack the above conditions. Your legal obligations vary considerably depending on the laws specific to where you are located. For example, many nations (e.g. the USA and the UK) encourage volunteering through Good Samaritan laws which protect off-duty volunteers from civil liability so long as they did not cause the harm and act in good faith. In other countries (e.g. France, Germany and Spain), however, everyone is obligated to provide help to people in need. Those who do not may face criminal penalties.

Once you have a patient under your care you cannot cease treatment unless someone else takes over their care. To do otherwise is to abandon your patient which is legally and ethically unacceptable.

Table 37.2 EMS ethical principles

These principles assist in the process of ethical decision-making by providing guidance in moral deliberation as to what questions to ask and what ideas are most important in a specific case.

Safety

Preventing and limiting harm to oneself and others

What actions could minimize morbidity and mortality?

Does a proposed course of action keep you safe from harm?

Does a proposed course of action go outside accepted bounds of security?

What actions will help protect your patient from harm?

Have you taken all safety precautions?

Has the patient's privacy been respected and protected?

Have you checked in with your partners?

Have you checked in with your chain of command?

Virtue

Goodness; excellence; character necessary for one to perform his/her duties

What is your desired outcome for this patient in this situation?

What are your options to lead to the desired outcome?

What option is most likely to be successful?

Does the choice or option fall within your scope of practice?

Do you have the skill or competency needed in this case?

If you do not, have you received instructions from medical command or the senior medical officer as to how to proceed?

Have you thoroughly documented the case and your actions?

Dignity

Treat all individuals with respect

Have you treated your patient as you would want to be treated?

Do your proposed choices acknowledge the individual human rights of all people?

Have you met the physical and emotional needs of the patient?

Does the patient have status and ability to make decisions?

If yes, did the patient consent or refuse?

If no, is someone with the legal authority to make a decision identified and available?

Is the patient at risk of death or serious harm if immediate action is not taken?

Fairness

To treat all people justly and equally. To distribute scarce resources in a just manner

Have all patients been treated equally as human beings and not discriminated against by age, sex, race, religion, sexual orientation, national origin, socioeconomic status, or other arbitrary category?

Have all co-workers been treated equally according to their ability and skill training?

Have you applied triage without bias, if necessary?

Have you followed all rules, laws, and policies?

Have you acted in good faith?

In general, you do not have the freedom to pick and choose whom to treat. Discrimination laws vary by location. Many countries have laws which prohibit discrimination in the providing of health care to someone based on their age, race, sex, colour, sexual orientation, religion, socioeconomic status or national origin. Even if there is no legal requirement regarding discrimination, ethics requires you to treat all patients who require your services.

Case 1: A person in need

You arrive beneath a bridge responding to an emergency call. No one is present except for an adult male. He is wearing torn and dirty clothes, appears malnourished, and has not bathed in several weeks. He appears to be the victim of an assault as he is bleeding from a 10 cm laceration on his scalp and is unconscious. His breathing is dyspnoeic. He does not respond to commands and has no identification.

Table 37.3 Patient's decision-making ability

Status (competency)	Ability (capacity)
The assumption that all adults can make their own health care decisions	A health care provider's determination that a person is able to make a specific decision at a particular time.
Competency is assumed if a person is over the age of majority or is an emancipated minor	Ability to understand questions asked of care provider
Competency is not all or nothing, but can be gradated	Ability to understand implications of decisions made
In some areas, being pregnant or giving birth may give some level of competency such as making decisions regarding the pregnancy or the child	May not be possible in cases of intoxication, drug ingestion, serious injury, or mental incompetence
Minors may also have limited rights to consent to certain reproductive services, as well as alcohol and drug abuse treatment	

Table 37.4 Consent

A competent individual's right to make his or her own health care choices. A patient giving permission to receive treatment or be examined.

- A patient with status has the right to refuse medical treatment for any reason. In the case of refusal, see Table 37.6
- If a person physically resists what you believe to be urgently needed care, you should call law enforcement

Informed	Presumed	Substituted
An adult patient with status and ability	An adult patient who lacks the ability and status to consent is	With a child or adult lacking status or ability
• Is informed of his or her condition	• Treated based on the notion that most people would want to receive emergency care	• Try to obtain consent from the parent or guardian
• Is informed of the treatment options including risks, benefits, and alternatives	• Assessed, stabilized, and transported	• Where parent/guardian is not available <u>and</u> the patients' life is in imminent danger (i.e. at risk of dying in the next few minutes), then children can consent to emergency treatment
• Understands the situation and makes a deliberate choice		• Refusing care but the legal parent/ guardian demands care, then care should be given
• Voluntarily gives permission free from coercion		
• Expresses the choice verbally or in writing		

Table 37.5 Minors

The age of majority and the laws concerning delivery of health care to minors vary significantly depending on the country.

In many countries, minors can seek emergency care without parental permission. There are significant differences concerning what information a parent can be told about the health of a minor

You must get proof of age if there is a possibility the patient is a minor

Consent for non-emergency treatment must be given by a parent or guardian

Mature minors

Many countries have provisions for giving minors the rights of adults in regards to medical care.

Using the ethical decision-making tool from Table 37.2, you would first look at what you can do ensure the safety of yourself and the patient. Then under virtue, you should assess the patient and come up with a care plan. Third, under dignity, you must assess whether the patient has status and ability to make decisions while keeping fairness in mind (Table 37.3). The primary principle in this case is dignity. Since the patient is unconscious and appears to be in need of immediate care he lacks the ability to consent to treatment or refuse it. Consent is permission to treat a patient. If you touch a patient without consent, you may be guilty of assault or battery even if your intention in touching was appropriate. If the need for treatment is not urgent, your next step would to be locate a family member or legal surrogate who can give consent for you to treat the patient (Table 37.4). Since no decision-maker is available, you can assume that the man would want to be assessed, stabilized, and transported as you would do for anyone else.

What if the patient was not an adult, but was a child? If possible you need the consent of a minor's parent, guardian or legal surrogate before rendering any care. However, since this is a child whose life may be in danger (dyspnoea and the possibility the assailants could return), treating and transporting the child is permitted (Tables 37.4 and 37.5). In our scenario, someone needs to contact the police to look around the bridge for identification and to try to locate the child's parent or guardian.

Case 2: Refusal of care

You are called to the home of Ms Weiss, a 69-year-old woman with terminal cancer. She has lapsed into unconsciousness and has bilateral decrease in breath sounds. Her daughter called emergency medical services because of their concerns. Her husband meets you at the door saying 'She doesn't want this. It was a mistake. Leave her alone.'

In regards to safety, you and your team do not seem to be in any danger and Ms Weiss does not face any external harms. You next consider virtue by assessing the patient (arrhythmia and rales) and creating a treatment plan which probably includes oxygen, electrical cardioversion, and transport to the nearest hospital. Under the principle of dignity, the patient lacks status and ability. Dignity is the primary issue in this case. The husband is the closest next of kin and can offer informed consent. However, Mr Weiss refuses to give consent. Table 37.6 shows the process for patients who refuse care. At this point you ask Mr Weiss whether he has legal documentation of his authority to refuse care on behalf of his wife (i.e. a healthcare surrogate). Mr Weiss then pulls a bag from the wall above his wife's bed and hands it to you. This bag contains an advance directive naming him as the Durable (otherwise called Enduring) Power of Attorney for Health Care and the living will which states that Mrs Weiss has a terminal disease and does not want resuscitation (Table 37.7). It also contains an Out-of-Hospital-Do-Not-Resuscitate Order. This legal document tells prehospital emergency staff that the patient does not want resuscitation. Continuing with dignity, you apologize to Mr Weiss, assess his state of mind and ask if there is anything you can do to

Table 37.6 Refusal of care

Patients with status and ability have the right to refuse emergency medical care at any time

Patient (or surrogate decision-maker) must:
- Be informed of and understand risks of refusing care
- Give informed consent of the refusal

Prehospital emergency personnel should:
- Ask if the patient has a written out-of-hospital do not resuscitate order
- Try to persuade the patient to accept care
- Determine if the patient has the ability to make decisions
- Explain the risks of not accepting care
- Try to get advice from a physician
- Document your medical assessment of patient, care provided, patient's refusal, and all attempts to convince patient to accept care

Table 37.7 Advance directives

Legal documents that establish an individual's desires regarding treatment when he or she has a terminal illness or irreversible condition AND the patient is not capable of making a decision.
Patients have the right to refuse resuscitation.
One must have status and ability to create these documents.
One can lack status or ability to waive or destroy these documents.

Directive to physician/Living Will	Durable Medical Power of Attorney/ Proxy/Surrogate	Out-of-hospital do not resuscitate order
A document that establishes what care a patient would or would not want when he/she is unable to make a decision or participate in decision-making.	*A document that appoints a person or person(s) to make health care decisions for the patient.* The proxy should make choices that the patient would have wanted.	*The OOH-DNR gives instructions regarding resuscitation of a patient in emergency situations, in long term health care facilities, and in transport.*

assist him. Make certain that you properly document this call as well as Mr Weiss's refusal for care using his wife's medical order.

Case 3: Disclosing death at an accident scene

You arrive at the scene of a motor vehicle accident. A couple are mechanically trapped in their car. The driver is a middle-aged woman who seems competent but has apparently broken her femur. She is turned so that she cannot see the male passenger whose body is halfway through the windscreen and is obviously dead. While you are helping the woman she yells at you, 'I'm fine, please help my husband first.'

The ethical dilemma in this case is whether you tell the woman that her husband is dead. Note that in many countries, there is no legal requirement that you inform her of the death. Some Prehospital emergency personnel may not be legally authorized to make a legal declaration of death however in most countries you can assume a person is dead if there is decapitation, advanced decomposition, or rigor mortis with significant dependent lividity. You have no legal obligation to provide any treatment to the

husband. Dignity would suggest that you tell her the truth since she is able to make her own choices. However, if she is told of her husband's death, then her safety may be at risk. Her grief may cause her to move or lash out and aggravate her injury. Thus, the primary principle in this case is safety. A small deception is justified for the greater need of protecting her from further harm. Once she is stabilized at the hospital, her husband's condition can be shared. At this point, your best response is, 'We are doing all we can for him, and we have to concentrate on you right now.'

Case 4: Keeping secrets

You arrive at the scene of a motor vehicle accident. The driver has multiple contusions on his torso – likely from an airbag – may have broken ribs, and is bleeding from a cheek laceration. While loading the patient onto the ambulance, the police request that you take a blood sample to test for a blood alcohol level. The driver is a local celebrity and is very concerned about his public image if anyone knew about the accident. He asks you not to tell anyone about the 'crash.'

This case has two main issues: confidentiality and the blood draw request. The principle of safety suggests that one must take action to protect patient's privacy. Also, the privacy laws of many countries require that you protect patient privacy and cannot tell anyone unrelated to the patient's care about his private health information (Table 37.8).

The issue of the blood draw is an issue of virtue as it is a question of scope of practice. As shown in Table 37.9, the laws on prehospital emergency personnel participating in blood draws for driving under the influence vary by country. Even if you are permitted to draw blood for these purposes, you may not be required to, which means

Table 37.8 Confidentiality

Maintaining the privacy of a person's health information.

Some countries have specific laws governing the confidentiality of patient medical information
- United States – Health Insurance Portability and Accountability Act
- United Kingdom – Human Rights Act, Common Law Duty of Confidence, Section 60 Of Health and Social Care Act, and Data Protection Act
- Australia – Privacy Act
- Canada – Personal Information Protection and Electronic Documents Act

Private information includes
- Patient history gained through interview
- Assessment of findings
- Emergency medical care rendered
- Any records you create or view

You may share information with
- Anyone involved with the care of the patient
- A parent or guardian
- A legal health care surrogate or durable power of attorney
- Law enforcement when legally required
- Required reporting situation (child or elder abuse; violent crime or sexual assault)

Do not share information with anyone else unless you have the patient's authorization in writing.

Table 37.9 Blood draws from drivers under the influence

A major exception to the rule of consent is in countries that require anyone suspected of driving under the influence of drugs or alcohol to submit to a blood test. These tests are required whether the driver consents or not. Some countries involve prehospital emergency personnel in drawing blood for motorists suspected of driving while under the influence. However, being allowed to do such a draw does not necessarily mean that one is required to do so. You need to know the law in your location.

that the choice is up to you. In regards to the blood test, privacy law may not apply, but you cannot disclose the results with anyone other than law enforcement.

Case 5: Duties to treat

You are flying internationally on an airplane heading on vacation. A flight attendant makes an announcement asking for anyone who may be a doctor to press the call button. As you are flying over international waters, there is no possibility for other outside assistance for many hours.

In this scenario, you are clearly off-duty. If a physician answers the flight attendant's call, then it is your personal moral choice whether you also want to announce yourself and provide assistance. The patient is already being helped and you have no further obligation to provide aid. However, what if no one rings the call button and no other trained healthcare providers are available?

Legally, this area is ambiguous at best and depends on the area where you are currently flying (international airspace, country of origin, country of current airspace). Under many nations' laws, you have no requirement to act but would be protected if you did. Under other countries' statutes, you have a requirement to assist people in distress unless such action puts you in danger. Remember that the law provides a minimal baseline saying what you must do, but does not say what you should do. The most important thing is to consider these situations in advance and decide how you would choose to act.

Ethically, the answer may be clearer. Drawing on the values of prehospital emergency medicine (especially altruism and compassion) and the principle of Virtue (Table 37.2), if a person is in need of help and you have the ability to provide assistance (assuming proper training, current capacity to think clearly, and danger of harm to the patient), then you should provide it. This ethical duty is not affected by whether you carry supplies with you. Thus, this scenario is not a legal problem, but rather an ethical one.

If instead of an airplane you were in a boat and learned of someone needing help, then you would both ethically and legally (under International Admiralty and Maritime Law) be required to provide assistance. If instead of an airplane you were approaching a motor vehicle accident, the law would depend on the country where you are, but the ethics is clear: if you can help without putting yourself in danger, then you should offer assistance.

In summary

The ethical landscape in prehospital emergency care requires you to be skilful at following the standards of practice, knowing your scope of practice and following the rules, regulations and laws of your region. The law and ethics provide you with guidance for your practice to help you provide safe, ethical, and legal care to your patients as well as to protect you and your family from legal problems in the line of duty.

Tips from the field

- Making an ethical decision in a healthcare emergency is a process. You are obligated to know and follow the laws where you work. Laws establish what you must do and what you cannot do. They do not always tell you what you should do
- In making ethical decisions, you need to consider safety, fairness, virtue and dignity
- Codes of ethics define appropriate behaviours and actions for healthcare professionals
- It is always important to get consent when possible. This can be the written or oral agreement of a capable patient or legal decision maker. Most countries' laws assume that someone at serious risk of death or injury who does not refuse treatment has consented to be treated
- Consent to treat minors comes from their parents/guardians unless the danger to the child's life is imminent
- Confidentiality means that you maintain privacy of a patient's healthcare information and only share it with other healthcare providers involved with the patient's care
- Advance directives consist of a patient's directive to physician and family as well as appointing a surrogate decision-maker. These documents guide a patient's care in the hospital and medical settings but not in the prehospital setting. Out-of-hospital do not resuscitate orders permit prehospital emergency medical personnel to withhold or withdraw resuscitative efforts
- Always maintain accurate and complete patient records to protect the patient and yourself
- Legal duties to treat vary by jurisdiction but ethically one should assist those in need if other care is not immediately available, danger is imminent, and you are able to safely provide help.

Further reading

Gillespie CB. 1978. EMT Oath & Code of Ethics. National Association of Emergency Medical Technicians (NAEMT). http://www.naemt.org/about_us/emtoath.aspx (accessed 25 February 2013).

Klugman CM. Why EMS needs its own ethics. *EMS Magazine* 2007; **35**:114–122.

Larkin GL, Fowler RL. Essential Ethics for EMS: cardinal virtues and core principles. *Emerg Med Clin North Am* 2002;**20**:887–911.

Touchstone M. Professional Development: Parts 1–5. EMS Magazine 2010; January-May http://www.emsresponder.com/publication/bio.jsp?id=366&pubId=1.

U.S. Department of Transportation National Highway Safety Administration. 'Standard Curriculums.' http://www.nh.gov/safety/divisions/fstems/ems/documents/National_EMS_Ed_Standards.pdf.

CHAPTER 38

Research and Development in Prehospital Emergency Medicine

Suzanne Mason[1] and A. Niroshan Siriwardena[2]

[1]University of Sheffield, Sheffield, UK
[2]University of Lincoln, Lincoln, UK

OVERVIEW

By the end of this chapter you should know more about:

- How prehospital and emergency care developed
- Research priorities in prehospital care
- Barriers and facilitators to prehospital research
- Emerging new technologies
- Future developments.

Box 38.1 **Priority areas for prehospital research**

1 Identification of clinically relevant performance measures for use across the whole emergency medical service system and not just the ambulance service
2 Development of alternative methods of patient management to reduce transports to emergency departments
3 Need for research evidence to underpin the delivery of clinical care in the prehospital setting.

(Source: Snooks H, Evans A, Wells B *et al. Emerg Med J* 2009:**26**:549–550.)

Historical perspective

Although the principles of evidence-based practice are supported in prehospital medicine, traditionally there has been a lack of evidence supporting prehospital practice. In recent years there has been a steady development of multicentre prehospital care research that utilizes robust methods in order to answer some of the more challenging questions about interventions in prehospital care.

Challenges continue to exist in undertaking research in the prehospital arena. Prospective studies and especially randomized clinical trials are extremely difficult to conduct because of the transient and seemingly rather chaotic nature of patient care in this setting. In addition, ambulance services have always perceived themselves as having research 'done on' them by outsiders rather than instigating and executing their own research. This has largely been due to a lack of research capacity and expertise in ambulance services. This situation is slowly changing due to increased numbers of paramedics gaining an undergraduate degree and postgraduate qualifications also being achieved. Improved funding and stronger collaborations between prehospital care and academic institutions is also making prehospital research possible.

Research priorities

Research priorities identified through in the literature can be found in Box 38.1.

In many priority areas, such as service (re)design or user involvement in service development, evidence varies with the context of the healthcare setting or clinical problem and is dependent on the needs and scope of the wider health system. For example, alternatives to ambulance transportation to emergency departments have been investigated for some clinical conditions but there is less evidence for patient groups such as children and those with mental illness.

Even in areas where there is more published research, this is limited to certain conditions such as acute cardiovascular conditions or trauma whereas there is little evidence on assessment for many other acute or chronic conditions.

Although progress is being made in some areas such as development of performance measures for ambulance services, this is constrained by limited information. For example, patient outcome-based measures will require better information sourced from elsewhere in the emergency care system.

As in other areas of practice, implementation of research and knowledge translation is slow. For example, safety in emergency settings has been evaluated in some research studies but is not measured widely or routinely used to assess service quality.

Barriers and facilitators

Historically there have been a number of barriers to undertaking research in emergency settings (Box 38.2).

As in many areas of health care, there are tensions between delivering services and undertaking research. However, this is particularly so in prehospital and emergency care where challenging response time targets (for example the 8-minute response for

ABC of Prehospital Emergency Medicine, First Edition.
Edited by Tim Nutbeam and Matthew Boylan.
© 2013 John Wiley & Sons, Ltd. Published 2013 by John Wiley & Sons, Ltd.

emergency transport in the UK) may be affected by delays due to recruitment, consent or additional processes required as part of a study.

The context of diverse or rapidly changing health systems or organization of care is another barrier, particularly when studies involve the development and evaluation of new pathways of care. For example, studies involving emergency care for falls may be hampered by local and regional differences in pathways, the numbers of organizations involved and changes in systems and processes of care due to national guidance. This may also compromise the research methods employed – for example a randomized controlled trial evaluating a service or pathway may be impossible if that service is already fully established.

Consent for clinical trials is governed by legislation which will vary from country to country. Normally where capacity for consent is not present the legislation allows for personal or professional legal representatives to give consent on behalf of the patient. In emergency situations where capacity is present but the patient has little time for fully informed consent as a result of their condition (e.g. acute myocardial infection), provision may be made for assent (agreement) to participate with full consent at a later point in the patient journey.

Specific methods such as cluster randomization, where randomization of groups of patients treated by one or more ambulance clinicians rather than randomization of individual patients may reduce some of the requirements for individual patient consent in the acute setting. However, in many such studies individual consent is still required for individual level data such as quality of life or data requiring review of subsequent clinical and service utilization records. The knowledge and expertise needed to consent patients by front line staff is often lacking, particularly in ambulance services where many paramedics have not had a background or training in research principles or methods. Such training requires resources and considerable effort but should be considered as an investment in future capacity for research.

New systems for ethical review and approval of research studies have been developed to enable more efficient processes but many ethical and other complexities of prehospital research are problematic for research ethics committees and health organizations responsible for research governance.

New technologies

Evaluating the clinical and cost effectiveness of new technologies in order to inform their integration into healthcare is essential. In the past, the evidence for what we do has been scanty. Technologies that require evaluation fall into three main categories:

Workforce

Evaluating new pathways of delivering care to patients is an important aspect of planning services. The ambulance service is no longer seen as a 'scoop and run' service and has expanded its scope of care to include the assessment and treatment of patients on scene with appropriate signposting to services where required. Numerous studies have shown that this can be effective, for example paramedics with extended skills can provide minor injury care to older patients. However, further evaluations are required in order to develop a workforce that is evidence based and fit for purpose within a modern healthcare system.

Systems

Prehospital care should not be considered in isolation. In practice, it forms part of an emergency care system that contributes to the wider aspects of patient care. Although patient outcomes are dependent on the whole system rather that the component parts, the process of care within the prehospital setting is an important contributor to these outcomes. The ability to evaluate process and outcomes in the emergency care system is challenging, but appealing. System performance, quality and safety of care are key drivers for change, and having a robust set of evidence-based indicators would be considered a world-leading achievement. Currently the focus is on the impact on patients and services of bypassing local emergency departments in favour of specialized centres such as trauma centres or stroke units for appropriate patients. While policy is driving the changes, the evidence supporting it is lacking and research is needed to address these deficiencies.

Drugs and devices

The use of new technologies within prehospital care should ideally be evaluated within that setting. It is no longer sufficient to translate findings from other clinical settings and assume the effects will be similar. However, as outlined above, the prehospital environment proves one of the most challenging for researchers and therefore drug or device trials are rarely undertaken in these settings. Previously successful trials demonstrated the benefit of interventions such as prehospital thrombolysis, and more research of this quality should be undertaken.

Future directions

There are continuing challenges for prehospital care research worldwide. The setting and often urgent nature of the clinical conditions presented make research in this area challenging. However, this should not act as a deterrent, but be utilized to develop strong and effective collaborations that can deliver a sound research evidence to inform healthcare professionals and managers.

The future of prehospital care should focus on developing a diverse service that takes healthcare to the patient and directs ongoing care from that point. This means that healthcare professionals will need to have a range of skills, equipment and pathways open to them in order to deliver the most appropriate and cost-effective care to their patients. In order to do this efficiently, it is essential that commissioners and service providers work with researchers to gain the knowledge and tools required to optimally reconfigure and monitor prehospital care.

Key points

- Despite the growth of prehospital care research, there is still a dearth of robust evidence to guide service providers.
- Recent evidence reviews have highlighted priorities for future research in prehospital care.
- The context of prehospital medicine makes research challenging; especially clinical trials where interventions can have a significant impact on service delivery and client groups may be hard to reach.
- New technologies and future directions of research should focus on delivering high quality and cost effective healthcare close to the patient with the ability to provide treatments where appropriate and refer on when required.

Tips from the field

- Prehospital research presents many individual challenges which can seem insurmountable – it is however, essential!
- Participate and support projects whenever feasible, form filling and data collection may seem arduous but it will lead to improvements in service delivery and patient care.

Further reading

Coats TJ, Shakur H. Consent in emergency research: new regulations. *Emerg Med J* 2005:**22**:683–685.

Mason S, Knowles E, Colwell B, *et al*. Paramedic Practitioner Older People's Support Trial (PPOPS): A cluster randomised controlled trial. *BMJ* 2007;**335**:919.

Pantridge F, Geddes S. A mobile intensive care unit in the management of myocardial infarction. *Lancet* 1967;**2**:271–274.

Siriwardena AN, Donohoe R, Stephenson J, Phillips P. Supporting research and development in ambulance services: research for better health care in prehospital settings. *Emerg Med J* 2010:**27**:324–326.

Snooks H, Evans A, Wells B, *et al*. What are the highest priorities for research in emergency prehospital care? *Emerg Med J* 2009:**26**:549–550.

Stiell IG, Wells GA, Field BJ, *et al*. Improved out-of-hospital cardiac arrest survival through the inexpensive optimization of an existing defibrillation program: OPALS study phase II. *Ontario Prehospital Advanced Life Support*. *JAMA* 1999;**281**:1175–1181.

The European Myocardial Infarction Project Group. Prehospital thrombolytic therapy in patients with suspected acute myocardial infarction. *N Engl J Med* 1993;**329**:383–389.

Turner, J. and University of Sheffield Medical Care Research Unit. *Building the Evidence base in Prehospital Urgent and Emergency Care: A Review of Research Evidence and Priorities for Future Research*. London: Department of Health, 2010.

Index

ABC of Pain

Lesley A. Colvin & Marie Fallon
Western General Hospital, Edinburgh; University of Edinburgh

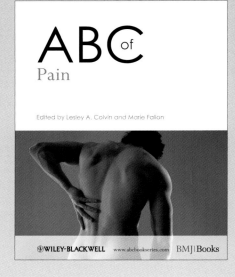

Pain is a common presentation and this brand new title focuses on the pain management issues most often encountered in primary care. *ABC of Pain*:

- Covers all the chronic pain presentations in primary care right through to tertiary and palliative care and includes guidance on pain management in special groups such as pregnancy, children, the elderly and the terminally ill
- Includes new findings on the effectiveness of interventions and the progression to acute pain and appropriate pharmacological management
- Features pain assessment, epidemiology and the evidence base in a truly comprehensive reference
- Provides a global perspective with an international list of expert contributors

JUNE 2012 | 9781405176217 | 128 PAGES | £24.99/US$44.95/€32.90/AU$47.95

ABC of Urology
3RD EDITION

Chris Dawson & Janine Nethercliffe
Fitzwilliam Hospital, Peterborough; Edith Cavell Hospital, Peterborough

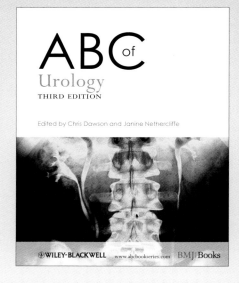

Urological conditions are common, accounting for up to one third of all surgical admissions to hospital. Outside of hospital care urological problems are a common reason for patients needing to see their GP.

- *ABC of Urology, 3rd Edition* provides a comprehensive overview of urology
- Focuses on the diagnosis and management of the most common urological conditions
- Features 4 additional chapters: improved coverage of renal and testis cancer in separate chapters and new chapters on management of haematuria, laparoscopy, trauma and new urological advances
- Ideal for GPs and trainee GPs, and is useful for junior doctors undergoing surgical training, while medical students and nurses undertaking a urological placement as part of their training programme will find this edition indispensable

MARCH 2012 | 9780470657171 | 88 PAGES | £23.99/US$37.95/€30.90/AU$47.95

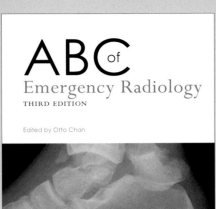

ABC of Emergency Radiology

3RD EDITION

Otto Chan
London Independent Hospital

The *ABC of Emergency Radiology, 3rd Edition* an invaluable resource for accident and emergency staff, trainee radiologists, medical students, nurses, radiographers and all medical personnel involved in the immediate care of trauma patients.

- Follows a systematic approach to assessing radiographs
- Each chapter covers a different part of the body, leading through the anatomy for ease of use
- Includes clear explanations and instructions on the appearances of radiological abnormalities with comparison to normal radiographs throughout
- Incorporates over 400 radiographs

JANUARY 2013 | 9780470670934 | 144 PAGES | £29.99/US$48.95/€38.90/AU$57.95

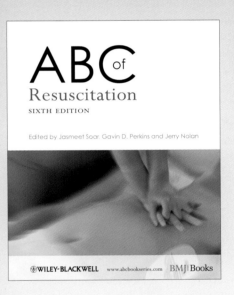

ABC of Resuscitation

6TH EDITION

Jasmeet Soar, Gavin D. Perkins & Jerry Nolan
Southmead Hospital, Bristol; University of Warwick, Coventry; Royal United Hospital, Bath

A practical guide to the latest resuscitation advice for the non-specialist *ABC of Resuscitation, 6th Edition*:

- Covers the core knowledge on the management of patients with cardiopulmonary arrest
- Includes the 2010 European Resuscitation Council Guidelines for Resuscitation
- Edited by specialists responsible for producing the European and UK 2010 resuscitation guidelines

DECEMBER 2012 | 9780470672594| 144 PAGES | £28.99/US$47.95/€37.90/AU$54.95

ABC of Ear, Nose and Throat

6TH EDITION

Harold S. Ludman & Patrick Bradley
King's College Hospital, London; Queen's Medical Centre, University of Nottingham

This new edition of the established text:

- Provides symptomatic coverage of the most common ear, nose and throat presentations
- Includes additional chapters on tinnitus, nasal discharge, nasal obstruction, facial plastic surgery and airway obstruction and stridor to reflect recent changes in the practice of otolaryngology and new content on thyroid disease, head and neck cancer, rhinoplasty, cosmetic and therapeutic scar
- Has been restructured on a symptom based classification for quick reference
- Incorporates guidance on assessment, treatment and management, and when to refer patients

NOVEMBER 2012 | 9780470671351 | 168 PAGES | £28.99/US$47.95/€37.90/AU$54.95

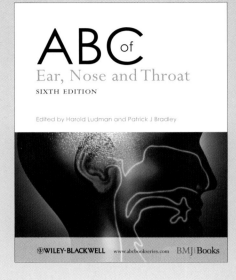

ABC of Major Trauma

4TH EDITION

David Skinner & Peter Driscoll
John Radcliffe Hospital, Oxford; Hope Hospital, Salford

Prehospital care is a growing area in medicine, and emergency treatments are becoming more sophisticated as the potential to save lives grow. This practical book:

- Is a comprehensive guide to the management of the multiply injured patient during the initial hours after injury
- Includes new chapters on major incidents and nuclear and biological emergencies
- Provides clear and concise guidance with accompanying photographs and diagrams
- Is edited and written by leading UK trauma authorities for everyday use by emergency medicine staff, nurses, hospital doctors, paramedics, and ambulance services

DECEMBER 2012 | 9780727918598 | 224 PAGES | £29.99/US$47.95/€38.90/AU$57.95

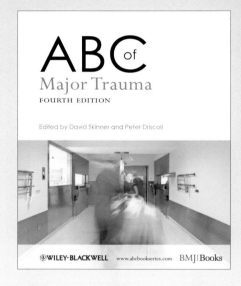